A Guide to Child Health

Michaela Glöckler and Wolfgang Goebel

A Guide to Child Health

Anthroposophic Press
Floris Books

Dedicated to the memory of Eugen Kolisko (1893-1939) physician and educator

Translated by Polly Lawson
Edited by Christopher Moore
Illustrations by Ronald Heuninck (1–7, 25–56) and
Walther Kraft (57–60)
Nutrition tables by Lotte Boelger-Kling
Colour photos by kind permission of Verlag Georg
Thieme GmbH from Helmut Moll, *Pädiatrische
Krankheitsbilder, Farbatlas,* Stuttgart 1983.

Originally published in German under the title
Kindersprechstunde
by Verlag Urachhaus in 1984. Seventh German
edition 1988.
First published in English in 1990 by Floris Books,
Edinburgh,
and the Anthroposophic Press, New York.

Printed in Great Britain
by Billing & Sons Ltd, Worcester

Floris Books, 15 Harrison Gardens, Edinburgh
EH11 1SH
Anthroposophic Press, RR4, Box 94A1, Hudson,
NY 12534

British Library CIP Data available

ISBN 0-86315-104-3 (Floris Books)

ISBN 0-88010-298-5 (Anthroposophic Press)

Contents

Foreword

This book takes as its starting point an insight which is of great significance for paediatrics: the connection between education and healing. Ideally speaking, by recognizing causes or sources of possible damage in good time and working actively on defects which have already appeared, we can succeed in providing a comprehensive prophylaxis against illness.

The choice of topics and emphasis given to them have been largely determined by our twenty years' experience in the children's out-patient ward of the Herdecke Hospital in Germany, a hospital run on anthroposophical lines. These sick children and their parents with their worries, questions and wishes have given us the inspiration for this book: parents have so often asked us where they could read for themselves what they have heard in the consulting-room.

The first part of the book describes the illnesses of childhood and gives basic guidance for home-nursing. In the second part we describe the best conditions for a child's healthy development and examine how these conditions can be created. In the third part we look at the significance of education and upbringing for later life. Here we try to show which educational influences work most positively on the growing child and which others run counter to a healthy development of mind and will. Typical situations of conflict and crisis in upbringing are discussed and suggestions for their solution are offered. If the book is read as a whole a comprehensive picture of the physical, psychical and spiritual development of the child emerges.

Medical advice is limited to general remedies. Preparations and prescriptions are mentioned, but it must be emphasized that there should be no delay in consulting a doctor when the situation requires. In addition, we do not wish the reader to look upon the present work as an absolute authority. Our intention is not to dictate, but to stimulate the reader's own judgment in the search for a dialogue between doctor and parent.

In paediatrics, a great number of medical, educational and religious questions overlap and a sharp distinction between them cannot be drawn. In this work, then, we have taken into account not only the findings of orthodox medicine, complemented by anthroposophical medicine, but also educational and psychological considerations, and references to the teaching of the New Testament. In the search for the meaning of illness in a given individual and in the attempt to further the individual's spiritual development, it is essential for us to study the human being as a whole: as body, soul and spirit. In this regard, we have been much inspired by the writings of Rudolf Steiner.

For the preparation of this edition, we should like to thank William Forward for his assistance in reworking some of the more philosophical passages into a style more accessible to the English-speaker; also the many doctors, teachers and parents, too numerous to mention in full, who have provided comment and advice on conditions in the UK, the USA, Australia, New Zealand and South Africa, especially Dr Jenny Josephson in Sussex, Margaret Shaw in Sydney and Dr Uwe Stawe in California. Our thanks must also go to the editorial staff at Floris Books, above all to Christopher Moore for his tireless and careful work in reshaping the book into a form appropriate for the English-speaking world.

With this book goes the wish that the connection which we have shown between education and the art of healing may help to promote awareness of our common responsibility for the future of civilization on earth. For the world of tomorrow depends on how we bring up the children of today and on all that we do for them.

We shall be happy to receive any comments which could help to improve and develop what is presented here.

Michaela Glöckler
Wolfgang Goebel

Introduction

Medicine and education have the common aim of furthering the development of the growing person. A closer look shows us that the two life processes of healing and learning are in fact intimately related. We find a similar pattern of development in both. Becoming ill, wrestling with illness and overcoming illness; these stages are paralleled in the act of learning by receiving a task, wrestling with the problems and finally gaining the ability or knowledge. In both areas, too, we seem to find experiences which correspond. We can, for instance, experience the inability to solve a particular problem as a kind of illness which leads to the feeling of being unwell and literally causes headaches. Equally, understanding something and feeling enlightened can be experienced as health-giving. We all know the feeling of relief when we suddenly "see the light." The characteristic of a healthy organism is to be constantly wrestling with the tendency to become ill and overcoming this tendency; so in the same way the characteristic of a healthy soul is to be unceasingly working to increase knowledge and insight into reality.

Through an approach of this kind, we can begin to understand illness at a deeper level. We can see it as a challenge to the organism which, to be overcome, involves us in a kind of bodily process of learning. But this then leads on to further questions: can illnesses arise when something which hasn't been actively learned by the soul now manifests itself on the physical level and has to be "caught up with" there? Is it possible, through an education which stimulates the ability to learn and work through one's own initiatives, to acquire at the same time a defence against illness? Questions like these take us even further into exploring the meaning of illness within the destiny of an individual.

For a better understanding we would like to explain, at this point, what we mean by the words *destiny, I, spirit, soul, body* and *constitution.*

By *destiny* we mean everything that a human being meets throughout life, both good and bad. Included in this is our experience of our own body, the whole range of mental and emotional experiences and reactions, the way the world works on us but also the fact that each of us experiences self as *I.* It is characteristic of our experience of *I* that it either affirms or negates destiny. The "I", as we shall refer to it, offers us the possibility of identification with our self, the possibility to work on self, to become clearer about self. The affirmation of one's own destiny has a scope for development tailored entirely to the individual, leading ultimately to a state of self-perception which is revealed by an inner harmony and peace with oneself. Before the "I" achieves this harmony, it is not united with itself. In the opposite direction, through negating destiny the "I" can become "hard" and "closed off" or else unstable and undirected.

Affirmation and negation, then, are the two possibilities of expression of the "I." Within the body it experiences itself as a unique being, closed off from the world around. Through the body it enjoys the possibilities of egotism, exclusivity, antipathy, and the experience of "now." Through thought, however, the "I" can reach beyond its own boundaries towards an interest in the "whole world"; it can say "yes" to what is not itself. The more we focus our thought on the eternal truths of life, the more strongly our "I" becomes aware of its spiritual nature and of its potential freedom of decision between "yes" and "no."

Spirit in this context is obviously not only the ability to think, but also the actively working will which is apparent at every moment of human decision. The way in which the spirit works in human beings is very different from the way it works in non-human nature, for in human life thinking and will are relatively independent.

We can all observe clearly that our thoughts and actions are separate. We do not always act immediately upon our thoughts. Often we act before we think whereas, in non-human nature, the relationship between thought and action is different. Human beings have a special ability. They can act in ways where they cannot control or even sufficiently foresee the consequences. Thus they can also — consciously or unconsciously — cause destruction and despair. On the other hand humans have the possibility through thought to stand outside everyday things and reflect on which thoughts they would like to turn into action. They can ponder on laws and truths without letting them ever become actions. Through this facility, humans have the freedom to distance themselves from the world around them, even to the point of doubting in all reality. They can even put *spirit* itself in question because they can consciously put themselves outside its working.

If however, we recognize the indestructibility and potential in thought, concepts, ideas and ideals, then we can become aware of the spiritual connection of the world. The thought of our "I" is just as eternal and indestructible as any law in physics, for example. In nature the spiritual works through natural laws and in an unfree way. In human beings it appears consciously and freely in the polarity of thought and action. The spirit, therefore, is manifest in the indestructible natural laws and their operation and thus is the very essence of nature.

The *soul* encompasses everything which is experienced individually. Thoughts can be thought in the same way by all people — they are of a supra-personal nature. What, however, the individual actually experiences while thinking, which feelings and emotions are evoked by ideals such as freedom, these are coloured quite individually. The soul-life is made up of the entire horizon of experience during a whole life on earth. It is the space for development of the personality and mediates between what is physical and self-centred and what is spiritual and supra-personal. Its nature is composed of the feelings of sympathy or antipathy which are the fundamental elements running through all manifestations of the soul.

The "I" is the centre of soul-life and through thinking has its own part in the universal laws. In its feeling life it experiences itself as individuality. In its action it expresses where it is in its development. Thus it has three areas of activity: spirit, soul and body. As it works actively in all three, we see it as the creative spirit of the human being. By "soul," we mean the more individual development.

The *body* is the third area in which spirit and soul operate. When we are fully awake, the body serves as instrument of the unfolding consciousness of actions. In sleep it only shows the manifestations of life. In death it maintains for a few days the form which it had in life. Then it disintegrates irreversibly because without life, soul and spirit it has no subsistence of its own. Thus the body depends on the working together of natural laws and those of human soul and spirit-life. This way of considering the body requires a wider look at the concept of *organism*. The reader will notice that in this book phrases like *organism, organization* and *body system* are used almost synonymously. This shows that we are not only looking at the individual symptoms which we see with our senses but also at the supersensory connections, apprehended only through thought, which we call "life."

Through the life-functions the soul and "I" of the human being are connected with the body in organizing and maintaining it in an individual way. This working together we call *constitution*. The physical features of the so-called constitutional types (pyknic, leptosome, athletic, and so on) are only aspects of a one-sidedness of life style. Through bad nutrition, shocks, stress and environmental damage, the sensitive balance of the constitution can be disturbed and so become more open to illness. The constitution can also be weakened by over-exertion or by severe emotional stress. On the other hand, it is strengthened by a life style which corresponds to the requirements of body, soul and spirit. The reader will meet the concept "constitutional remedy" in various parts of this book. What is indicated are possibilities of homoeopathic and anthroposophical medicine which through mineral, plant and animal remedies balance out one-sidedness of the constitution if an illness is prognosticated or has started.

These areas of work of the "I," the body, soul, and spirit as described above, are referred to as "worlds" by Rudolf Steiner in his book *Theosophy*. The "I" works in a world of the senses, in a soul-world and in a spiritual world, each having their own laws. As these laws are accessible to human beings through thinking, they are in a position to grasp the conditions of existence and future possibilities. Present-day events challenge us to do this: a culture threatened with nuclear destruction, environmental catastrophe and unbridled economic growth calls for answers to the whole question of our existence on earth and its purpose. New forms of culture more suited to our future development will become possible if more and more people think through the conditions of their humanity and pursue the consequences of their actions out of this. Contributing to this, it is necessary to see that illness is not a meaningless event, or something which should not exist. Illness is in fact the great educator in life which can lead to insights and abilities which will be of immense significance for the further development of humanity.

Part I

Childhood Illnesses and their Symptoms

Joys are gifts of destiny
And their value is in the present,
But sorrows are the source of knowledge
And their meaning is in the future.

Rudolf Steiner

1 Fever and its treatment

1.1 Typical examples of fever

To begin with, let us look at some different ways that a fever can run its course:

A four-year-old boy had been outside playing most of the day. He did not eat much for supper and, at bedtime, his mother noticed he was rather pale and that his hands were cold. Unlike his usual self, he was quite glad to go to bed. At about nine in the evening, he was sleeping rather restlessly and was tossing about on his pillow. On looking in and checking at eleven, the mother found him burning hot. He was talking in his sleep, woke up suddenly and looked rather surprised when he was put into his parents' big cool bed. He now had a temperature of 40°C (104°F). His voice was thinner and quavery, but gentle, as if he had grown older and more mature.

His parents had experienced this kind of incident and thought it was a harmless fever. They also knew the boy's tendency to be delirious, so they took their usual action: cool calf compresses and some herb tea. The boy immediately fell asleep. The fever ran its course and by morning the boy's temperature was down again.

A school-age girl did not feel well all day during her lessons. She was querulous, shivery and finally brought up her lunch which she had not really wanted to eat. By evening she had a headache and stomach-ache and she asked to go to bed early with a hot-water bottle to comfort her stomach. She slept only a little and, on waking, had a temperature of 38.5°C (101.5°F). But she had stopped shivering by this stage and felt a bit better. She took a few sips of herb tea but did not want anything else to eat or drink.

Next day the girl's temperature went up to 39°C (102°F). When the mother spoke to the doctor, she commented that her daughter had not been quite right for three days: she had been easily upset and prone to start crying. The doctor noted that the child's throat was a bit inflamed, but did not prescribe antibiotics or antipyretics (drugs to lower the temperature). He diagnosed it as a fever associated with flu (see Chapter 3.2). The fever lasted another two days. The following week the girl was allowed back to school.

A young girl had a cough which got worse over two days and on the third day there was a steep rise in her temperature. Her breathing was rapid, she had rather blue lips and her nostrils distended with her breathing. The doctor was called. He examined the child and diagnosed bronchial pneumonia. He showed the parents how to treat her with chest and leg compresses and without using antipyretics and antibiotics. The fever lasted for another few days in which both parents continued the treatment with much patience. Finally the girl coughed up a lot of mucous and after that she recovered rapidly. The whole family remembered this illness as a special event in her life.

Another child of about six had a sudden colicky stomach at fairly regular intervals. Then he began to vomit, which continued for a day or so until a high temperature developed. Then he felt a bit better and was able to keep down the herb tea with glucose which he was given. His parents realized that he had had an attack of gastric flu with vomiting (see Chapter 4.2).

A young child showed a high fever and complained of a headache and feeling unwell. The child seemed very sensitive to touch and was not comfortable sitting down. Within a few hours the condition and appearance worsened, and the parents called the doctor immediately. The doctor sent the child to the hospital where a suspected meningitis was confirmed and the essential antibiotic treatment administered straightaway.

The above examples show some typical ways in which fever runs its course and how sometimes parents are faced with alarming symptoms. How should they react? Confidence in assessing feverish conditions only comes with experience, insight and trust. Fear and anxiety are never helpful for the child so if you are at all uncertain, consult your doctor. It is always satisfying in paediatrics to see how parents' confidence grows with experience and how, with time, they need to turn to the doctor less and less.

Figure 1. Taking the temperature under the arm.

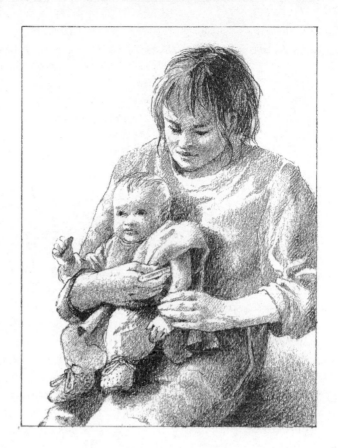

1.2 General diagnosis and treatment

In order to overcome an illness, the most effective action which the child's organism can take is to react with fever. By raising the body's temperature, all the metabolic processes are speeded up. This not only helps to eliminate bacteria and viruses, but also strengthens the body. It is the child, not the symptom that is to be treated, so there is no ready-made course of treatment for all cases.

Taking the temperature

Under the arm

This gives the least reliable measurement of temperature. Measure for at least five minutes making sure that the bulb of the thermometer is tucked well into the armpit (Figure 1). Cover the shoulder. The reading will be 0.5°C (1°F) lower than the internal body temperature. A reading of

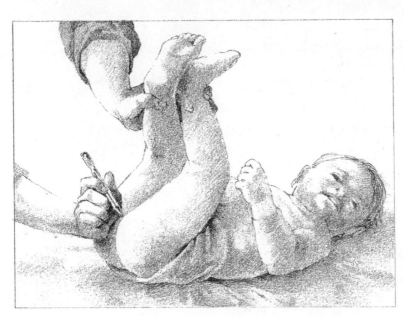

Figure 2. Taking the temperature in the rectum.

37.5°C (99.5°F) taken under the armpit will mean a body temperature of 38°C (100.5°F).

In the mouth

This method gives an accurate reading. Generally two minutes is long enough with a mercury thermometer. Put the bulb of the thermometer under the tongue. With children the danger of this method is that they may bite on the thermometer. For this reason, it is advisable to use the rectal method, described below, with children. Travellers abroad should ask before putting borrowed thermometers in their mouths!

In the rectum

This gives an accurate body temperature after two minutes if the thermometer is inserted properly. The bulb should be inserted right inside the anus. With restless or very young children, the adult should hold the thermometer in one hand and the feet of the child with the other (Figure 2). This ensures that the thermometer remains still even if the child wriggles a bit. The advantage of this method is that you can watch the mercury rising and coming to a halt during the measurement.

Note that in a suspected appendicitis, the temperature difference between the armpit and the rectum is more than 0.5°C (1°F).

In judging the progress of a fever, it is important to remember that the behaviour of the child is more significant than the actual temperature itself. Watch the child closely to observe any change in behaviour or unusual behaviour. Observe the child's movements, eyes, gestures, nostrils and breathing. Feel the forehead, back of the neck, compare body and limbs for warmth. Continue to take the temperature at intervals. If there is a stomach-ache, take the temperature also under the armpit and compare the difference (see above). Watch for breathing difficulties requiring urgent medical attention (for a full description, see Chapter 3.5). If at any time you do not recognize what is wrong or if you are concerned call the doctor. He will ask a number of questions not only about temperature but also, for example, about appetite, bowel movements and any vomiting.

If the limbs, particularly the calves, feel cold but the thermometer registers only 38.5°C (101.5°F) the temperature will rise. The body cannot spare any warmth yet for the periphery. Calves and feet will only become warm before the temperature has stopped rising and the body is ready to disperse warmth. Therefore do not apply leg compresses before that stage has been reached. Cover the child warmly and give liquids, for instance, hot herb tea or any non-stimulating drink.

If, however, the skin is hot right down to the calves and the temperature is over 39°C (102°F), leg compresses are called for. This helps the body to disperse surplus heat through the skin (Figure 3, and see Appendix).

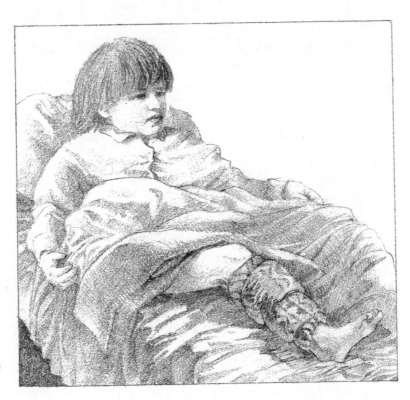

Figure 3. Using a leg compress.

A cool wash tepid sponging is effective if the child likes it. The child must be well covered but not as warmly as when the temperature is rising. At this stage, do not let the child become too hot.

If the temperature rises above 40°C (104°F) and the skin remains cool, or if there is **a seizure,** always call the doctor. If you cannot get hold of him give an antipyretic such as paracetamol (but not aspirin) and take the child to the hospital.

While the temperature is rising, children usually feel unwell and are inclined to vomit. Often they have headaches and stomach-aches, which ease off once the fever has reached its peak. The child should not be urged to eat but encouraged to drink liquids like warm herb tea.

If headaches persist after the temperature has risen and there is retching or vomiting, there is a possibility of **meningitis**. Meningitis is an infection of the membranes covering the brain and spinal cord and is indicated by a marked change in behaviour during the course of a fever and, in older children, by a stiff neck. A stiff neck can also be associated with other illnesses in which there is high fever. Also an inflammation of the deep cervical lymph nodes or a muscle-spasm may underlie this symptom.

There are two types of meningitis. The more harmful **bacterial meningitis** normally requires a lumbar puncture (an extraction of fluid from the spinal cord) to be carried out in the hospital so that it can be distinguished with certainty from an **aseptic meningitis**. An aseptic meningitis sometimes arises as a complication of another illness, for example, mumps, and does not always require a lumbar puncture in order to be diagnosed. Our experience in Germany shows that in certain cases where mumps has preceded the condition, a doctor may be reasonably certain that an aseptic meningitis is involved and may not carry out a lumbar puncture.

The parent can carry out the following simple tests at home with older children to eliminate the possibility of meningitis:

1. Can the child sit up in bed with legs straight out and raise the outstretched arms? (Figures 4 and 5).
2. Can the child sit up and, bending the knee, touch it with its mouth? (Figure 6).

Figures 4–6. Checking for meningitis.
This child has definitely not got meningitis: she can stretch her arms and body forward while keeping her legs straight and bending at the hips without feeling any pain (Figure 4).

When told to sit up and keep her legs straight, this child cannot sit up properly (Figure 5). She props herself up with her arms behind her back and her head tilted back. She cannot bring her arms forward without feeling pain in her head and back. She has probably got meningitis.

When told to bring her knee up to her chin or kiss her knee, the child cannot manage it even with the help of her arms because of the pain in her head and back (Figure 6). Meningitis is even more likely, and she should be examined by the doctor as soon as possible.

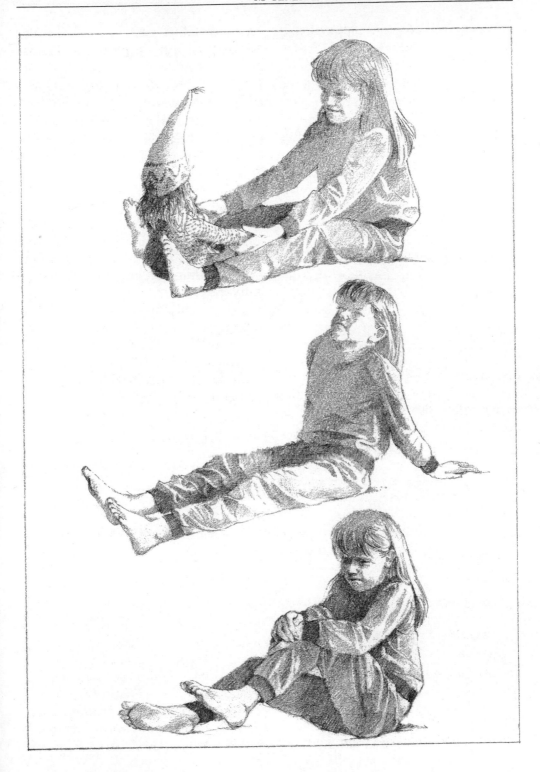

If both of these tests can be carried out successfully, then meningitis is almost certainly excluded. Remember, though, that the tests will be inconclusive if the parents try to carry them out in an anxious atmosphere in which the child gets upset or refuses to cooperate. If the child fails either test, or is too small to do them, it is better to call the doctor.

If meningitis is excluded by the doctor's diagnosis, the child should be given some herb tea (see Chapter 14.4) with glucose to sip. Follow with general treatment for fever as described below.

Nourishment during a high fever

It is important to keep up a child's nourishment during a fever. In cases where there is no diarrhoea, give plenty of liquids (herb tea, milk diluted with water and sweetened a little with sugar, fruit juice diluted half and half with water), light foods, no potatoes, very little fat or protein, no nuts, chocolate or sweets. The child may lose weight but any weight that is lost at this stage will be regained very quickly later.

For treatment in cases of fever with diarrhoea, see Chapter 4.

1.3 Febrile convulsions and seizures

Look at the following two cases:

A girl was playing outside as usual. There was a sharp change in the weather that day, and she may have been too thinly dressed. Suddenly as she was going home she turned pale, fainted and went rigid. Her lips were opening and closing. She was quickly *carried home. There the girl lost her rigidity but retained the marked paleness. Then she regained consciousness. She seemed to feel cold and was put to bed warmly wrapped up. The mother phoned the doctor and told him that her daughter felt cold so she had not thought it worthwhile to take her temperature. The doctor, howev-*

er, advised her to take the girl's temperature. She was surprised to find it was 39°C (102°F). The doctor came, found the girl asleep, examined her and did not think there was any immediate cause for concern. The child was allowed to go back to sleep.

In a case of suspected meningitis, the doctor would have sent the child to hospital, but here the problem was a "febrile convulsion." About two weeks later, the doctor arranged for an electro-encephalogram (EEG) as a further check on the child.

A boy was in bed on the second day of an illness with a temperature of more than 40°C (104°F) when his face suddenly began to twitch. In a few seconds the convulsions extended over the whole body. He lost consciousness. His parents were distressed at this frightening experience and their alarm diminished only when the convulsions eased off by themselves.

In a case of this sort, if the convulsions do not ease by themselves after one to five minutes, the child should be rushed to hospital.

Febrile convulsions in a child's early years are not an unusual occurrence because the child's brain, being immature, reacts much more sensitively to raised temperatures than it does later (doctors speak of a lower convulsion-threshold in childhood). An electro-encephalogram (EEG) taken immediately after the febrile convulsion can show up more or less serious pathological changes which however revert to normal within about fourteen days.

In most cases, a febrile convulsion is not an indication of anything serious and usually occurs only once. In only two per cent of children is a febrile convulsion a first symptom of a later proneness to seizures. It is sometimes thought that epilepsy can be produced by febrile convulsions. This is certainly not the case. It is rather the other way round: if there is a disposition towards epilepsy this can show itself for the first time in a febrile convulsion. This means that if an antipyretic is given in order to prevent a febrile convulsion, it will not prevent epilepsy later on. The onset of epilepsy is not related to the feverish infections of childhood.

In the USA until very recently it was usual to prescribe treatment with phenobarbital over a long period to prevent seizures. But a new study has shown that children treated in this way do not suffer fewer seizures and, in addition, tend to show more behavioural disturbances.

We recommend therefore both for children who are inclined to have febrile convulsions and for those who are subject to seizures, that they should have preventive treatment tailored to the individual.

For a child with a history of straightforward febrile convulsion, we recommend the following precautions:

— make sure that the child is always warmly dressed. The temperature

may suddenly and unexpectedly shoot up and if the child is already warmly dressed, this will guard against the accompanying shivering phase becoming too violent.
— the child should be given a constitutional remedy prescribed by a doctor to control the organism's way of reacting.
— when the child has a high fever, cool the head with a wet face cloth and follow the general guidance given above. Do not let the child get upset or worried.

1.4 Fever as the expression of warmth

Physically and mentally, we need a temperature of ideally around 37°C (98.5°F) to function properly and the body's warmth regulatory system has to maintain this. Perspiration releases excessive warmth, and shivering and chattering teeth are the body's way of generating warmth when we are cold. At neither extreme of our body's possible temperature range are we really capable of concentrated thought or action.

But warmth is not only something that can be measured with a thermometer. It is also the expression of activity of soul and spirit. We feel a warmth towards someone who is dear to us. We speak of a "chilly atmosphere" or a "lukewarm reception" but also of the "human warmth" which affects us when we meet someone who is interested and open-minded. Equally, the dawning of an idea or enthusiasm for something can make us feel warm right to the tips of our toes. Anger or shame can bring a flush to our cheeks or make us blush, often quite involuntarily. Fear, hatred, envy, dissatisfaction or anxiety can all cause the blood to run cold in our veins. We may quite literally go cold and pale in the throes of certain emotions.

The processes of nature are all characterized by differing degrees of warmth. These determine, for example, whether an element appears in solid, liquid or gaseous state. Only warmth is capable of penetrating all forms of existence and can bring about a metamorphosis from one condition to another. In the human organism we find that warmth regulated by the blood circulation is a decisive factor in the metabolic processes. Whether something remains in a state of flux or is deposited, whether a substance is absorbed or burned up, will depend on the level of surrounding warmth.

In this, warmth is not only the expression of our physical and emotional activities but also their vehicle. The stirring of our emotions can quicken the rate of circulation of the blood. Conversely warmth generated by the metabolic system can heighten our awareness and vitality.

We may refer to all these warmth-related physical and emotional processes together as a "warmth organism" since they are connected and interact in the same way as the living organism. The undivided nature of warmth — whether experienced emotionally or physically — means that a person can experience self as an integrated being through warmth. Warmth in body, soul and spirit enables us to be active in each of these three areas. Hence Rudolf Steiner wrote that "the warmth organism is the bearer of the "I" in the human being." Since every illness is accompanied by a change in the warmth organism, the "I" is also affected by and involved in illness.

Fever is a change in the warmth organism that comes to a crisis and may be brought about by a whole variety of causes. In children, fever may be provoked by a birthday, a long journey, a change of weather, a sudden chill or a tooth breaking through. All these events can temporarily weaken the organism and lead to illness. Individual children react in different and typical ways: there is the child who "never" has a temperature, the child who has long and relatively mild temperatures or the child with short and very intense bouts of fever. There are families whose children are regularly the first to go down with something while the somewhat slower neighbours are still playing out and about. Then they swap roles and sometimes the child that became ill later suffers a particularly heavy bout of the illness.

Adults, too, have their own different ways of reacting to fever: a person who works hard and regularly and enjoys it may be much less often affected by flu than someone who carries a lesser burden of work. Could it be that the first type is more able to generate warmth within himself? Is fever an attempt by the organism to increase soul activity in the body where it is proving insufficient?

How often do we hear people say of a new-born child: "She's just like her grandfather." Later they may start to say: "Well, now she looks rather more like her aunt." Later still, after an illness with fever, the parents may notice that the child's features have acquired something new and individual which cannot be attributed directly to any of its relatives. And now the parents are delighted to see the personality of their child more clearly. The fever has helped to make the inherited body a "better fit" in which the soul can come to expression more easily.

Anyone who sees this connection will take quite a different interest in their children's feverish symptoms and will no longer regard them as a misfortune. Feverish illnesses can be seen as an opportunity for the child to use its own warmth to individualize the body. Outwardly one can see this in the fact that weight loss which accompanies any attack of fever is subsequently regained. It is as though the child has demolished and rebuilt part of its inherited body, using its own resources of warmth. We have observed countless times in sick children how a flu accompanied by a high temperature, or an attack of pneumonia from which a good recovery has been made, or even measles, can herald a new and more stable phase in the child's development.

The effects of a fever on the body are directly comparable with the effects of good teaching in the realm of the soul: the child learns something by means of its own efforts. It would, for instance, be quite unpedagogical to say continually: "Do this, do that, don't do this, don't do that." Unfortunately, many parents do the equivalent of precisely this in the case of feverish infections when, on medical advice, the child is given something to take care of its temperature the moment it goes over the 38.5° (101.5°F) mark. And if there is an inflammation of any kind, out come the antibiotics too. This leaves the organism no possibility of dealing with the sickness in its own way. If the body continues to be treated in this way, later on it will lack the resources and "practice" needed to deal with anything more serious than a fever.

It is of course well known that some illnesses can result in dramatic and extreme reactions such as febrile convulsions or seizures. Indeed the course of some illnesses can be harmful to the child's development. Dealing with these dangers is a real concern of medicine. One should not overestimate, however, the risk of a simple attack of convulsion during fever. Out of one hundred children only five are likely to suffer from fevers leading to convulsion in their entire childhood. These hundred children are likely, together, to have had about five hundred infections accompanied by high temperature. Thus, to prevent five attacks of convulsion one would have to treat five hundred bouts of fever. In some cases, too, fever is only noticed after the convulsion. In such cases, treatment with drugs would be too late anyway.

Anyone who takes the child's development into account when treating an illness will avoid indiscriminate use of fever-suppressing drugs just as they will be careful not to exclude their use on principle. Every case of a child with a temperature needs to be treated with due regard to the child's own needs and capabilities. While one child may "need" a temperature to increase the activity of its metabolism and to allow it to "work at" its physical constitution, so another may need protection from being weakened by an excessive febrile reaction.

It is very heartening to see how, when parents have found confidence in their child's own resources after an attack of convulsion, the child is subsequently able to withstand fever up to 40°C (104°F) without suffering a convulsion. The child has now learned how to cope with fever.

2 Pain

The smaller a child is, the harder for us to find out where it is feeling pain. Let us look at a typical example of pain in a small baby:

A five-month-old baby has been rather fretful all day, and even during bathtime which it usually loves. When put to bed, it begins to cry. This is unusual as it normally goes down quietly for the night. The mother lifts it up again in case it has wind but the baby continues to be miserable. She has already changed its nappy (diaper) and the bowel movement was quite normal. Though the child does not seem hot, she takes its temperature (rectally) and the thermometer shows just over 38°C (100.5°F). When she lays the baby down again, it cries more than ever. The mother begins to get anxious. Why does the baby have a slight fever? Perhaps she should get it to drink. But by now the infant is so agitated that it refuses the drink she offers. So she picks it up again and rocks it in her arms — no use. She dances with the baby — it usually likes that — but soon its yelling becomes unbearable. By this stage, the mother is so worried that she takes the child to the doctor.

She tells the doctor her story but, with the baby in its present state, any sort of examination is impossible. So the doctor takes the child from the mother and walks very slowly and calmly up and down with it, almost to the rhythm of breathing. The mother watches and begins to relax. The child in the doctor's arms becomes quieter and quieter. Slowly the tension recedes. After all that crying, a great burp of swallowed air escapes from the baby's stomach. The little head droops exhausted; there are a couple of sobs and a deep sigh.

Now the doctor can examine the infant carefully. One by one the stomach, limbs and ears are checked. And then the doctor feels the lower gums at the front, finds them slightly swollen and knows at once what is wrong. The baby is teething.

Back at home, the child cries again twice during the night but mother, now enlightened, remains calm, and in the morning they both sleep a little longer. At nappy-changing (diaper-changing) time, the baby's behaviour is back to normal, and the mother is delighted to see that the first tooth has just appeared!

It is clear from this story that the way the baby reacted to its discomfort was influenced by the mother's anxiety. A child's response to its pain is frequently affected by what is around it. Let us look at another common example:

A toddler has fallen and badly scraped his knees and hands. He clenches his teeth and totters away from his playmates heading for home. The nearer home he gets the quicker he walks or runs, and only when he sees his mother does he begin to cry. He sobs out his pent-up feelings.

Both these stories illustrate that the way in which a child shows it is in pain is influenced by surroundings. As adults, we are supposed to come to the rescue calmly and confidently. If we cope calmly with the situation, the child can bear the pain much better than if we get into a panic. Worry, anxiety and noisy reactions in the adult are transmitted to the child and will only increase its distress.

2.1 Headache

Headaches without fever

Migraine
Headaches without fever can indicate a number of causes and need medical diagnosis. Spasmodic attacks with or without nausea or vomiting may indicate childhood migraine. Treatment will be prescribed by the doctor, and will depend on the individual case. In general, it is recommended that the patient's digestion is not overloaded: a light diet with not too much protein, but plenty of vegetables and salads should be given. Be sparing with sweet things. Generally four to five smaller meals are better than three larger ones. Allow regular and not too long periods of sleep; a regular routine of bedtime and getting-up time, even at weekends, is preferable. Sufficient physical activity and plenty of fresh air are essential. Once an attack of migraine has started, the best remedy is for the child to sleep it off in a darkened room. During the attack herb tea with lemon may be given, but nothing to eat except possibly dry crisp-bread. Patience, rest and quiet will help to ease the migraine.

Eyestrain
If headaches comes only with reading or watching TV, this type of headache is usually caused by eyestrain. The problem may be short- or long-sightedness or some other form of impaired vision. The eyes should be tested.

In school-age children

If a child complains of headaches before or after school or towards the end of school, the teacher should be consulted and the doctor also if necessary. Bear in mind that children — especially between the ages of nine and twelve — not uncommonly suffer from headaches or stomach-aches during the school-day. At that age the circulation of the blood is adjusting itself to the rapid growth of the body before puberty, with the result that the blood is redistributed to meet the higher demands of certain parts of the body.* If the head is receiving too little blood, this will cause a headache. But if there is a good supply of blood to the head, then the intestine may be temporarily deprived, resulting in spasms and colic pains.

If headaches appear mainly at home and particularly at weekends, the family situation should be looked into. It may be that at weekends, the usual rhythm of getting up, meal times, exercise and going to sleep is interrupted. Recurring headaches can be helped by maintaining a regular schedule over the weekend. Avoid sweets between meals. Check that the action of the bowels is regular, and treat any flatulence (see 2.7 below).

It is important that the child should not become the centre of family concern when complaining of headaches. It is better for the child to be bundled off to bed and put "out of commission" because if too much fuss is made, the child can easily start using the headache to get its own way with the adults. On no account should pain-killers be given without a doctor's advice, and there are many alternatives to chemical painkillers. For example, we have found Biodor-on 5% effective. The child should take two tablets morning and midday before meals every day for about three months. When the headache is acute, two tablets may be taken every half-hour.

Headaches with fever

Headache with rising temperature

A child complains of a headache during the morning and does not feel well. By evening he is running a fever of 39.5°C (103°F). The headache appears before or during the rise in temperature, and is probably associated with a bout of flu or other illness. Once the fever has reached its highest point the headache usually disappears. Additional symptoms may be shivering, pains in the limbs, stomach-ache and nausea.

Headache with fever and vomiting

If a headache persists after the temperature has risen and there is retching or vomiting, the child should be checked for a possible **meningitis** (see Chapter 1.2). If meningitis is

---

* The rapid shunting of blood to vital organs is a normal bodily response known as the "diving-reflex." It can appear with any reaction to stress and was first researched among deep-sea divers. In situations where exceptional demands are made, the body first provides for the most important organs: brain, heart and kidneys, restricting the flow of blood to the periphery and in the intestines.

excluded, the child should be given some herb tea (see Chapter 14.4) with glucose to sip, and follow on with treatment for fever as described in Chapter 1.2. If the headaches or vomiting persist for more than eight hours without signs of improvement, a doctor should be consulted.

Headache in babies

If a baby shows pain or discomfort after being put down to sleep, the cause may be **teething troubles, earache** or **headache**. The pain is felt at bedtime because the veins in the head fill more when the infant is lying down. Examination can confirm suspected teething troubles (see 2.2 below) and earache (see 2.3 below), but headache can be inferred where other obvious causes are eliminated. Fever may occur in all three situations, and is usually present in acute inflammation of the middle ear.

2.2 Teething pains

A continuous edge of pale whitish mucous membrane along the gums will show there are no teething pains. If there is a swelling or increased reddening and signs of the teeth showing through the gums, all these can indicate teething pains. The baby may also be continually rubbing his finger over the gums. Discomfort can be eased by allowing the baby to bite on a hard teething crust or a teething ring. An effective remedy is to massage the gums with diluted Weleda mouthwash, or with sage tea.

The teeth usually come as shown below in alphabetical order:

G E F C B B C F E G

G E F D A A D F E G

A and *B* are the middle front teeth, *C* and *D* the two side front teeth, *F* the eye-teeth, *E* and *G* molars.

2.3 Earache

To confirm a suspected earache press the tragus (ear-flap) shut to see if this causes discomfort (Figure 7). If the child is constantly rubbing the area around his ear, the trouble is much more likely to be seated inside the mouth, for instance, teething (see above).

The recent occurrence of a cold may suggest a middle ear infection *(otitis media)* as the cause, in which case fever is usually present.

Acute pains accompany an otitis due to flu, in which blisters rapidly form on the ear-drum. When these burst they release a drop of secretion often blood-coloured. Pain may last for a day.

With certain kinds of acute inflammation, the ear drum may rupture and discharge pus and mucus. This occurs in ten to twenty per cent of untreated cases. After the pus has burst through, the pain quickly disappears. If there is no rupture, the pain often disappears after one or two days. However, if the condition lingers, the other ear will often be subsequently affected.

Pain can be relieved in all these cases by applying a warm camomile or onion bag (see Appendix).

There should be a marked drop in temperature within three days. If the fever persists, the patient should be examined by a doctor in case complications develop. Reducing the fever does not in itself clear up the problem. Inflammatory discharges from the middle ear usually last from five to ten days. Even earaches which last longer do not necessarily entail damage to the hearing.

Babies often get "runny ears" without warning and the ears heal just as quickly again. In our experience, it is seldom necessary to pierce the eardrum to let out the discharge. There can easily be a relapse if the ears dry up too quickly because this may lead to their becoming gummed up and then pus building up behind the blockage. In such cases, the temperature usually rises again to above 38°C (100.5°F) and the doctor should be consulted.

As a rule a rupture of the ear-drum

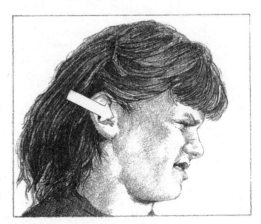

Figure 7. Checking for inflammation of the ear. Press the cartilage over the earhole (as indicated). If there is inflammation the child will react by screwing up his face or pulling his head away, and babies will start crying.

heals up well. But in the rare cases when it does not, and there is a chronic discharge from the ear, the cause is nearly always due to an inherent weakness of the membrane. From our experience we consider that the inflammation of the middle ear rarely needs to be treated with anti-biotics. If a suitable constitutional remedy is given, this will encourage the body to combat the illness and the whole hearing system will be streng-thened. Relapses will then occur much less frequently. Treatment of the middle ear should always be supervised by a doctor, and related colds and infections of the upper air passages and adenoids will then be treated simultaneously.

A quite harmless "runny ear" re-sults from tears or from bath-water getting into the ear-passages and melting the wax *(cerumen)* so that it runs out and looks like a discharge. A brownish "bloody" stain on the pillow is often only a dark lump of wax that has been dissolved and run out.

Vomiting is not a symptom of a simple inflammation of the middle ear, and if occurring in conjunction with earache should be referred to a doctor.

When cleaning the ears with a stick of cotton-wool clean out only the external ear (auricle) and the visible part of the ear-passage. Deeper prob-ing disturbs the self-cleansing action of the ear. As the mucous membrane of the air passages and the deeper ear-passages are served by a common nerve, coughing and sneezing may occur if the ear-passages are cleaned out too deeply.

2.4 Sore throat

A child with fever lies crying in bed. When asked where it hurts, the child points to his stomach. He has not eaten anything today and has drunk only a few mouthfuls of herb tea.

If children complain of stomach-ache and food is refused, parents should first examine the abdomen to see if it is rigid or soft. If the abdomen shows no signs of rigidity, they should then examine the mouth and throat as that is where the problem may lie.

Before calling the doctor parents can have a look at the mouth of a feverish child and see whether the tongue is coated, whether there are spots, ulcers or coating on the mucous membrane. Finally get the child to say "Ah" or press about two thirds of the tongue down sharply and firmly with the back of a spoon or tongue depressor (Figure 8). This makes the child gag and the tonsils and the back of the throat become visible momentarily. Triggering the vomiting-reflex must be avoided. You can see whether the tonsils are inflamed, coated or merely slimy. If the child has lost his voice or has difficulty in breathing or is seriously ill leave this examination to the doctor.

The most common appearance is tiny glassy red spots round the edge of the palate, more or less inflamed tonsils, a temperature of over 40°C (104°F), coated tongue, and nausea. This is a **virus infection*** which is mostly harmless.

If white spots are found on flaming red tonsils accompanied by a temperature, it is usually a discharging **tonsillitis (or "strep-throat")**. Fortunately this is no longer as serious as it used to be. We have been able to treat it in most cases without antibiotics. Tonsillitis can lead in exceptional cases to complications with the heart or joints, and sometimes with the kidneys. This is the reason why the majority of doctors insist on antibiotic treatment and see its omission as unprofessional. Therefore a course of treatment without antibiotics should only be undertaken by agreement after all concerned have been made fully aware of the risks. A further consideration is that, even with antibiotic

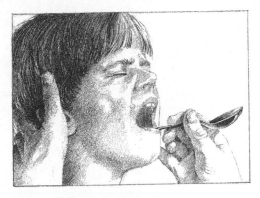

Figure 8. Examining the throat.

treatment, complications can set in, though they are more rare and have nothing to do with the severity of the throat infection. Streptococci bacteria* are found widely in the population (up to 30% of throat swab tests in nursery classes are positive) even where there are no symptoms. As a result, the risk of reinfection is extremely high.

Home treatment for tonsillitis: wrap the neck with hot lemon compresses (see Appendix), give warm sage tea with honey and lemon, and gargle with strong boiled sage tea. Sweat-baths (see Appendix) can sometimes help. Mouth disinfectants do not help. Give internal medicine only on a doctor's advice. The patient should stay in bed for at least three days after the temperature has subsided. The doctor should be asked to

---

* Viruses are minute cell-parasites, visible only in an electron-microscope. Viruses cannot multiply outside a living cell. Antibiotics have no effect against viruses.

* Bacteria are visible under a normal microscope as the smallest living creatures. They can be bred in an organic culture. They induce the pus in a living organism. Antibiotics are effective only against bacterial infection.

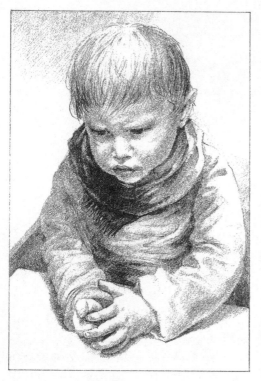

Figure 9. Treating a stiff neck.

check progress every two to three days until the child is completely better. A further check should be given one to two weeks after the illness, and possibly again one to two months later. For **chronic tonsillitis** or repeated infections of this kind a fourteen day treatment with mustard footbaths before bedtime has proved highly successful (see Appendix).

Quinsy, though not very common, appears as a complication of tonsillitis. Symptoms: high fluctuating temperature, feeling very unwell, inability to open the mouth properly. Requires prompt medical attention. Thicker coating spreading out over very red tonsils should be urgently examined by a doctor. This is usually caused by a **glandular fever** *(mononucleosis)* or, in rare cases, by diphtheria.

Thrush *(candidiasis)* is more often on the inside of the cheeks of infants and toddlers and does not cause pain (see Chapter 5.10). For aphthous ulceration on the inside of the mouth, see Chapter 6.9.

Swollen lymph nodes in the neck *(cervical lymphadenitis).* In almost every child you can feel small lymph nodes which may appear during harmless infections or without any signs of illness at all. A visit to the doctor is only necessary if the nodes continue to increase in size over some weeks and especially if they are painless.

Symptoms requiring attention: a lumpy swelling, painful when pressed, at the side of the neck. Slow development of the condition allows time to keep it under observation. There are two ways in which the problem resolves itself:

1. The lumpiness slowly disappears after leaving somewhat rougher lymph nodes which can be felt for months afterwards, and which gradually become smaller.

2. The painful nodes daily become bigger and harder, until the skin over them becomes red and there is a general swelling over an area of lymph nodes. This is a sign that an **abscess** has formed, which will either burst of its own accord, or must be lanced by the doctor, leaving only a small fine scar.

In both cases the body itself will take care of the healing process. As a result, many children will acquire a good resistance against future pus-forming illnesses. In our experience, therefore, it is worth trying to manage without using antibiotics.

Pains in the neck and throat may be caused by a **stiff neck:** a stretched muscle can present a pain similar to lumbago. The trouble lasts for some days and can be relieved considerably by applying heat to the affected part. Stimulating ointments or an oil compress can be applied at the same time (for throat compresses, see Appendix). Cover with a woollen cloth (Figure 9). Sunflower oil, olive oil, lavender oil (10%, Weleda) or eucalyptus oil (5%) are all effective.

2.5 Eye disorders (conjunctivitis)

Pink or sticky eye, **conjunctivitis**, is one of the most common eye troubles. It is recognized by the reddening of the mucous membrane that covers the white of the eye and the inside of the eyelids *(conjunctiva)*. The child may also experience an aversion to light or the sense of a foreign body in the eye and itching.

Conjunctivitis can be caused by several things: cold or dusty wind, allergies, infections, or measles. In new-born babies, it may be caused by the preventive eye-drops administered by the hospital after birth.

If there is ever pain in either or both eyes, consult a doctor. The following forms of conjunctivitis can be treated at home.

New-born babies: Blocked tear ducts
In a new-born baby, the tear-ducts leading into the nose can be blocked by mucous for months. This and other congenital adhesions in the tear-ducts can be recognized by watery eyes with no apparent cause, and by drops of yellowish-white pus in the corner of the eye nearest the nose. Sometimes a careful pressure-massage with a clean finger on the part above the tear-duct will help. It is only rarely necessary for an eye-specialist to clean the passage with a probe.

Treatment: *Calendula D4* eye-drops (Weleda) under a doctor's supervision.

Reddened eyes with discharge (sticky eyelids)
After birth or in the first four weeks, a baby's eyelids are inclined to stick, and there can be marked reddening as described above.

Treatment: clean the eyelids using a paper tissue with boiled lukewarm water (do not use camomile as it contains irritants which can lead to an allergy). *Calendula D4* eye-drops

(Weleda), three to four drops hourly in each eye will wash the eyes out.

If there is no improvement after two to three days, consult the doctor.

Both eyes watery and reddened without discharge
Usually this condition is caused by wind, dust or smoke, or is connected with hay fever.

Treatment: give *Mercurialis* eye-drops (Wala) three to four drops hourly in each eye. For hay fever use Gencydo 0.1% eye-drops, one drop in each eye several times daily.

One eye reddened, with or without discharge
Observe with care, as a foreign body may be lodged in the eye, or the reddening may be a side symptom of an infection of the cornea. It is best to consult a doctor.

For a foreign body in the eye, see the first aid section.

2.6 Chest pains

Sudden and sharp pains in the chest may be felt when the muscles are irritated locally during influenza, rather like muscular rheumatism. The patient cannot breathe properly but gets enough air and there is no cough. If the trouble is situated near the heart, the patient may complain of "heart-pains" and here the treatment is a warm oil compress.

Chest pain on the left side when breathing can be caused by flatulence. This occurs when air gets into the intestine below the left dome of the diaphragm. The patient can also have difficulty in breathing, and feels a dull intermittent pressure on the left side near the heart.

Actual **heart pain** is extremely rare in children and will usually be associated with grave preliminary illness. Serious general upset, a racing pulse and the desire to lie down are signs of a grave disorder, and are always grounds for calling the doctor.

Treatment for flatulence: relief can be obtained from caraway tea and other remedies for flatulence (see 2.7 below). Another remedy is to gently massage the abdomen with warm hands moving clockwise so as to release the trapped air. Often an older child can do this itself.

A sharp pain, or **stitch**, in the muscles of the stomach wall is usually due to cramp when running with a full stomach.

Treatment: get the child to hold its breath, press on the upper part of the stomach with its forearms, progressively increasing the pressure, and squat.

Chest pains felt **behind the breast-bone** when breathing or coughing are mostly due to irritation of the mucous membrane of the air passages. For treatment, see Chapter 3.5.

Pains felt in the general region of the chest **when breathing or coughing** are frequently experienced at the beginning of a flu. For more detailed coverage of breathing difficulties, see Chapter 3.

Pains in the chest **with a high temperature and interrupted breathing-out** are a clear indication of pleurisy which is usually preceded by pneumonia and requires hospital treatment (see Chapter 3.2).

2.7 Stomach-aches

Parents tend to conclude that the baby has got a stomach-ache when they see symptoms that worry them: "My baby keeps doubling up with pain." "She keeps crying, but then quietens down in between." "His stomach is distended and hard." "She looks so pale." "His stomach rumbles so." "She's been sick twice today." "He won't eat anything." "She hasn't had a bowel movement since yesterday." And so on.

Such worries are often heard at the doctor's consulting-room. However, if parents carried out their own examination calmly, they would in most cases be able to distinguish the harmless from the dangerous and save themselves much anxiety.

Wind in babies (flatulence)

A very young baby cries after each feed but less often while feeding. If it has not drunk too little or too much, if the bottle was not too cold or the contents too thick, if it has brought up its wind properly, then the problem is usually flatulence or too strong a movement of the bowels. Possible accompanying symptoms are: some regurgitation a taut stomach, straining when passing stools, whether hard, normal or soft. "Crying time" in the evening between 6 and 9 pm has nothing to do with flatulence. Stomach-aches due to flatulence will normally disappear by themselves after about eight to twelve weeks.

Vomiting (that is more than one or

two mouthfuls), paleness, distended stomach, diarrhoea (that is, several thin movements between the feeds), generally not thriving, or sudden devastating screaming, will all indicate disorders other than flatulence and require medical attention.

Even breast-fed babies often suffer from flatulence, for example if the mother eats a lot of wholemeal bread, legumes (pulses) or cabbage. In the case of babies who are not breast-fed, a change of diet should be tried in consultation with the doctor or nurse (see also Chapter 14.3).

Treatment: the following remedies give relief:

Apply *warm* (wet or dry) compresses to the stomach. In addition, the stomach can be rubbed with lemon-balm or diluted caraway oil* in a clockwise direction. Woollen vests reaching down over the stomach, thicker nappies (diapers) and a hot-water bottle are recommended.

Give some teaspoonfuls of warm fennel or camomile tea just before meals

Lay the baby on its stomach after feeding, or walk up and down with it for ten minutes.

Take the baby on your lap after feeding, lean it back against your chest and gently knead-massage its feet, heels and lower leg.

* In some countries, 5% diluted caraway oil can be obtained ready prepared. If this is not available, use pure etheric caraway oil and dilute it yourself: 5% caraway oil: 95% cooking oil.

Control the amount of milk (see Chapter 14.3).

If breast-feeding, avoid eating coarse bread and oats for breakfast. We believe a breakfast of fresh fruit (such as apples or pears) causes less flatulence.

Avoid being in a rush, under stress, constantly distracted and upset, and eating hurried meals, as this makes the baby's condition worse.

Appendicitis

Appendicitis is generally recognized in children through a continuous pain lasting for some hours, slowly growing stronger and concentrating in the lower part of the child's abdomen. In addition, we can also observe apathy, nausea, coated tongue, rejection of hot-water bottles and pain felt when walking or jumping.

The child should be seen by the doctor. Before calling the doctor, take the following measures:

— give the child nothing to eat or drink;

— take the temperature in the armpit for five minutes, making sure that the thermometer is properly lodged, and cover the shoulder with a blanket (Figure 1). Then take the temperature in the rectum and note both readings. With a suspected appendicitis, the difference may be more than 0.5°C (1°F). See Chapter 1.2 for a full description of taking a temperature.

In babies and young children, appendicitis can be less easy to determine.

It often shows very slight and uncharacteristic symptoms or may suddenly develop into the highly dramatic acute abdominal illness (see below: Violent stomach pains with vomiting). Even for a doctor, the diagnosis in a baby is often not straightforward, and of course he will wish to avoid an unnecessary operation.

Colic

The main symptom of colic is a sudden intense pain at the navel. The child is glad to go to bed. Usually the pain eases off after an hour and do not return at first. The child is pale, but feels no special pain when the stomach is pressed. Nevertheless the problem calls for the doctor's diagnosis, but if he confirms that the child is only suffering from this harmless but unpleasant condition, a course of hot stomach compresses after either the midday or the evening meal for four to six weeks will be found helpful (see Appendix).

See also urinary infection (below), and violent stomach pains with vomiting (below).

In certain cases, worms can cause stomach-aches. For a full treatment of this problem, see Chapter 4.

Urinary infection

Stomach-ache, back-ache with or without fever, lack of appetite, paleness, general weakness, and a burning sensation when passing water can indicate an infection of the urinary tract. The cause can be inflammation either of the bladder or of the renal pelvis (pyelitis), or both. Sometimes the burning sensation is so strong that the child holds back its urine with the result that it may wet itself during the day or in bed at night. It is important to know that the burning sensation disappears before the inflammation has completely cleared up.

Treatment: if urinary infections occur frequently, they can cause severe damage to the kidneys. Diagnosis and treatment should therefore be supervised by the doctor who will normally arrange a urine test. Even slight infections can be determined from the test.

For initial treatment at home, a steaming hot cloth — well wrung out — and/or a hot water bottle, can be laid on the bladder. Take care not to scald the child though! (See Appendix for bladder compresses).

Hernia

A protrusion ranging in size from a hazel-nut to an orange which can be seen and felt above the groin is an inguinal hernia (Figure 24, page 98). Large protrusions can contain a portion of the intestine. In girls an ovary can slip forward into the protrusion. In boys the rupture can extend right into the scrotum and involve the testes. Any painful swelling in this area requires urgent medical attention for not only may the hernia become nipped but torsion or inflammation of the testis may also occur which will be extremely painful. An inguinal hernia is only in some cases cured without an operation.

An umbilical hernia, causing similar swelling at the navel, usually goes back by itself in time. Using a plaster to hold in the rupture can cause skin irritation.

A swelling in the groin or scrotum can also be caused by a **hydrocele,** a sac filled with fluid next to or above the testis. Hydroceles mostly occur at birth but they can appear at any age. When the testis descends from the abdominal cavity through the inguinal canal into the scrotum, it takes with it the delicate inner covering of the abdominal cavity. In this tubular covering the testis may ascend and descend as in the case of a retractile testis. Before this sac obliterates completely, remnants of fluid may be left behind and form a new hydrocele.

In babies these hydroceles usually disappear by themselves and can generally be left alone so long as there is no pain. In case of pain, they should be seen by the doctor. If they do remain or grow bigger, they are normally operated on in early childhood, especially if there is accompanying hernia.

Violent stomach pains with vomiting

Colicky or continuous violent stomach pains with vomiting, paleness and usually a painful rigidity of the abdominal muscles (stomach as hard as a board), found by pressing on the stomach, are signs of an **acute abdominal condition.**

Treatment: this condition requires immediate medical attention even where the pain subsides after a time. The child should be taken straight to the hospital in case an immediate operation is necessary.

This condition can be confused with the less serious **acetonemic vomiting** if this has not been seen before (see Chapter 4.2).

Stomach-aches with shivering and headaches

Stomach-aches together with shivering, indisposition, headaches, aching limbs can be indications of the start of **gastric flu (flu with intestinal irritation)**. Even vomiting can occur at this stage. Usually the pains disappear after a sharp rise in temperature. The difference between a gastric flu and appendicitis is the following: there is no local pain when the lower abdomen is pressed; the temperature difference between rectum and armpit is less than 0.5°C (1°F); there is marked shivering and a rapid rise in temperature to over 38.5°C (101.5°F); warmth applied to the body is felt as pleasant, whereas with appendicitis it is not and is even harmful. Cold arms and legs indicate that the temperature has not finished rising. In case of doubt call the doctor or take the child to the surgery despite the fever.

Recurring stomach-aches

Recurring stomach-aches before or during school indicate **overwork or emotional stress**, and the case should be discussed with the teacher. The doctor's advice may be sought for a mild prescription or other measures. Chemical sedatives and pain-killers are generally uncalled-for. Recurring stomach-aches can also result from an imbalance between the demands made on the child and his capacity to meet them. Possible causes can range from the excitement of a birthday party to bacterial food-poisoning, from a parent's or teacher's anger to nervous impatience, from the child's hurt pride to secret jealousy.

By way of contrast, it is astonishing how much work children can take on when they have enthusiasm, interest and love for the matter in hand.

We recommend that you think through the child's day in order to see how far you yourself may be involved in the cause of stomach-aches. Compare the following two situations:

1. *"Now I've got to feed Stephen,"* the *mother says.*

"Mum, may I eat an apple?"

"You mustn't always think that you've got to eat something when Stephen gets something."

"Mum, you were going to go on reading me the story."

"Now leave me in peace and let me finish feeding, then I must change Stephen's nappies, and when he's asleep I'll have to go shopping. I'll ask Mrs Green to come over and look after you both."

"Mum, I've got a tummy-ache."

"Oh heavens! Not again!"

2. *"This little glutton's hungry again. Please, Clare, go and fetch me Andrew's bottle off the heater,"* mother asks.

Clare goes and gets it.

Mother, singing away to herself: *"Now we're getting something to eat. Baby's got his bottle to drink and Clare's eating her apple ... Will you give me a bite?"*

Clare gives her a bite.

"Once you've both finished, I'm going shopping quickly."

"I want to come too!" Clare cries.

"Not today, because it's too late. But you can help to look after Andrew. See that the sun doesn't shine into his face. I'll tell Mrs Brown next door I'm going out, and she'll pop in as usual and look after you both till I get back. Now when the big hand and the little hand of the clock are together I'll be in the supermarket and I'll think of you both, and this afternoon I'll tell you the story I promised you."

Clare is happy watching the big hand creeping over the little hand and seeing that Andrew is quiet and not crying.

In the first situation, Stephen's mother does not fully identify with what she is doing. She is being dragged along by her work, and is struggling to get free. She is probably overtired. Perhaps some member of the family is critical of her. She feels tied to her children by invisible strings which they are constantly tugging. Once the stomach-ache stage has been reached the mother might try to regain control of the situation in the following educational way:

3. *"Mum, I've got a tummy-ache."*

"So you've got a tummy-ache. Well, fill your hot-water bottle with hot water, not too hot mind, and go to bed. I'll be along shortly to have a look at you."

And a little later: "Now you're nice and cosy. Is your tummy a bit better now? I'll ask Mrs Brown to come and stay with you both while I'm out."

Unless the mother takes the initiative there will be no end to the stomach-aches. Only by taking the initiative will she be able to contain the problem, and she should not let herself abandon her original intention unless the child is really ill. The child says: "I've got a tummy-ache." But the message is really: "You haven't given me proper attention today," or, "You're working in such a rush and not enjoying it," or, "I can't find anything to imitate in what you're doing," or, "You've built up a wall between us."

In the second situation, Andrew and Clare's mother shows initiative and imagination. She goes halfway to meet Clare's demands and offers care beyond the physical needs.

In the last example, once the mother is aware of the stomach-ache, she begins by bringing warmth to the child's body, following up with warmth of feeling and her own nearness. Soon the child will not need the hot-water bottle any more.

Children do not produce stomach-aches just for effect, unless they have already seen examples of deceptive behaviour. Children experience their surroundings so strongly that what they cannot digest emotionally is manifested in their bodies. Whether or not the child then consciously uses the pains to achieve something will depend on circumstances. In no way should the child's behaviour be seen as "bad."

Other kinds of stomach-ache

When a child complains of a stomach-ache, first look into the mouth; it is not infrequent to find tonsillitis (see 2.4 above) which affects also the large abdominal lymph nodes.

Strained stomach muscles resulting from sport or play can give rise to needless anxiety, and will clear up by themselves.

More sensitive children are subject to colicky abdominal pains some hours or half a day before the outbreak of **vomiting** (see Chapter 4.2). Here hot stomach compresses with essence of oxalis or milfoil (yarrow) tea, possibly even a course of these, will afford relief.

Unusual thirst and increased urination over several days would lead to suspected **diabetes.** Consult your doctor.

For **stomach-aches with diarrhoea,** see Chapter 4.1.

2.8 General aches and pains

A two- or three-year old child was going for a walk with her parents. At the end of the garden, she suddenly stopped and would not go on. She wanted to be picked up and carried. The parents wondered if she could possibly be tired so soon. What was the matter with her? Was it a stone in her shoe? Was she cold? Was she playing a game? Or did she have a pain somewhere?

General aches and pains are so varied in cause and appearance that we can give very little general advice. For a case of limping, see the first aid section at the back of the book. In general, parents should try to get as complete a picture as possible of the period and events leading up to the pains, for instance, whether or not there has been a recent accident or knock.

Before taking the child to the doctor, check its temperature. Also check whether there are new or temporary swellings or warmth in the painful areas. Knowing the history and time of appearance of these symptoms can be useful information for the doctor as they may indicate serious constitutional illnesses like rheumatism, inflammation of the bone and marrow *(osteomyelitis)* and others. These illnesses are not discussed here as they are only diagnosed by means of a thorough medical examination and fortunately they do not belong in the category of common ailments.

Broken collar bone in new-born babies

If a new-born baby seems to show pain when turned over or when its shoulders are moved, it is possible that the child suffered a broken collar-bone during birth. This may have escaped the initial medical examination, but will become apparent later as a swelling around the place where it is healing. The bone always mends of its own accord, and the trouble is over after a few days. Special treatment is not necessary.

Another small problem at birth which can make a baby hold its head slightly on one side for a time is a haemorrhage in the side neck muscle. Make sure that the baby continues to sleep in different lying postures so that the head does not become malformed. If this is not possible, the doctor or physiotherapist will show how to exercise the baby with slight turning movements of the head.

2.9 Boys' disorders

Tight foreskin *(phimosis)*

Seventy per cent of all boys have a tight foreskin at birth, that is to say the foreskin cannot be pulled back over the head of the penis, but this declines to four per cent at puberty. In most cases, then, the problem resolves itself in time and therefore, in our opinion, automatic circumcision (an operation to remove the foreskin) for medical reasons is unnecessary. The exception is when repeated painful inflammation of the foreskin leads to scar tissue contracting the foreskin even further. Stretching the foreskin inexpertly or slight chronic irritation of the foreskin are two other causes of a scarred contraction. In these cases circumcision under a general anaesthetic is recommended. For treatment consult your doctor.

A partial adhesion of the foreskin to the penis can lead to an accumulation of secretion *(smegma)* and eventually to a suppurative inflammation. With this condition, the foreskin may come unstuck by itself or the doctor may release it with a probe. Such adhesions however can last for years without giving any trouble and do not require treatment. We recommend regular cleaning of the penis under the foreskin only when puberty sets in or when there is considerable secretion.

Occasional erection of the penis, with or without a tight foreskin, takes place naturally from babyhood onwards. It occurs mainly in the morning before waking. The child may complain of pain or a feeling of tightness. This has nothing to do with masturbation (see Chapter 17.10).

Undescended testicle

At birth the testicles may not yet be in the scrotum but usually they descend soon afterwards. If a testicle only comes down into the scrotum in a warm bath and goes back up when cold or being washed, it is called a retractile testis and does not need an operation. Any other form of this problem requires medical assessment.

Some paediatricians and surgeons recommend hormone treatment before resorting to an operation. We do not recommend this treatment as it constitutes an unnecessary interference with the body's own hormonal control and produces undesirable side-effects on the physical and emotional nature of the child. Instead we usually suggest that, before deciding on an operation, a constitutional remedy with anthroposophical or homoeopathic medicines is tried. If this has no success, we usually recommend the operation in the second year and we have had good results from surgical intervention without previous loosening up of the tissue through hormone treatment.

2.10 Fear and emotional stress

Both fear and stress are common in children. Children experience injustice and unfair punishments. They can be torn between their parents during a divorce. Some find themselves outsiders at school and are not accepted in their circle of friends. They may even be tormented or teased because of their clothes, appearance or disabilities. Younger children may weep bitterly or become frightened when they notice their parents are going out in the evening (despite all the efforts to get a good baby-sitter). Older children experience pangs of conscience, a sense of shame, profound depths of sadness, hopelessness and despair.

All of these experiences can be described as suffering. Children of all ages experience suffering, and with it begins their shadow-life which accompanies all their happy and positive experiences. Suffering is basically the experience of separation. In suffering, the child's soul is prevented from opening up joyfully and engaging with the world around it.

Children are much more deeply affected by suffering than adults, many of whom believe that children have no real problems at all! The adult, after all, is in a position to distance himself from his own problems, to think them through and thereby dominate them. With children it is quite different. Depending on their age, they are delivered up in varying degrees to what goes on around them. Their suffering is of a quite different intensity for they cannot see beyond it. Only by forgetting or being distracted can they find relief.

As children grow older the possibility of talking their emotions through with an adult gains in importance. How the adult stands towards the experience in question is then crucial. One-sided expressions of sympathy or indignation at the event which caused the anguish will be of little use. What will help, however, is for the adult to make clear to the child, with or without words, that he or she is genuinely concerned with the child's distress, and takes it seriously. For dealing with handicapped and chronically ill children, see Chapter 9.

Before the age of ten, the child is unable to come to terms consciously with emotional stress. However, if he experiences that the adult is concerned with his problem, accepts it, and does not repress it, then he may feel that his suffering has a purpose and represents a kind of task to be accomplished. He senses that even negative experiences, if they can be worked through, have positive consequences later on. If a child plagued by fears comes into contact with an adult who has acquired a deep trust in destiny, then in the soul of the child a longing takes root, consciously or unconsciously, to acquire the same trust. Later he will find it easier to work on his own fearful attitude to the world.

Here too, we find what we have already noticed in dealing with physical pain: the adult must take on that part of the burden which the child cannot yet deal with and, in place of the child, work it through and overcome it. In the final analysis, the real remedy for all suffering is genuine interest in the other — namely, love.

3 Breathing difficulties

3.1 Colds

Colds in babies

With a very young baby, a cold can lead to problems and should therefore be checked and treated by a doctor. Young babies normally breathe through the nose; they breathe through their mouths only when they are crying. As a result, a cold can lead to a severe obstruction of breathing even to the point where the skin can turn blue *(cyanosis)*. Obstructed breathing is most apparent when they are drinking at the breast. The baby fixes hungrily, sucks a gulp, chokes or tries helplessly to breathe, lets go of the nipple, cries, becomes pink again and fastens on again; and this goes on until the child is exhausted.

When a baby's nose is obstructed, it must therefore be cleared, and this can be done in the following ways:

Fresh air in the room moistened with steam prevents the mucous membranes from drying out so that mucous can be more easily cleared from the narrow passages by sneezing and swallowing. With central or floor heating, extra humidifiers can be used, or damp cloths can be hung up. These should be renewed frequently.

Fresh air will often have a soothing effect. Wrap the baby up warmly in pure woollen clothes and shawl. Cover well, if necessary adding a hot-water bottle at the feet and put the pram or bed by the open window or outside.

Oily nose-drops and ointments should be applied only to the entrance of the nostrils. For the inner mucous membrane only water-soluble preparations are recommended. One cannot always avoid using nasal decongestants, but make sure that they are intended specially for babies. They should not contain ephedrine, and should not be used for more than a few days. The nose can be washed out by careful use of a medicine-dropper filled with a salt solution (1% sodium chloride concentration) which you can make yourself.

Dissolve one level teaspoon of salt in half a litre (one pint) of water. Boil the solution and it will keep for up to two days. Boil the dropper daily to sterilize it.

After its first cold, a baby may regularly snort or snore for months. As long as the baby is not unduly troubled, the cold can be left to clear up eventually on its own, and any attempt at treatment is usually pointless.

Sneezing in a young baby does not usually mean the beginning of a cold. By sneezing, a baby expels from the nasal passages any crusted flakes of mucous, resulting normally from dry air in the room rather than from an inflammation.

Colds in older children

Even with older children, the use of nasal decongestants should be treated with caution; a cold has its reason and follows its natural course, and will clear up. The use of drugs contracts the vessels of the mucous membranes and the ensuing flaccidity hinders the natural processes. Constant use of nasal drops may eventually dry out and damage the mucous membrane of the nose. If the nostrils do become dry or chafed for whatever reason, a soothing herbal ointment (such as Weleda *Balsamicum* or *Calendula)* can be applied.

For severe colds, we recommend inhalation with camomile infusion (see Appendix). In addition, a 2% solution of salt in lukewarm water, sniffed up through the nose and spat out of the mouth, has proved very effective. The salt solution is more concentrated than mucous, thus causing the membrane to shrink and at the same time absorbing excess secretion and clearing the entrances to the nasal sinuses. Although this is not a very pleasant exercise, it is extremely effective.

3.2 Catarrhal infections and influenza

A runny nose usually develops at the beginning of or during a catarrhal infection *(catarrh* means "downflow"). Inflammation of the sinuses may occur and extreme inflammation may cause ear problems as well. The throat with its lymphatic tissues is always affected: specifically the tonsils and lymph vessels at the side and back wall of the pharynx (the cavity behind nose and mouth). These lymphatic organs at the very frontier of the body develop the organism's immune system and are its first line of defence.

A catarrhal infection often brings with it an inflammation of the mucous membrane   of   the   wind-pipe *(tracheitis)* and of the bronchial tubes *(bronchitis)*. When the entrance to the air passages and larynx is affected, the patient becomes hoarse. When deeper parts are affected, a cough ensues. These infections are accompanied by a more or less high fever for one to three days, and can develop into flu quite easily.

Flu (influenza) becomes acute when, in addition to the above symptoms, aches and pains are felt in the head or limbs. Sometimes these infections are characterized by a double peak of fever: a short rise in temperature (often undetected) occurs over two days or so, followed by a pause, followed again by a fresh bout of high temperature lasting about three days. If fever over 38.5°C (101.5°F) continues for more than three days, it is possible that the original infection has developed into a more serious illness. By then it is high time to contact the doctor.

Most catarrhal infections and flu will clear up after a few days without any other treatment than nursing. During this kind of illness, treatments that merely suppress the symptoms such as antipyretics (for example, paracetamol and aspirin), codeine, decongestants, analgesics and antibiotics, are only an unnecessary hindrance for the organism. A child who is otherwise healthy will cope with a mild flu infection unaided and will acquire resistance for a time against further infection.

Increased immunity from colds, flu and similar infections may not be immediately apparent. Often parents complain that no sooner has their child started pre-school nursery than he is at home in bed again, and this can happen to the same child again and again. However, generally the child acquires the necessary immunity after a couple of winters; his body has "learnt" to deal with common infections.

We can see, too, how common children's diseases play a part in this "learning" process. After catching measles or chicken-pox, for instance, a child is often not so affected by colds, coughs and similar ailments. The effect of common children's diseases can be even more striking when younger members of the family catch an illness from an older brother or sister. At first this can be worrying for parents as younger children who have not yet developed strong powers of resistance may contract the illness in a more severe and at times alarming form. Later, however, they generally grow more robust than their older siblings and their immunity is stronger.

The whole process of building up immunity starts with contracting an illness, and we should understand that this may be due not just to the prevalence of the illness or to lack of resistance but to a whole range of circumstances affecting the child. Illness can be a reaction of the child's whole organism to an overtaxing experience. The temperature can shoot up after a birthday party or a long car journey, or after watching an exciting film. What is happening here is that the organism "seeks" and contracts the illness in order to compensate for being overtaxed. Experiences such as a grown-up's anger or a severe telling off, can similarly overtax the child's psyche. In cases like this, the child's soul "freezes" into itself, and cries out for comfort.

To help a child through illness, we must provide soul-warmth, to make the child feel loved and cared for, as well as physical warmth and comfort. A complete therapy will be directed not at suppressing the symptoms of the illness but towards calming and strengthening the child's whole being.

With these considerations in mind, we can now turn to practical measures in a case of flu:

Provide fresh (not too dry) air in the room.

Spray a little eucalyptus oil or Oil of Olbas on a cloth or put some on a warm saucer and place in the room.

Give steam inhalations (see Appendix).

If the child is shivering, keep it warm. To bring out sweat, give hot herb-tea and wrap the child up well. Once the child is hot, it can be put in the parents' pleasantly cool bed.

Sick children should be allowed to sleep a lot and should not be subjected to excitement. Don't give them mechanical or electrical toys (see Chapter 12.8). A woolly dwarf, peeping out from under the blankets, or going mountaineering on top of the blanket, will keep a child happy for hours (Figure 10).

A chest rub is usually very pleasant and soothing (for instance, a 10% lavender oil rub).

For general treatment of fever, see Chapter 1.2.

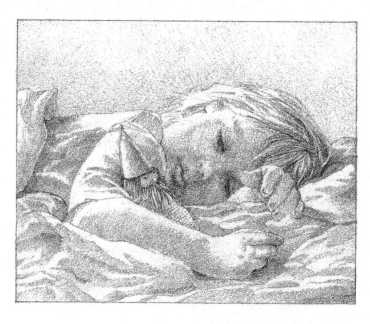

Figure 10. A soft toy is a comfort during illness.

3.3 Adenoids

In childhood, chronic blockage of the air passage at the back of the nose is usually due to enlargement of the lymphatic tissue of the adenoids. In older children, an ENT (ear, nose and throat) specialist can see adenoids clearly with a special mirror. In exceptional cases the adenoids can be felt with a finger, but this is not pleasant for the child. We do not recommend that adenoids be X-rayed because of the exposure to radiation, and in any case the clinical symptoms are quite clear. Pronounced cases of enlarged adenoids are easily recognizable from the child's characteristically somewhat sleepy facial expression, the open mouth, blocked nose, defective hearing, and snoring at night.

These lymphatic enlargements tend to become smaller later on, but even so they often prevent the child from acquiring the desired resistance to infection by the age of five. Being badly ventilated, the local area becomes an ideal breeding ground for all kinds of "bugs" and the sufferer is subject to repeated inflammations of the middle ear or the nasal cavities, or to bronchitis. Sometimes the hearing is affected as the enlargements obstruct the entrance to the Eustachian tubes, preventing aeration of the middle ear. This may lead to a delay in the development of speech.

With enlarged adenoids, it is always worth trying simple natural treatment at home in the first instance. Start by giving the child regular sea-salt baths two to three times a week. Give steam inhalations twice a day, a cup of equisetum (horse-tail) tea to be taken three times daily, and mustard poultices under the soles of the feet three times a day (see Appendix). It is recommended that a lot of singing and humming is done with the child. Continue the whole treatment for four to six weeks. If there is no improvement, the doctor should be consulted. A holiday by the sea is often beneficial.

An operation to remove the adenoids is always advisable where the complaint represents a real physical and mental impediment to the child. Nevertheless the swelling can grow again after an operation. As the palatine tonsils are important protective organs, they should be removed at the same time only in really pressing cases, and not merely because of a danger of tonsillitis.

3.4 Hay fever

Hay fever is nearly always associated with an allergy to the pollen of flowering grass, trees or flowers. Often it is animal hairs or even house-dust (more specifically the excrement of the acarina, or housemite) which irritate the mucous membrane of the eyes and nose. Bacteria and fungi can cause the same symptoms. Sufferers from this complaint, especially if they are also inclined to be asthmatic, should seek long-term treatment. Sea air with its low allergy content has a good effect, and prolonged or repeated visits to the sea are generally strengthening. There are three possible therapies, all of which must be carried out regularly and consistently:

Desensitization
This consists of regular injections of specially prepared allergen-extracts which are injected under the skin in increasing doses. The patient is tested for allergies beforehand. Good results are obtained when the problem arises from a specific plant allergen. Results are not so good when several allergens are involved, or in the case of house dust which is not completely avoidable. Disadvantages of this treatment are: it can last three years or more; it requires frequent injections; and there is a certain risk that the patient may react badly to them. A bad allergic reaction can be so violent that it induces a circulatory shock requiring immediate medical treatment. Finally, it is not unknown for a change of allergy to take place during or after desensitization, with the result that hay fever returns but now brought on by a different allergen. Therefore we recommend the second and third treatments.

Honey treatment
One spoonful of *honey* must be taken regularly each day for a whole year. The honey should be pure *local* honey, eaten straight from the comb, including wax and all, as this contains local pollen.

Gencydo inhalations
Sufferers are given regular inhalations of Gencydo, an extract of lemon and quince (Weleda). It is normal for Gencydo treatment to start in spring so as to provide protection during the coming season. Additional treatment for the constitution will usually be necessary. Many patients obtain relief with this treatment and return a year later to consolidate the improvement.

For older children, Gencydo injections can be used as an alternative to inhalations.

3.5 Illnesses of the lower air passages

For a better understanding of illnesses in the lower air passages, it will be useful to take a general look at different breathing noises and their origins.

Coughing
Coughing is the body's defensive reaction against mucous or inflammatory irritation in the air passages or bronchi, and more occasionally against an inhaled foreign body.

Barking cough
A barking cough with air hunger and inspiratory wheeze (stridor) due to swollen or inflamed vocal chords indicates what is called croup or laryngitis (see below).

Hoarseness and loss of voice
Inflammatory irritation of the vocal chords can also come about through overstraining the voice. Chronic hoarseness can be the result of lumps, known as singer's nodules, on the vocal chords, a condition which needs to be diagnosed by an ENT (ear, nose, throat) specialist.

Harsh noise when breathing in, air hunger, indrawing of the skin between the ribs and at the neck above the breastbone
Any of the following can be involved:
A reflex closure of the vocal chords, caused by small particles of food after choking. Calm the patient and slap his back.
Croup or acute laryngitis (see below).
A lack of calcium sometimes occurring between the ages of three and eighteen months. A visit to the doctor is urgent (see Chapter 15.2 on calcium deficiency and rickets).

Snoring noise when breathing in
The limp tongue lies on the lower throat. Lay the child on one side and the snoring will stop.

Muffled noise and very little air entry when breathing
This constricted throaty noise is not the same as normal snoring as it occurs on breathing in and out. If this symptom appears with a high temperature, sore throat, and a feeling of being very unwell, often with a flow of saliva, as well as the lips and fingernails turning blue, then it is likely to be a **swelling of the epiglottis**, which can lead to suffocation. *Get the patient to the hospital immediately.*
At the hospital, a plastic tube will be inserted through the nose or mouth into the air passage to get through the blockage (intubation).

Hawking, rasping noise when breathing in
This is harmless as long as there is no high fever or "flaring nostrils" (see

below). Some mucous has collected somewhere in the throat.

Fine singing high-pitched noise when breathing out

This comes with longer out-breathing in relation to in-breathing, and there may also be a shortness of breath. It indicates a wheezy bronchitis or asthmatic bronchitis (see below).

Flaring nostrils

The sides of the nostrils distend when the child breathes in and fall back in when he breathes out. This indicates lack of air, that is, the supply of air is obstructed or parts of the lungs are not functioning due to some illness. Together with normal but heavier breathing, high fever, coughing and dark lips, this is often an indication of pneumonia (see below). Call a doctor.

Various types of cough

A cough which lasts for a week or two after a bout of catarrh or flu can in most cases be regarded as normal and treatment can be continued on the same lines as before. Cough-suppressing medicines are not called for, but we recommend a soothing tea consisting of sage leaves or plantain *(Plantago lanceolata),* or a mixture of both. Infuse one teaspoon per cup, add honey and lemon and give to the child as hot as possible. This infusion works like a good cough mixture.

A cough persisting longer than two weeks needs watching for fever. Take the child's temperature morning and evening for one week and if there is still no change in the cough, consult the doctor.

With a **cough occurring increasingly in bouts,** whooping cough may be suspected. The bouts are fairly short and at intervals of more than half an hour. The cough sounds hard, staccato, and is often accompanied by a wheezing intake of breath. The face may turn blue. Eventually a glassy mucous is coughed up. If however the bouts come more frequently or there is constant constricted coughing, the problem is less likely to be whooping cough and is probably a **bronchial irritation.** Whooping cough is usually worse at night and may be accompanied by vomiting. (For a full description of whooping cough, see Chapter 6.11).

Coughing, a cold and a temperature ten to thirteen days after the child has been exposed to measles is a sign that he will probably get measles too. He should then be isolated from other children who are liable to catch measles, unless the parents particularly want them to get it. Also do not bring the child to the doctor without prior permission, otherwise other children in the doctor's waiting-room may be infected. (For a full description of measles, see Chapter 6.1).

Coughs going on for hours at night only, *without* any other complications, are usually due to a minor irritation of the wind-pipe. Treat as for catarrh (see 3.2 above). The child is usually less affected than the parents whose sleep has been disturbed.

A sudden fit of coughing without warning by day, possibly accompanied by a desire to vomit, difficulty in breathing, wheezing intake of breath, a high-pitched or a squeaky jerky noise, especially when breathing out, suggest that a foreign body has been swallowed and is lodged in the windpipe. Likely candidates are small nuts, beads or bits of plastic toys. Particularly dangerous are marbles and pellets which can totally block the air passages.

Where a child's airway is completely obstructed, you will hear high-pitched noises as the child tries to breathe, and the lips may start to turn blue. In this case, with an infant, hold the baby supported on your arm with its head lower than its body (Figure 11). Support the head with your hand around the jaw and chest. Give four rapid blows between the shoulder blades. Turn the baby over on to its back, continuing to support the head and neck, and lay it on your thighs with the head again lower than the rest of the body. Give four chest thrusts with the heel of your hand.

In the case of an older child with completely obstructed airway, kneel on the floor and lay the child across your thighs, keeping the head lower than the rest of the body (Figure 12). Deliver four sharp back blows between the shoulder blades. Supporting the head and back, roll the child over and give four chest thrusts using the heel of the hand.

If a child or infant has only partial airway obstruction, that is, some air is being breathed in and out, do not

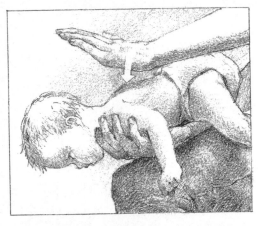

Figure 11. Clearing airway obstruction in an infant.

turn the patient upside down. This may cause complete obstruction. Do not carry out abdominal thrusts on an infant or child, and do not stick your fingers blindly down the child's throat.

If you suspect that a **foreign body is in the lung,** phone the doctor or take the child into hospital. As a precaution do not give little children nuts

Figure 12. Clearing airway obstruction in an older child.

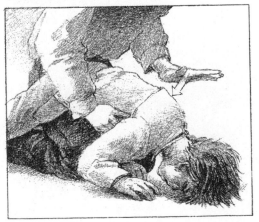

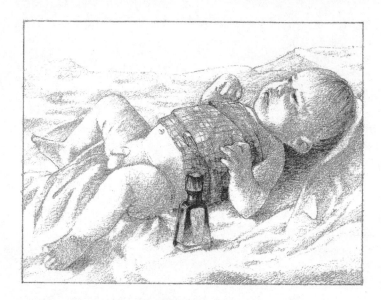

Figure 13. Using a chest compress.

(unless they are ground), or toys with small parts. (See also the section on first aid at the back of the book).

Pains felt behind the breastbone when breathing or coughing are mostly due to irritation of the mucous membrane of the air passages and can be treated by steam inhalation and drinking appropriate herb teas (see Chapter 14.4) with honey, and with oil compresses on the chest (Figure 13 and Appendix). For an effective oil compress, use 10% lavender oil or eucalyptus oil, adding one part of the oil to nine parts olive oil.

Croup (acute laryngitis)

Croup begins with a hard barking cough, often accompanied by a noisy intake of breath (inspiratory stridor). The symptoms are brought about by an inflamed swelling of the vocal cords and the surrounding mucous membranes, due to a viral infection. This cough usually begins during the night between 11 pm and 1 am, and rarely during the day. It is often preceded by a walk on a windy day, excitement or a change of weather. In early winter the number of cases increases. Children between the ages of two and four are particularly affected as they are learning to speak and heavy demands are being made on the larynx at this stage of development.

Croup can be a frightening experience for children, made worse when attacks happen, as they frequently do, at night and in the dark. With severe difficulty in breathing, the child may become afraid of suffocating and will need a lot of reassurance. Take the child out of bed into your arms or your lap. Check the child's breathing difficulty and repeat ten minutes or so later to assess the stage of the illness (see below). Moisten the air in the room with a humidifier, or damp cloths hung round the bed, or a basin of hot water placed in a safe spot on the floor. The bathroom shower turned on hot will produce steamy air. Keep a watch on the child's temperature and give any medicine prescribed by the doctor for such an emergency. Encourage the child to drink sips of sweet herb tea (see Chapter 14.4). When the child is put back to bed again, an adult should sleep in the same room or in a neighbouring room with the doors open in order to listen for any worsening of the condition.

The first time an attack of croup occurs, it is best to bundle the child straightaway into the car and drive to the nearest hospital or doctor. With experience of the condition, you will learn to divide the attack into four stages, and this will help in assessing the severity of any future attack:

Stage 1: barking cough.

Stage 2: slightly noisy intake of breath (stridor) when resting, stronger when agitated.

Stage 3: stronger stridor when resting, flaring nostrils, indrawing of the chest wall between the ribs and the base of the neck, exertion of the auxiliary breathing muscles in neck and shoulder.

Stage 4: symptoms of stages 1-3 now more pronounced, the child becoming noticeably more restless, lips and fingernails turning blue, pulse increasing to 150 to the minute and faster, possible collapse.

Stages 1 and 2 can be safely treated at home. If stage 3 lasts longer than ten minutes or goes into stage 4, the child should be taken instantly to the hospital. If other methods fail, it will be necessary to insert a plastic tube through the nose or mouth into the air passage to get through the blockage (intubation).

In home treatment, do not use strong sedatives as these can mask the condition. The best way of reassuring and calming the child is for all involved to respond to the situation coolly, calmly and efficiently. Because of the obvious dangers of this illness, advice at a distance may be less reliable than in other cases.

Asthma and wheezy (spastic) bronchitis

"Is it asthma or wheezy bronchitis?" We often get this question in the consulting-room when a child has frequent bronchial coughs. It is worth looking at wheezy bronchitis and asthma in more detail.

With wheezy (sometimes known as obstructive or spastic) bronchitis, a child breathes out with long drawn out breaths and lies listlessly with inflated chest and flaring nostrils. When the child breathes out, you can hear a mixture of soft whistling and thin blowing sounds from the nose, rather like water murmuring in a kettle or the asthmatic breathing of older people.

Wheezy bronchitis usually develops from a mild infection of the upper air passages, resulting from a cold or sore throat. The infection then spreads down into the lower air passages. Mucous accumulates in the bronchi, the mucous membrane swells up, the bronchi become blocked and breathing is obstructed. Spasms of the bronchi can occur in both older infants and children. The illness can run its course either with or without fever.

Wheezy bronchitis often affects fatter babies, particularly in winter and when the seasons are changing. Children tend to grow out of it and by no means every child sufferer of wheezy bronchitis later becomes asthmatic.

When symptoms appear for the first time, the doctor should be consulted. With experience, you will learn how to assess the condition yourself. There are mild forms which hardly affect the children's general well-being; indeed, they become very lively and up to all sorts of tricks. In other cases, they whistle badly in their breathing, can hardly drink and show a slightly bluish colouring. These cases need medical attention, sometimes even hospitalization.

The best home-remedy apart from fresh moist air is the mustard compress (see Appendix). This compress is so beneficial that it is well worth the trouble involved in its preparation. The effect of the compress is powerful, so it should be used only if you know exactly how to apply it. Seek a doctor's advice first. The compress is generally suitable for children over four months old whose skin is not too sensitive and who are not allergic to it.

The efficacy of the mustard compress lies in the powerful stimulus which it gives to the blood circulation in the skin of the chest, which in turn stimulates breathing and encourages the flow of secretions (thus making it easier to cough) and the relaxation of the bronchial muscles.

Asthma sounds very similar to obstructive bronchitis and is distinguishable only by its persistence. It can be provoked by external allergens (such as pollen, animal hair or house-mites) or by infections, exertion or psychological causes. Therapy is easier in adults than children, and the problem sometimes clears up of its own accord during puberty.

As asthma is a serious chronic illness, it requires careful long-term treatment. The affected child and those around him have to learn how to cope with the suffocating and frightening symptoms of an attack. How serious an attack is must be learned by parents through experience. Just as an asthma attack can be brought on by excitement and emotion, so it can be eased and soothed by calmness and by breathing and relaxation exercises. An extensive talk with the parents of younger children is often necessary here, and later with the child, too. Accepting and learning to live with asthma will help positively towards an improvement in the condition.

Treating an acute attack of asthma is normally a matter for the doctor. Taking a longer view, the doctor must decide whether the condition can be controlled with homoeopathic or anthroposophical medicines together with treatment for relief of the symptoms. Sufferers should have plenty of liquids and possibly hot foot-baths with lemon, lavender oil or equisetum. If the patient is not allergic to it, mustard compresses (see Appendix) are useful in attacks caused by infections. In other cases, compresses with lavender oil or hot equisetum (see Appendix) should be tried first. Massages can also be helpful if correctly applied. With some children, rubbing the area of the kidneys with Cuprum met. 0.1% ointment every evening can bring relief. Teas containing tannin (India or China) in the morning, and bitter teas in the evening, can help to strengthen the rhythm of waking and sleeping.

Internal medicines should always be prescribed specifically by the doctor. Your doctor may recommend broncho-dilators, cortisone, and other drugs which are commonly used. In our practice, we try to manage with as few such drugs as possible, as they have considerable side-effects affecting the whole hormone metabolism as well as the cardiovascular system. On the whole, we recommend homoeopathic and/or anthroposophical constitutional remedies with which we have had good results.

Pneumonia

If, after three days of flu or bronchitis, the child's fever is still high and there are signs of shortness of breath, flaring nostrils and dark red lips, then pneumonia has set in. The diagnosis of pneumonia usually sounds frightening to parents, though in the majority of cases where school-age children are involved, the illness is not really dangerous. Only with babies and very delicate children do we have to be particularly careful.

Treatment of pneumonia should be supervised by the doctor who, with a vulnerable child or where home nursing is inadequate, may recommend hospital admission. Specialist knowledge is needed to treat without antibiotics, but in our experience, managing without antibiotics has the advantage that pneumonia is very rarely caught a second time. If we block the normal course of the illness with antibiotics, the body will be unable to use its own resources fully to tackle the infection and therefore will not be strengthened to resist new infections. Those who regard illness as something to be got rid of as quickly as possible will prefer antibiotic treatment, but if we understand illness as the body's learning process, we will choose a treatment which has a harmonizing and soothing effect on the course of the illness rather than one which merely suppresses it and weakens the organism.

Home treatment of pneumonia is basically the same as for flu, but modified to suit the child's condition.

If the cough is predominant, especially with thin children, we recommend rubbing the chest with 10% lavender oil (see Appendix) or balsam which contains other etheric oils such as camphor, eucalyptus, plantago bronchial balsam (Wala) or plantago lanceolata 10% ointment.

If there is a considerable accumulation of fluid in the lungs, use a warm damp compress with equisetum (horse-tail) tea or a thick quark (curd cheese) compress (see Appendix).

If there is also asthma-like breathing as described above, a mustard compress could be used. Care should be taken with clothing and covering the patient. It is not enough to clothe only the upper part of the body with a sleeveless vest and cover the rest of the body with a warm quilt or eiderdown. In most cases a long-sleeved

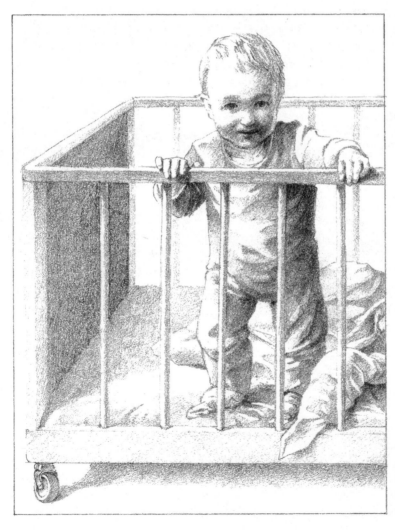

Figure 14. A cot on wheels can be moved easily around the house.

pure woollen vest or woollen pullover that covers the kidneys and elbows is recommended. Even in the warmest weather, it is necessary to cover the whole body, and this can be done by means of a cotton or linen sheet in bed or a long-sleeved cotton night-gown. The feet and ankles, however, may be allowed to stick out from below the covering as long as the child is awake and feels comfortable. In general, it is preferable to use natural textiles such as pure wool, cotton, linen or silk, for the simple reason that natural textiles allow the child's body to manage its warmth and liquidity much more flexibly.

The air should be as fresh as possible without causing a draught.

But the child should never be allowed to shiver or be at all cold. So long as the rest of the body is warmly clad, exposing the face to the cold will do no harm.

Restless children who, in spite of their fever, are always throwing off their covering, jumping out of bed, or wanting to run around the room, should be calmed down and encouraged to stay in bed. An asset here is a cot on wheels which the mother can push around the house with her (Figure 14). Give the children simple toys to play with which will allow the imagination plenty of scope and encourage creative play (see Chapter 12.8).

3.6 Breathing as the expression of soul

Nothing is more revealing of a person's feelings than to observe how they are breathing. If we watch the breathing of a new-born infant, we can already see a delicate variation between excitement and rest. In a baby or a small child we notice a full breathing out and relaxation as they fall asleep and a deep breathing in as they wake up. In the everyday life of children we observe the indrawn breath of pain, of anxious anticipation, of sudden cold; and then the exuberant outpouring of happiness, of letting go in resignation, of high spirits. All these moods are conveyed by a rhythm of breathing that is responsive to the slightest change.

Breathing is a part of the rhythm of daily life. In the waking state, the soul is fully drawn into the body ready for sensation, movement and experience, the urge to act, love and hate. In the sleeping state, a peacefully resting "remainder" is left behind: the body lies there relaxed and heavy and the breathing continues now only as a part of the life processes in a gentle in and out. It is no longer the bearer of any conscious thought-life and it is no longer the vehicle for any expression of feeling.

Illness and other disorders in the body can affect the breathing. For example, with heart, lung or kidney disease, a small change in the acidity of the blood alters the rate and depth of breathing. Certain medicines and drugs can also change the pattern of breathing as in the case of barbiturates which have a dampening effect on breathing.

Just as we were able to speak of a warmth organism in connection with the activity of the "I" (see Chapter 1.4), we may also refer to the body's relationship to air, regulated by breathing, as an organically distinct air organism. On the one hand it is linked with the whole metabolic system by means of gaseous exchange and various buffer systems in the blood circulation. On the other hand it allows the soul-life of the human being the possibility of coming to physical expression. The characteristics of the soul-life (sympathy and antipathy, joy and sorrow, laughing and crying) correspond to the laws determining the behaviour of air (compression and expansion, heating and cooling). Whatever the "I" experiences in its soul has an immediate effect on the warmth and air systems and so exercises a helping or hindering effect on the body's working. Conversely, of course, the physical disorders we have mentioned can also have a powerful effect on our soul-life. The interaction between body and soul is thus a very concrete example of principles which are at work in warmth and air. On the one hand, these are the vehicle for experiences which are purely in the soul and spirit and on the other hand they regulate the metabolic processes. Seen in this way, the material world and the soul are only different areas in which spiritual activity takes place. In the course of life a human being can develop spiritual powers to an ever higher degree of perfection and may express these through the body.

By its very nature, the soul wishes to be preoccupied with itself only temporarily, thereafter to open itself to its environment. That is why the soul's connection with air is also the basis for fellow feeling. As we listen to and share someone's joys and sorrows we experience a corresponding ease or constriction in our breathing. By the same token much of what someone is wishing to tell us is conveyed to us through the medium of air in the sound of what is being said.

The alternation of sleeping and waking is a rhythm we find on a small scale in every breath we draw: as we give back the breath we have drawn and breathed out there is a falling asleep and as we breathe in, a waking up. And we can also see how the great alternation of birth and death is expressed through breathing. With the first breath that is drawn the consciousness-bearing soul is drawn into the dark-coloured body of the newly-born child. At that moment the skin becomes pink, the eyes open and the child's first cry is heard. In the last indescribably delicate and long exhalation of the dying human being, we experience the final departure from a now unusable body.

4 Stomach and bowel disorders

It will be helpful to indicate what we mean by vomiting and diarrhoea as parents are often worried by perfectly normal events which do not indicate anything wrong.

Vomiting is when at least a quarter of the nourishment taken is brought up again. It should be distinguished from *regurgitation*, sometimes called possetting or spitting, which is when babies bring up mouthfuls of food for a variety of reasons.

Diarrhoea does not mean a couple of soft bowel movements a day. The things to look for in helping the doctor to decide if diarrhoea is present are as follows: first, frequency (how many bowel movements are there a day? More than six?); second, amount (do the movements amount to a few squirts or a cupful?); third, colour (is the movement yellow, grey, green, brown, black, bloody?); fourth, consistency (is the movement runny, slimy, or paste-like?).

Take the child's temperature in a case of diarrhoea to see if there is fever. By fever we mean a temperature of over 38°C (100.5°F) measured in the mouth.

Chronic digestive disorders

Chronic disorders of the digestion in babies are indicated if the child does not thrive over a period. Such problems must be treated by a doctor. One possible disorder may be a gluten allergy (see Chapter 14.3).

The doctor will be helped considerably in making the diagnosis if the parents can tell him whether the total daily motion is more than a large cupful, and can bring a small specimen of the stools.

4.1 Vomiting and diarrhoea in baby's first year

Occasional vomiting

Occasional vomiting can occur in young babies for a wide variety of reasons and is not always to be taken as indicating a disorder. It can be caused by overfeeding or eating food which has been stored too long, stomach wind, over-excitement, a cold, a sore throat, or teething. Try to find out the cause but, regardless of what it is, give the baby some liquid, for example mineral water or herb tea (see Chapter 14.4).

Frequent vomiting

If a young baby, frequently brings up its milk in a spurt which runs down its chin, or constantly spits out while drinking, it may be that the entry to the stomach is malfunctioning. When the stomach contracts, the milk flows back to the oesophagus instead of onwards. To help this problem, the doctor may recommend laying the child more on an incline with the head higher than the feet. This can be done either by tilting the bed or by putting an extra cushion under the head of the mattress. Normally the entrance to the stomach will start to function correctly after some weeks. By laying the baby down regularly in the correct position, an operation can usually be avoided.

Look out for reddish-brownish streaks of blood in the vomit which rather resemble banana fibres. This is a sign that the oesophagus may have been irritated by the stomach's juices and the doctor should be informed straightaway. Another possible cause of blood in a child's vomit is a Vitamin K deficiency in the child which has to be treated immediately.

Projectile vomiting

In the first few weeks of life, a baby may begin to spew up like a fountain away from the mouth (projectile vomiting) after most meals. The vomiting can become more pronounced after a few days, and in many cases there is a considerable loss of weight. The baby is inclined to cry but there is no fever **or diarrhoea**. This is **pyloric hypertrophy** or **stenosis**, a condition caused by narrowing of the exit of the stomach.

Action to be taken: check the weight two or three times a week; give smaller feeds more frequently; the mother must get more rest during the day; give baby plenty of time to bring up his wind. If baby loses weight, or even if he does not gain, consult the doctor without further delay. Some children's stomachs can be settled by rubbing copper ointment into the upper stomach, or with a warm stomach compress (see Appendix) or a hot-water bottle. Others need medicine or even a minor operation. In case of hospitalization, the mother should be admitted along with the baby.

Diarrhoea

Diarrhoea in babies under one year requires professional help whether or not it is accompanied by vomiting and fever. Babies at this young age can very quickly dehydrate and collapse.

There are many possible causes of diarrhoea: stale milk or food, local or general cooling of the body, viral infection, bacterial infections (such as E. coli bacteria which affect only babies, or salmonella which can also make adults ill).

Breast-fed babies rarely get this condition. If your breast-fed baby does get diarrhoea, continue to breast-feed and replace what has been lost by mother's milk. You can also give fennel or camomile tea, but do not give anything containing dairy products (see also Chapter 14.3 and 14.4).

With *bottle-fed babies,* follow your doctor's advice. A possible course of action is as follows:

First day: during the period normally covered by the first two feeds, give only fennel tea as often as the baby demands, even hourly. The fennel tea (or fennel-camomile 50:50) should be mixed with 5% glucose (5 grammes to 100 ml tea, or 1 teaspoon to a small teacup) with a few grains of salt. For the third meal in the evening, give thin soup made from rice, cooked until soft and passed through a sieve (about one heaped teaspoon of cooked rice to a cup) with about 5% added glucose. The addition of a little glucose will not do any harm as it can easily be absorbed by the intestine. Recent research has shown that the addition of sugar is of considerable help in the regeneration of the mucous membrane of the intestine.

Second day: Rice soup as above. For babies over three months old add strained mashed carrots to the bottle-feed or feed it as porridge (see Chapter 14.3). Add 5% glucose as before. Increase the mashed carrot with each feed; between three and nine months of age, give between 100-400 grammes a day (4-14 oz) depending on the age of the child. For babies under three months who have not yet been weaned, give only the rice soup, but you can make it a bit thicker. You can also add some strained apple or, where available, blueberry juice which has a binding effect on the diarrhoea, although commercial varieties may contain syrup which acts as a laxative. Do not give any milk products as yet. Any vomiting should have stopped by now. Bowel movements should have become less frequent, and after the carrots the stools should look firmer, the mashed carrots looking much the same coming out as when they went in. Without the carrots the stools usually look unformed, rather slimy and have little substance.

Third day: If all has gone according to plan and any fever has started to go down, you can start to feed with a little milk. If the stools have become more solid or have stopped, mix a quarter to a third boiled milk (or powdered milk if that is what the baby is used to) to every carrot or rice soup feed.

Occasionally the diarrhoea can start again on re-introducing milk to the diet. In this case, professional advice should be sought.

When to call the doctor
If the stools are still runny on the third day or if the baby is very delicate, consult the doctor. You should also let the doctor know if at any stage the baby's tongue becomes dry, dark circles appear around the eyes or fever reaches 40°C (104°F). When a fever first starts to rise, babies will not always drink as much as they should and often react with vomiting. But do not panic. What is the total impression? If the baby looks just a little upset, just keep a watchful eye. If there is blood in the stools, contact the doctor. If you ever observe a total change in the baby's condition, always take the child to the hospital.

4.2 Vomiting and diarrhoea in young children

Simple vomiting and diarrhoea

Vomiting and diarrhoea without fever or appreciable colic and where the abdomen remains soft can be treated at home. In all other cases, consult your doctor.

For home treatment, put the child to bed and nurse as follows:

For the first day give only fennel tea with perhaps a little oatmeal cereal, or thin soup made from rice cooked soft and passed through a sieve, slightly salted. Children who have a history of frequent vomiting should have 5% glucose added.

On the second day, the vomiting should have ceased. Give fennel tea, mashed carrots, grated apple, and possibly mashed bananas, rice cereal or oatmeal cereal, unsweetened blueberry juice, and rusks (zwieback) soaked in water.

By the third day, the diarrhoea should have cleared up, and now you can give thick potato soup or thin oatmeal porridge, toast or crisp-bread.

Children's favourites like sweets, puddings, chocolate and ice-cream should really be avoided until forty-eight hours after vomiting or diarrhoea has stopped. Relapses are often caused by your patient wanting (and getting!) what the other children are eating. The child can start eating normally again after three days without vomiting, diarrhoea or fever.

If vomiting has not stopped on the second day (or in the case of diarrhoea, on the third day), the doctor should be consulted. Similarly you should let the doctor know if the child still cannot take a light diet by the fourth day.

Vomiting or diarrhoea with fever

In cases of vomiting or diarrhoea with fever, see Chapter 1.2.

Acetonemic vomiting

Children between the ages of two and ten are prone to attacks of acetonemic vomiting. This problem occurs when the digestive system temporarily fails to break down fats properly, and acetone is produced. The exact cause is not known. The child's stomach is soft and not painful when pressed, but strong colicky stomach pains can occur before the attack of vomiting, even several hours before.

People with an acute sense of smell can detect a smell of fresh apples or nail polish remover: if you detect this smell, inform the doctor. What the child needs urgently is glucose and plenty of liquid so that the digestion regains its balance.

The following treatment has proved effective: every ten minutes give a mouthful or two of herb tea with 5 to 10% added glucose (1 to 2 heaped teaspoons to a cup). Suitable teas are fennel, camomile and weak apple-tea. Mallow and peppermint are less suitable. Place a warm camomile or sorrel compress (see Appendix) on the stomach.

If the child continues to vomit do not worry. Try to comfort the child, saying that the stomach will soon get better. The patient should sip the tea slowly. Some of it will stay down. After one or two hours, the amount can be increased gradually up to a whole cupful.

Instead of pure glucose-tea, you can give mineral water with glucose. This will make up for the minerals lost.

Every now and again check the stomach carefully to make sure that it is still soft. Once the vomiting has stopped, add rusks (zwieback) to the diet, but nothing else. Next day the child can have light food with no fat. For the third and fourth days, keep fats to a minimum. There is no further need for medicine.

If vomiting continues longer than a few hours, or if the child develops rings round his eyes and a dry tongue, consult the doctor.

Acetonemic vomiting has no connection at all with diabetes, except that in both cases acetone is produced.

Occasional vomiting with headaches

If you notice an increasing occurrence of vomiting, especially with headaches, the symptoms suggest that neurological examination is required. Consult the doctor as soon as possible.

Vomiting after a head injury

Vomiting after a head injury means that the child should be taken to the hospital immediately.

Vomiting after a fright

If a child vomits after a fright, calm the child and keep it warm. In serious cases, take the child to the doctor.

4.3 Chronic constipation

Chronic constipation can have a number of causes. Something in the child's constitution or organs, or even a mental or emotional condition can bring on constipation. It is often triggered by painful anal fissures. The first thing is to see the doctor who will give guidance on treatment. Cases where there are no organic causes are rare but can be cured.

The best and most gentle remedy for chronic constipation is to give an enema with camomile tea (see Appendix). This can be done with a prepared enema or a glycerol suppository, but these do not always soften the stools sufficiently. It is important that the whole colon and not just the rectum is emptied. By feeling the stomach, you can tell how effective the enema has been. As this method of clearing the bowel is habit-forming, it is good to ask the doctor's advice about how often the enema should be given.

Next, a suitable diet should be provided. A number of foods, such as cocoa, bananas, apples, ordinary tea, blueberries and too much milk, are constipating and should be avoided. Peppermint tea may be a useful substitute for the usual glass of milk. Laxative foods are rhubarb, soaked prunes, buttermilk, sour milk, and mineral water. In addition, ground linseed is a universal remedy for constipation in children; give one teaspoonful twice a day before meals, either with a little honey and three drops of lemon, or in sour milk or soup.

The child who prefers a macaroni-white-bread-chocolate diet needs to be introduced to wholefood nourishment such as muesli, honey, wholemeal bread, brown rice and fresh fruit. A diet which contains plenty of natural fibre is to be preferred. But where a child is already getting plenty of high-fibre foods, including coarse wholemeal bread, and is suffering flatulence and stomach-ache, we recommend that you go over to a less bulky diet.

If older children have already experienced constipation, parents will not begin worrying when a child has missed a day. Nothing is more constipating than worrying about it! On the whole, a lively interest in life keeps the body's systems working regularly and so, if the day offers nothing to look forward to, some little surprise should be arranged.

4.4 Worms

Threadworms (pinworms) *(Oxyuris)* arc fragile, threadlike creatures about 1 cm (½″) long. They live in the colon and lay their eggs at night around the anus. This causes itching and eczema in the anus, and children begin to scratch. Fingernails and towels become contaminated and the infection is easily spread to other people.

Treatment: For threadworms, there is a one-off chemical treatment available. But for those who prefer an alternative approach, we have found the following constitutional treatment effective and more long-lasting. Give the child *Allium/cuprum sulphuricum compositum* (Weleda) three times a day for two to three weeks, seven drops at age four to fourteen drops at age ten, diluted in water. Every member of the family must regularly and thoroughly wash hands with soap using a nailbrush, and each person should have a personal towel. Children's nails should be kept short and clean. To reduce itching, localized treatment of the anal area with a anti-itching cream is possible.

Roundworms *(Ascaris)* are common in warmer climates especially. They are about 20 cm (8″) long (the males markedly smaller than the females). They can cause stomach-aches.

Lettuce and raw vegetables fertilized with human excreta can carry the eggs of roundworms. The larvae take between thirty and forty days to develop from the eggs. They are taken into the body through the intestinal lining. They travel to the liver, then to the heart and then to the lungs. Eight days after entering the body, they break through the lung vesicles into the bronchi, and pass through the throat and down again into the stomach and intestine. In the intestine they grow into full worms. During this complicated migration, various symptoms and allergies can appear. The eggs of the worms appear in the stool only after this cycle has been completed.

Treatment: Treat roundworms as for threadworms but additionally give Weleda Quartz 50% three times a day. After about three weeks of this treatment, the itching should stop and no more eggs should be found in the stools.

5 Skin disorders

The skin reveals the state of health of the whole person. Diet, water, metabolism, circulation, liver, kidneys, adrenal glands, thyroid gland and nervous system are all involved in the appearance and condition of the skin. Our emotions, too, are rapidly reflected in the state of our skin: paleness from fright or fear, vivid blushing with shame, and the gentle flush of pleasure.

5.1 Birthmarks

Stork's beak marks or salmon patches

Level, pink patches of skin at birth, commonly known as stork's beak marks or salmon patches (*capillary* or *macular haemangioma*) normally result from a harmless distension of the fine vessels of the skin. When situated in the middle of the forehead or symmetrically on the forehead, eyelids, eyebrows or at the back of the neck, they will usually disappear in the course of the baby's first year. But the asymmetrical marks tend to remain for a lifetime.

Strawberry marks *(Naevi)*

Soft red round lumps known as strawberry marks (superficial *cavernous angioma*) often protrude above the level of the baby's skin. They generally appear and grow during the first year, and disappear slowly during or after the second year. They can be helped to disappear by using a thin application of antimony ointment daily.

Café-au-lait patches

These coffee-coloured patches are usually up to a few centimetres across, with irregular edges. Normally rather inconspicuous, they remain permanent. If there are more than about five of these patches or if they cover a large area of the skin, the doctor should be consulted as there may be an underlying serious disorder.

Dark pigment patches or port wine stains

These darker pigmented areas of the skin *(pigment naevi)*, with or without hair, last for a lifetime. Because of the wide range of sizes and shapes, they need to be assessed in every individual case. Pigment patches that change or grow should be examined by your doctor or perhaps a dermatologist.

5.2 Yellow skin (Jaundice)

Yellow skin *in babies* where the white of the eyes is not affected, is usually due to eating carrots and is quite harmless. If the whites of the eyes are affected, the condition is **jaundice**. Nearly all new-born babies have jaundice to some degree because the liver is being overworked in converting the foetal haemoglobin. Treatment of acute cases is done in the hospital by the use of blue light. Very severe cases are rare but when they occur (usually where there is a blood-group incompatibility between mother and child), the light treatment may be supplemented by an exchange blood transfusion.

Jaundice *in older children* is probably due to a disorder of the liver and will require urgent medical attention.

5.3 Milia (whitish pimples)

Milia often occur with new-born babies. They are small hard white pimples like pinheads, containing horny matter *(keratin)*. The pimples are generally situated around the nose and near the eyes, and will eventually disappear by themselves.

Milia also occur as rather more yellowy patches as big as lentils on the gums or on the border between the bony and the soft palate. Sometimes parents think these are thrush-fungi, but they are not.

5.4 Seborrhoeic dermatitis

There is no common general term for seborrhoeic dermatitis, a group of skin disorders which includes cradle cap. Seborrhoeic dermatitis is an inflammation of the skin due to an irregular flow of sebum, a naturally produced fat in the body. The skin becomes over-active, produces too much sebum, and becomes covered with scales. Rough pimples appear and begin to redden. The inflammation can start in the nappy (diaper) area, in folds of the body and the navel. The problem can slowly spreads and may affect even the whole body. If this happens, the skin must be specially protected so that the raw places do not fester. However, children with this complaint are not itchy and are usually cheerful.

It is not always easy for the doctor to distinguish seborrhoeic dermatitis from an attack of fungus. The two conditions can easily overlap. Seborrhoeic dermatitis usually clears up by the time the baby is four months old. It may, however, change location and character, finally turning into *atopic dermatitis*, meaning that the condition can now occur anywhere on the body. Treatment consists of oil-baths and ointments containing precipitated sulphur.

Cradle cap

Cradle cap is the name given to coarse greasy yellowish scales that harden on the scalp and eyebrows in the first months of a baby's life. When they appear, the scales can be removed by soaking with oil and then gently prising off with a fine comb. You need not be afraid of damaging the fontanelle, the soft spot on the top of the head. As the baby grows, cradle cap will gradually disappear.

Pimples on the cheek

Pimples commonly appear on thickened skin of the cheeks in the first weeks of a baby's life. The pimples are tough in texture and resemble cradle cap. They belong to the category of seborrhoeic dermatitis and are the result of hormonal changes similar to those of puberty. These pimples contain sebum and are not purulent or contagious. They need to be distinguished from pustules (see 5.8 below). Treatment is unnecessary but they are usually helped by a skin cream or camomile ointment.*

---

* *Unguentum leniens,* or cold cream.

5.5 Chronic eczema

In recent years, chronic eczema, otherwise known as atopic dermatitis or neuro-dermatitis, has become widespread. In our opinion, this is not principally because of environmental pollution with poisons and irritants, but is due to changes in modern living conditions.

Chronic eczema affects the skin chiefly in the creases of the joints, but also the face, neck, trunk, and even the whole body. Rough little papules appear, sometimes combining and forming raised patches, and sometimes becoming raw and oozy. Because of itching, the affected areas are often scratched so that they bleed and become crusty. In most cases consultation with the doctor is necessary.

In more than half the children suffering this condition, the problem runs in the family. Sufferers are prone to have food allergies (for instance to milk and other protein foods), and similarly there are frequent associations with hay-fever and asthma. Occasionally, there may be underlying causes: malfunctioning of the liver-gall system, of the kidneys, or of the digestive system.

As eczema is accompanied by severe itching, the complaint can become a test of endurance for the whole family. Much depends on how calmly the parents cope with the situation. Often parents are at the end of their tether because the itchy scratching child is not only suffering but can also be extremely demanding. The child wants attention. It will not settle in bed. It always wants the opposite of what everyone else wants. From being the darling of the family, the young eczema sufferer can easily become the tyrant. But it is precisely the most difficult children who should be treated as normally as possible. After you have attended to the itchy skin, let the child fit into the normal routine of the day without any further special attention.

Therapy should be internal as well as external. The following suggestions are only stopgap measures. When the itching is particularly bad, calmly and quietly get a bath ready. Baths or compresses with an equisetum (horse-tail) infusion will relieve the itching. Take a handful of equisetum leaves and boil for five minutes in one litre (a quart) of water, allow to infuse for fifteen minutes and use the strained liquid as a compress or else as a bath mixture in not too hot a bath. After the bath, apply fresh skin cream and cover all the itchy places with cotton underwear, ideally a one-piece suit which even covers the hands (see Appendix). *Hypericum/ Calendula* ointment (Weleda)* is re-

* A possible prescription is *Equisetum arv.* H 10% 50, *Eucerin cum Aqua ad* 200.

commended for the skin when dry. At other times when the skin is very itchy, it should be rubbed at frequent intervals with a soothing ointment such as *Combudoron* or *Dermatodoron* ointment (Weleda).*

These remedies are meant as a temporary measure until your doctor has been consulted and regular treatment is prescribed for the individual case. A common prescription is for the regular use of ointment containing cortisone. We have used this only when the parents or child could not cope with the extra demands of the other treatment.

Eczema tells us something about the child and its surroundings. The skin of an eczema sufferer is dry, dead and as if cut off from its environment. The scratching is an expression of the urge to break out of this shell. The child needs, in the first place, a more comfortable outer skin. We attempt to provide this through covering the affected areas with compresses or ointments, and by dressing the child in appropriate and non-irritable clothing. But we also need to awaken the child's interest in its surroundings, to draw attention away from the body and into the environment itself. If confident boundaries are set, for instance, if the parents know exactly what they want and express it clearly, then the personality of the child can be helped and its relationship to the outside world strengthened. This has a calming effect on what is happening to the skin and is a form of reinforcement which complements medical treatment.

For a fuller description of the meaning of children's illnesses, see Chapter 6.14.

5.6 Skin appearance

Mottled skin

Mottled red and blue skin over whole parts of the body or bluish colouring round the lips, fingernails or feet, can simply mean that a child is getting very cold. Dress the child in warm woolly underclothing and generally wrap the child up warmly, making sure that the limbs and extremities are well protected.

After a large meal children are more susceptible to this condition, as blood-flow to the skin is affected. Such patches can also appear in the early stages of a fever.

If the skin turns blue with, at the same time, faster breathing, a weak or fast pulse and a general feeling of

* A possible prescription is *Equisetum arv.* 10%, *Herba dec. aquos* 100, *Eucerin. anhydric. ad* 200.

being unwell, these may be signs of a lung or heart disorder. The doctor should be called the same day.

When young children have been too long in the cold without moving, **chilblains** can occur. These are red, doughy swellings especially round the finger and toe joints. It is wrong to apply intensive warmth from outside. The former common practice of rubbing the affected part with snow is also harmful. The best remedy is to give hot herb tea with honey and wrap the child up warmly with woollen blankets or in a duvet. Frost cream (Weleda) can be applied.

Flushed cheeks and frost-bite

Flushed cheeks can have a number of causes: fever, teething, scarlet fever, fresh air, excitement. Flushed cheeks can result from too long a walk in the cold wind. Chubby-cheeked babies sometimes suffer very slight frost-bite (see the first aid section at the end of the book). Under the dark red of the skin of the cheek you can feel a rough thickening of the tissue. The skin thus affected is for some weeks very sensitive to cold and should be specially protected with thick daubs of skin cream (Rosecream, Wala/Weleda), and if necessary covered with lint or gauze.

Cases where frostbite leads to increasingly painful swellings on the cheek need immediate medical attention.

Paleness

Paleness of the skin is probably not a sign of anaemia as long as the inside of the eyelids, the lips, ear-lobes and fingernails are pink. But if these are also pale and the child is listless and languid, see the doctor.

5.7 Inflammation of the navel

The navel of a new-born baby can still be moist after three weeks or, after apparently drying up, it can become moist again and sometimes even bleed a little where the umbilical cord was attached. If the skin around the navel is red and swollen, or if the wound is oozing and bleeding, seek medical advice. If there is only slight irritation round the navel, this is usually due to the small wound where the umbilical cord was severed. The rawness will heal in time but the wound should be kept clean and dry.

The doctor will usually help the umbilical wound to heal by dabbing the affected part with an silver nitrate stick. Follow-up treatment at home will be as the doctor prescribes, or as follows:

Clean the navel with cotton wool soaked in surgical spirit, allow to dry, or dab dry, then powder. Do this once or twice a day. The navel-bandage can generally be dispensed with, as a fresh nappy-liner (diaper-liner) is just as clean and is changed more often. Any minor irritation in the area of the navel will also disappear with this treatment. Surgical spirits can irritate the skin and should therefore not be used for longer than three or four days. Oil can be used after that. If the navel still continues to ooze, the doctor should be told.

Secretions, hardened skin, or old powder can irritate inside the navel and could even lead to slight bleeding. Most mothers are understandably not inclined to dabble around much with the navel, but the fear of penetrating inside the abdomen is quite unfounded. So after the baby is at least three weeks old, do not be afraid to give the navel a good clean with cotton wool soaked in calendula or camomile oil.

5.8 Pustules and vesicles in babies

Babies can suffer from a number of purulent skin diseases which cause rather flat pustules and vesicles, usually only about 2 mm (1/8″) wide and filled with a greeny-yellowish fluid. Staphylococci are to be found in the pus. The pustules appear singly or in groups, generally on the hairy skin of the head, under the armpits or in the nappy (diaper) area. But, unlike the rather more pointed, coarse, yellowish nodules of the seborrhoeic changes of the cheeks, these pustules can appear anywhere on the body.

In rare cases, large pus blisters about one centimetre across swell up in a matter of hours. If this happens, the child should be seen by the doctor right away. Even with the smaller pimples, medical treatment is desirable, but as long as the child otherwise feels all right and there is no fever, the situation is not urgent.

The most important thing in a case of this kind is to prevent any further spread of the infection. All the child's underwear should be changed daily and fresh towels used. The container for the baby's toilet things should be cleaned out and fresh articles used. Ointments should be applied only with a wooden spatula which is afterwards discarded. Wash your hands thoroughly with soap and a nailbrush before and after attending to the child.

Skin problems of this kind appear

not only where there is a lack of hygiene but also in households where there is excessive use of disinfectants for cleaning everything. Disinfectants destroy the normal skin-flora and leave the skin more exposed to bacterial growth. As babies have little resistance to this type of infection, it can easily spread to other infants, and even lead to inflammation of the mother's breasts.

People coming into contact with the baby should make sure their fingernails are kept short and clean. It is also important that hair does not brush over the child and so pick up the bacteria. By following your doctor's advice, the condition can usually be cleared up with careful disinfection and drying of the skin.

5.9 Nappy (diaper) rash

A variety of inflamed skin conditions can easily affect the baby's nappy (diaper) area where the skin is especially sensitive. Frequent changes of nappy and careful cleaning in this area are important to prevent irritation and infection.

During the baby's first weeks, skin irritation can easily occur in the folds and creases of the groin if this sensitive area is not kept thoroughly clean. Take care in cleaning, though, not to rub the skin too roughly. Clean gently using plenty of cooking oil and apply zinc and oil ointment well in the creases. Too much powder in this area cakes and irritates. Sometimes a coarse and greyish thickening of skin appears along the creases. This is simply the top layer of skin becoming encrusted with the cream and powder used. With regular bathing and oiling, this coating should disappear within a week.

Chafing of the skin by plastic pants or plastic nappies can cause a red strip around the baby's stomach or thighs. Protect the skin with a good coating of zinc ointment and change the way of putting on the nappy (see Chapter 12.2).

In the first weeks, you may find a rash of little spots or blisters mainly in the nappy area, but sometimes also on the upper part of the body. These could be an allergic skin reaction rather than resulting from a bacterial or fungal infection. Skin reactions can be caused by materials used in the baby's clothes or by washing powders and conditioners used in washing. We recommend washing nappies and baby-clothes without fabric conditioners and with plain soaps and detergents without enzymes. Also take care not to use too much washing powder. It may be a good idea to give the baby's clothes an extra rinse by hand in case the washing machine does not rinse adequately.

A sudden flaming **redness round the anus**, usually just in the crease between the buttocks, can simply mean that the nappy has remained unchanged too long after a bowel movement. But it can also be caused by the nature of the stools themselves: after the baby has had apple-juice, apples or citrus fruits; or because teething has upset the digestion; or simply at the start of diarrhoea.

Treatment: change the baby's nappy frequently to prevent irritation of the skin. If inflammation occurs, clean the area with a damp cloth, then cover with oil (cooking oil will do) and dab dry using the clean dry corner of a nappy. Apply a thick layer of protective cream that dries the skin, adheres well and is oily (for instance, zinc and castor-oil ointment).

Ammoniacal dermatitis arises when the urine begins to decompose giving off ammonia which irritates the skin. It indicates that nappies are not being changed frequently enough.

Seborrhoeic dermatitis (see 5.4 above) can also attack the nappy area. In this case, too, the area should be cleaned with oil rather than water. After cleaning, apply a good coating of zinc and oil ointment.

Small red spots around the anus or genitals with a fine white scaly ring round the edge suggest an infection with **thrush** (see the following section).

5.10 Fungal infections

Throughout the world, diseases caused by fungi continue to spread. Certain fungal skin diseases have become incredibly widespread since synthetic material in clothing came into common use. Diseases once mainly associated with particular occupations involving, for example, exposure to water, or diseases associated with poor nutrition or housing, are nowadays quite common. In spite of (and in some senses, because of) the increased use of antibiotics to combat them, fungal diseases are more and more of a problem.

Thrush in mouth and nappy (diaper) area

Thrush *(candidiasis)* usually establishes itself in the mouth and thence proceeds through the gut to the anus. It can therefore also be seen in the stools, which will tend to smell of yeast. If the child is having systemic treatment with an antibiotic at the same time (for some other condition), or in the case of very weak children, thrush can be very persistent.

With patience, local treatment of

the mouth and anus will generally be successful. This is also true in cases where antifungal treatment (normally with nystatin) has had only temporary success.

Thrush in the mouth can be seen as a white coating, solid or dispersed, especially along the inside of the cheek. Sometimes a furry coating extends right to the edge of the lips. White coating on the tongue alone, and not on the mucous membrane of the cheek, is not necessarily thrush.

Treatment: paint the mouth with a wash that will make the mucous membrane more resistant to thrush. At the same time, brush away some of the fungus coating. We use a diluted tincture of rhatany and myrrh in equal parts; Weleda mouthwash is made up in this way and can be used diluted, or you can get a solution of extract of echinacea and glycerine in equal parts made up by a pharmacist, and this can be used undiluted. Try it first on your tongue to test the strength. Apply with a cotton-wool bud dipped in the mixture. The fungus does not disappear as quickly with this treatment as with antibiotics, but recurrences are much less common.

Thrush in the nappy (diaper) area consists initially of small vesicles and oozing little nodules which quickly spread, sometimes joining together, with little rings of scales round the edges. The spots usually appear round the anus or genitals, grow together and can finally affect the whole of the nappy area up to the navel.

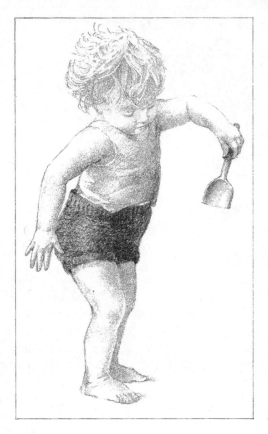

Figure 15. Woollen pants help to absorb moisture in the nappy (diaper) area.

In a case of thrush, it is especially important to change the baby's nappy frequently during the day, and at least once or twice during the night. In general, the smaller the child, the more often the nappy will be wet. During the period of treatment, the child should not have the usual bath but only a very quick wash or dip so as to prevent the skin from getting soft and thus allowing the fungus to get a deeper hold. After washing, the skin must be thoroughly dried. You can use a hair-drier for this purpose, being sure to set it on a low heat. After drying, oil the skin well.

Treatment: in nature, fungi grow where it is damp and shady, some preferring warmth, others coolness. So when fungus invades the nappy area, instead of giving it the dampness it loves, deprive it of its natural environment. The use of plastic pants and disposable nappies will hinder any healing measures taken. Plastic protects the outer clothes from getting soaked, but not the baby's skin which will continue to be affected by the wetness of the urine and the products formed as it decomposes. We recommend nappy-liners (diaper liners or home-made cotton diapers) and, for absorbing the moisture, woollen pants (Figure 15, and see Appendix for knitting instructions).

For the same reasons, be extremely sparing with water when cleaning the baby's skin, and instead where possible simply use sunflower oil (because it is a lot cheaper in the quantities required than commercial baby oil). Finish cleaning with an oil that contains an etheric oil, such as 10% lavender, calendula or camomile extract, or mixtures of any of these. Thyme oil and eucalyptus oil are too irritant and are therefore not suitable. On top apply a covering cream.*

* A possible prescription is *Sulphur. praec.* 3: *Kamillosan R* (ethanol, extract of camomile blossom) 10: cod liver oil 30: *Zinc. oxyd.* 30: *anhydrous lanolin* ad 100.

Additionally you can try the "open treatment" which permits the best possible ventilation around the affected nappy area. Fix a rod across the baby's bed to support the cover or blanket (Figure 16). Dress the upper part of baby's body only, leaving the bottom bare and lying on some nappies. Drape the blankets or covers over the rod to form a tent providing a warm space below. Make sure the covers are fastened securely so that the child cannot pull them down. Overheat the room and put a hot-water bottle (using only warm water and wrapping the hot-water bottle in a cloth) under the sheet to prevent the child from getting cold.

Improvement can be expected after three or four days even if at first some new patches appear. Complete recovery takes from two to three weeks. If there is no improvement, the problem may have been wrongly diagnosed as thrush.

Athlete's foot

Athlete's foot *(dermatophytes)* can be recognized by crumbling skin or layers of dead skin between the toes. Flaking and itching of dry skin on the soles of the feet can also be indicative.

Treatment: keep the feet well ventilated and use as little water as possible (though without incurring smelly feet). Have only quick showers or bathe the feet in a foot-bath of sage or oak-bark tea. Dry the affected parts thoroughly: a hairdryer can be used. Then rub the affected parts with oil of lavender, calendula, or camomile. A massage-oil containing no irritants but only natural etheric oils is also suitable. Let the child go barefoot as much as possible or just wearing socks or open sandals. Avoid nylon and other synthetic socks. Do not let the child wear rubber shoes or shoes with artificial lining any longer than absolutely necessary. Wearing pure wool socks, changed daily, is the best preventative.

Figure 16. Arranging a baby's bed for "open treatment" of thrush.

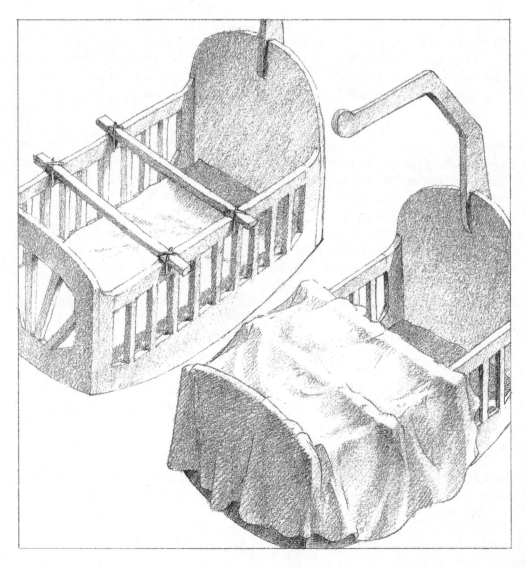

5.11 Purulent skin infections

Erysipelas (St Anthony's Fire)

Erysipelas shows as sharp irregular bright-red hot patches, spreading anywhere on the body, and is accompanied by fever and listlessness. This condition can occur at any age and needs a doctor's attention. It is hardly ever possible to treat this condition without antibiotics.

Infective impetigo

Infective impetigo *(impetigo contagiosa)* produces itchy single spots that spread quickly and are usually covered with thick yellow crusts. Scratching helps to spread it. The disease usually begins where there is a sore area, as for example under the nose with a cold. The disease mainly attacks young children in summer and is very contagious between siblings and children at play.

Treatment: medical treatment is required. Without using antiseptics, it is very difficult to clear up impetigo. Older remedies containing mercury are no longer used. If there are recurrences, try to locate the source. Cuddly toys, things which the child is likely to suck, and pillows should be washed or cleaned. The problem may be a sandpit and so sand in these should be changed regularly.

Folliculitis

Folliculitis, also called *staphyloderma,* can be recognized by little pustules sometimes with a hair in the middle of them. This condition is associated with greasy skin, heavy sweating, dirt, too much animal fat in the food, digestive irregularities (including constipation) or poor skin care. The problem occurs most commonly in puberty.

Boils and carbuncles

A large festering inflammation lying deep in the skin is called a boil. A very large boil is a carbuncle. Treatment is similar to the case of lymph node abscess (see Chapter 2.4). When pus has accumulated in this way, the abscess must be lanced by a doctor. The advantages of treatment without antibiotics are described in the section on lymph node abscess.

In a normal inflamed abscess, the body isolates the pus with a protecting wall of tissue. On rare occasions, the protective wall does not develop and the surrounding subcutaneous tissue becomes infected by pus. If this happens, hospitalization will be necessary.

If a child suffers several boils at the same time or if the problem keeps recurring (mostly in pre-school and school children), some kind of constitutional treatment is recommended.

Inflammations of the hand

Cracks at the base of the fingers and on the palm of the hand can lead to a deep inflammation spreading to the fingertips. The nail fold can become inflamed and may even develop a blister of pus (called a **whitlow**). If the inflammation worsens and begins to throb, seek medical help immediately. Delay, even of only one day, at this stage can result in permanent damage or even the loss of a finger.

Persistent whitlows *(panaritium* and *paronychia)* should be treated in the same way.

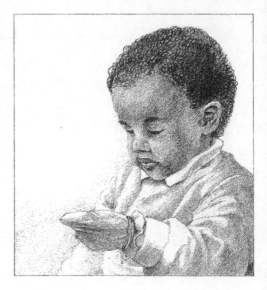

Figure 17. Using a mitten.

Inflammation of the nails

Young babies can easily get inflammations of the nails. These sometimes appear spontaneously but can also be brought on if the nails are cut too soon and too short. They usually heal with a suitable ointment but the doctor should see them if the inflammation starts to spread.

Treatment: first put a dab of *(Calendula* or *Mercurialis)* ointment on the affected finger. Cover all the fingers with clean gauze and tie round the wrist. Put a mitten over the gauze that can be tied loosely round the wrist (Figure 17). Change the dressing once or twice daily. Do not use sticking plaster on babies; it can constrict the finger or it can be swallowed.

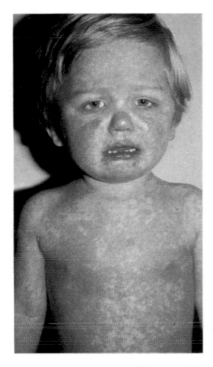

Figure 18. Measles (see Chapter 6.1).

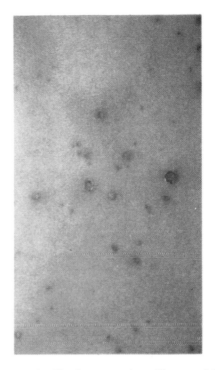

Figure 19. Chicken-pox (see Chapter 6.8).

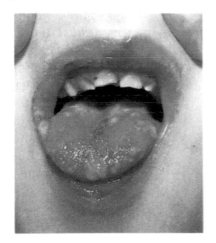

Figure 20. Aphthous ulceration: painful ulcers (aphthae) in the mouth with reddening of the membrane (see Chapter 6.9).

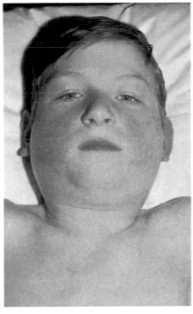

Figure 21. Mumps (see Chapter 6.10).

Figure 22. Scarlet fever: a fine spotty rash appears, looking like red goose-flesh, especially in the groin. The rash is often short-lived (see Chapter 6.3).

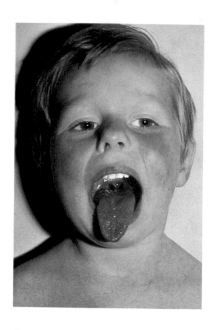

Figure 23. Scarlet fever: initially a thick white coating forms on the tongue. This disappears after two days leaving a raspberry-red surface to the tongue strewn with tiny "berries." The throat and tonsils are often inflamed bright red, and white pimples and coating on the tonsils are not uncommon. The cheeks are red leaving a pale triangle round the mouth (see Chapter 6.3).

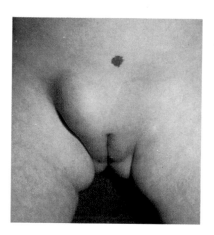

Figure 24. Hernia: a bulge can be seen above the right curve of the groin (see Chapter 2.7).

5.12 Blood poisoning

Blood poisoning, more correctly described as purulent inflammation of the lymphatic vessels *(lymphangitis)* is dangerous and must be treated at once. Infection can enter the body through a hardly noticeable scratch or a small cut that has been opened again. The first symptoms appear as rapidly developing red strips on the inside arm or leg. Soon afterwards, the lymph nodes in the armpits or groin will swell up and become painful. The child should be seen by a doctor without delay.

Treatment: usually the affected limb needs to be splinted and bandaged with a moist disinfecting pad. A booster injection against tetanus (lock-jaw) will often be given. Special care will be needed if there is already an onset of fever.

5.13 Cold sores *(Herpes labialis)*

Cold sores usually appear on the lips and are caused by the same virus as mouth ulcers *(aphthous stomatitis,* see Chapter 6.9 and Figure 20). They are not purulent.

Treatment: Do not expect the doctor to wave them away by magic. They can be helped with drying creams or melissa extract, but it is usually a question of waiting until they clear up by themselves in ten to fourteen days. *Mercurialis* lotion and ointment (Weleda) may also help.

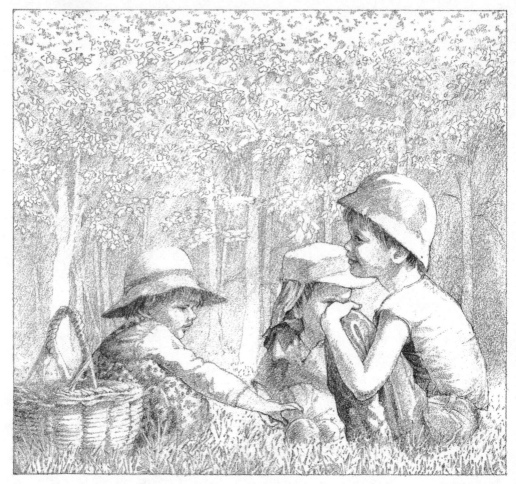

Figure 25. Young children need protection for head, neck and shoulders when playing in the sun.

5.14 Sunburn and sunstroke

A child's skin is more sensitive to the sun than an adult's, and it needs to be protected. The general rule is never to allow too much exposure to strong sunlight at one time. Rather than overdoing it at the beginning of your holiday, it is much healthier to be exposed to the sun for a short period daily over several weeks.

Like all good things, sunlight can be harmful in excess. The safety threshold may be passed well before there are any noticeable signs of sunburn or sunstroke. Parents should therefore develop an instinct for caution and remain alert to the dangers. In bright sunlight, always let the child wear a sun-hat and vest to protect the brain and spine (Figure 25). Never let the child sleep in the sun. If the child begins to tire, it is time to play in the shade.

Sunburn can be treated with a diluted solution of nettle and arnica (Weleda *Combudoron).* Note that some children are allergic to arnica and in this case it should be avoided. Frequent changing of the wet dressing or dabbing the affected part with cotton wool soaked in the solution helps the soothe the discomfort.

A child may already have had an overdose of the sun without any sign of sunburn, but the overdose may show itself in the form of **sunstroke**. Later that evening or next day, the child starts to shiver and has a temperature of up to 40°C (104°F). There may be vomiting and headache. If this happens, the doctor should be called in as there is danger of an encephalitis.

While waiting for medical attention, a child suffering from symptoms of sunstroke should be kept cool indoors or in the shade. A cool compress should be regularly applied to the forehead to remove excess heat.

5.15 Skin parasites

Scabies

Scabies is caused by a mite laying its eggs in the outer layer of the skin. It burrows tunnels which become visible where the skin is inflamed, but the mites themselves are hardly ever seen. After hatching, the mites easily pass from one person to another with the result that usually the rest of the family become infested as well. Traces of the mites' secretions in dust or clothes can continue to cause skin irritation for weeks.

Treatment: scabies needs to be treated by the doctor.

Flea-bites

Sometimes dog-fleas or cat-fleas lose their way and hop on to human beings. Flea-bites can show as small spots in a row, for instance along the end of the trousers. Midge-bites (see first aid section at the end of the book) are often mistaken for flea-bites.

If there is evidence of fleas in the house, shake out all used underwear, sheets and blankets over a bath filled with water. The house should then be sprayed with pyrethrum, then fumigated. Any domestic pets should also be treated for fleas.

Treatment for flea-bites: dab with diluted Combudoron.

Head-lice

Head-lice, the eggs of which are called nits, have become extremely common, being easily spread through contact between children at school. The first sign of head-lice is an itchy scalp. With experience, you can quickly find the nits and also the lice themselves, which are lively little creatures of varying sizes. Treatment consists of using an effective shampoo, for not only the carrier but also the whole family. We advise the use of shampoo containing pyrethrin lotion, and rinsing the hair afterwards with a small amount of vinegar in water. After the hair has been dried, the scalp must be checked again for nits. The best way to do this is to use a nit-comb. Begin at the hairline at the back of the neck, part the hair into very thin strands and search the whole scalp systematically through the hair, allowing at least five minutes for the task. Comb the hair right down to the scalp, because many nits stick close to the skin. After withdrawing the comb each time, push it through a piece of gauze to catch the nits. Pull off the gauze with the nits and throw away. If the child rebels against all this combing, you may have to cut the nitty hair off. This is no less work but it is painless.

Discuss further measures with the child's teacher. Also discuss the problem frankly with the parents of the child's friends, asking them to check their children's hair, as well. Only in this way can the spread be stopped and reinfestation prevented, for although your own children may no longer be carrying the lice, they can catch fresh lice the following day from the children sitting next to them at school. Reinfestation can also occur from their own bedding or clothing. To ensure this does not happen, change clothes and bedding completely and, after the usual wash, lay them out in the sun or in a well-heated room for two days. The larvae soon crawl out and die in the heat.

If a number of children are affected, for instance a class at school, the whole group should be examined by a qualified person. Where treatment has been started, there will normally be a thorough weekly examination of all the children's heads till the infestation has been eradicated. Children affected should ideally be kept off school and allowed back only when the head is completely clear of nits. This is because, if there is a fresh outbreak at school, any child with nits will be suspected of bringing in the lice. It is only possible to tell whether the nits are dead or alive by using a microscope.

5.16 Warts *(Verrucae)*

Warts appear as lumpy or flat growths, mostly on the hands or feet. They are due to a virus which penetrates to the lowest layer of the skin. They are easily caught from other people and passed on, and are often picked up at the public swimming-baths. Warts on the feet, commonly called "verrucas," tend to be flat and painful.

Treatment: warts can be treated with dry ice (frozen carbon dioxide or nitrogen) or removed surgically. Corn-plasters are no use, but a corrosive tincture prescribed by the doctor can be tried. We recommend an ointment containing bismuth and stibium (Weleda), to which many warts respond. This treatment lasts from one to three months and requires patience, but the results are good.

Molluscum contagiosum

These are more common than warts and tend to occur in groups of several together, particularly where the skin is soft. They are about the size of a pinhead, coarse, horny and sit on the skin as little lumps with a dimple in the middle. They can be squeezed out or removed by the doctor or treated with the above-mentioned ointment. They are spread by contact, also in swimming-pools.

5.17 Skin allergies

The variety and frequency of allergic skin reactions have grown in recent years with the abundance of synthetic substances now used in detergents, washing powders, hand-creams, cosmetics, textiles, and so on. Allergic reactions can take so many forms and appearances that we might almost say there is no skin disease which cannot be imitated by an allergy. Where a skin disease is suspected, the first sensible move may be to try avoiding contact with one or other of the synthetic substances mentioned, and see whether the condition disappears.

Certain foods, such as strawberries and cow's milk products, and even healing herbs like arnica may be the cause of a skin allergy. One group of skin allergies appear as undesirable side effects of a number of modern medicines, in particular drugs like penicillin and sulphonamides. These allergies often mean that an individual can no longer take the drug in question.

The body can also react with a skin allergy to an infection; for example, flu can cause a rash to appear. Here, too, the shape and form of the symptoms vary considerably, sometimes fine to medium-sized spots, sometimes humped and red patches like stinging-nettle blisters. Any part of the skin can be affected.

Treatment: with all skin eruptions caused by allergens, bathing in equisetum arvense (horse-tail) infusion (see Appendix) has proved effective. Once the skin has been dried thoroughly, apply a moisture-retaining cream.*

With normal skin or even slightly greasy skin, you can use an anti-itch powder after bathing, but only when the skin is very itchy.

Skin reactions to plants

On summer days out of doors, a child can easily touch poisonous plants or grasses such as hogweed or yarrow, and perhaps not even notice at the time. Afterwards the skin may become red and blistered very like after a burn. Treat as for sunburn (see 5.16 above).

Children should learn to recognize the characteristic leaves of **poison ivy** and avoid contact. The itch can be terrible. If there is contact, wash the skin well with soap as soon as possible. The liquid from blisters causes other blisters to erupt. Try Combudoron ointment, or compresses with Combudoron liquid or jelly, but you may need to seek the doctor's help.

* Following preparation can be made up by a chemist: *Urtica dioica* 10% *Herba, Dec. aquos* 80: *Eucerin. anhydric. ad* 200.

Nettle-rash *(Urticaria,* hives)

A nettle sting produces little whitish or reddish weals on the skin. The sufferer is likely to rub or scratch the affected part. The stinging sensation and the weals last for different lengths of time, usually disappearing by the next day, but sometimes lasting for weeks. The precise cause of the reaction to nettles is not known, but is generally thought to be allergic.

Treatment: minor cases can be treated at home with soothing powder or Combudoron lotion. If further and more widespread (systemic) symptoms are observed, such as swelling of eyelids, hoarseness, air hunger or general indisposition, the rash should be shown to the doctor.

Rash in new-born babies

New-born babies sometimes suffer from a kind of rash which disappears by itself after a few days. The rash appears as an irregular area of pinhead-sized lumps, surrounded by a larger irregular red ring. The cause is unknown.

Treatment: no treatment is required and the rash will clear up by itself.

6 Children's illnesses

In countries all over the world, it is now the normal practice to immunize children in their first two years against tuberculosis, tetanus, diphtheria, polio, measles, mumps, and whooping-cough; and, in addition, to immunize girls before puberty against German measles. Following the successful elimination of smallpox on a world scale, one of the current aims of the World Health Organization (WHO) is to eliminate measles completely by immunization. As a result of these programmes and other factors, there is a tendency for people to believe that children's diseases are not to be endured at all.

However, feverish illnesses present the child's organism with a chance of developing and strengthening itself, overcoming hereditary influences unsuitable for the child's own personality and building up a well-functioning immune system. Although there is the occasional risk that the illness will leave permanent damage, damage may equally well be caused by the wrong treatment, as for example the indiscriminate use of antipyretics (see Chapter 1.2). In our experience a child kept in bed through an illness, nursed with love and care, and given a chance to convalesce afterwards, will in the long run be better able to cope with common child ailments.

In this chapter, we give a straightforward account of the most common children's illnesses, describing the normal course of these diseases without the interference of antipyretics or antibiotics. In the following chapter, we shall discuss the question of immunization to enable parents to form their own judgment in each case on whether to immunize or not.

6.1 Measles

Measles is a common infectious disease found all over the world, mainly in pre-school children. The illness is passed on by "airborne infection," that is by tiny little water droplets carrying the virus. These droplets may be passed on in the open air when children are playing or they may blow in through open doors. Nearly all children are susceptible. Very few people escape getting measles as children and those few, if they contract the disease as adults, are more likely to have a severe bout.

It is rare, even in children, to find a mild case of measles and, when this occurs, it can usually be explained by a previous infection when the child was perhaps about five months old. At that age, the child still has a certain passive immunity derived from the mother and so is unable to develop typical measles, but becomes immune to a certain extent, rather like the effect of an immunization. The general question of immunization is discussed in Chapter 7.

Symptoms of measles

The illness starts with a harmless cold, slightly reddened eyes and a loose cough. A slight fever may develop, followed by a temporary improvement for a day or two. If you suspect measles, ring your doctor. Do not take the child to the hospital or consulting-room because of the risk of spreading infection (see below).

Even at this early stage, the doctor or nurse will recognize the first signs of measles in the child's mouth: little white spots and stripes on the inside of the cheeks. On the fourth day, the child will begin to feel cold and a high fever develops. At the same time, the characteristic rash of measles appears with merging spots beginning behind the ears and head, and spreading quickly over the arms and legs (Figure 18).

At this point, with the child looking so ill, parents often feel they need a further visit by the doctor, but this will only be necessary after another three days or so if the fever has still not gone down or if there have been further developments such as earache or vomiting. The child will generally be feeling much better after the three days but may continue to have a cough for a week or longer. After the fever has subsided, the patient should have a week's convalescence at home.

Treating measles at home

This illness runs a fairly typical course. The child with measles just wants to rest, so should be kept in bed and provided with plenty of liquids. The sufferer is likely to hide away under the blankets, listless and avoiding the light. Disinclined to talk, the child is prone to coughing — a loose and mucousy cough. The face is bloated with red spots and the patient can hardly see out of the slits of reddened eyes. Keep the sick-room quiet and with little or low light. The child should not have to look into strong light, or at TV or even at brightly coloured wallpaper, and should not have to listen to endless background music. (See Chapter 1.2 for treating fever at home).

Exposure to measles

Measles are contagious from the first day of the initial cold (that is, nine days after exposure) until about the fourth day of the rash. Children who were in contact with the patient during this period are infected and therefore need not be kept away. Other children should not be allowed in the same room until five days after the ras'ı started, and even then they should only be allowed quiet and short visits.

If your child has been exposed to measles and may be in the first stages of the disease, telephone your doctor in the first instance and explain the situation. Do **not** take the child to the doctor. Children with measles are sometimes brought to the doctor's consulting-room because the parents are not sure whether the symptoms are really those of measles or not. The family may be in the waiting-room for half an hour before the doctor can see them. It does not occur to them that every other child in the waiting-room has now been exposed to the disease.

Complications with measles
The most common complications with measles are pneumonia, inflammation of the middle ear (purulent *otitis media)* or sinusitis. Skilful nursing is generally sufficient to cure these complications without any after-effects, and without using antipyretics, cough-suppressants or antibiotics. In tropical and developing countries, however, the danger from measles is much greater. Decisions about treatment and immunization must be taken in the light of local conditions and experience.

Even febrile convulsions at the beginning of the illness normally cause no lasting harm. The greatest danger following a bout of measles is the possibility of an **encephalitis**, which is indicated by renewed fever after the rash has faded, with delirium and possibly convulsions. A child with encephalitis must be hospitalized as soon as possible.

Encephalitis is said to occur once in every one to two thousand cases of measles.* With our present state of knowledge of measles-encephalitis, there is a mortality rate of about fifteen per cent of children affected and about a quarter suffer permanent neurological damage, in some cases serious.

Children who have not had suppressive treatments for previous infectious diseases are likely to recover from measles better than children who have.

* At the beginning of the sixties, the frequency of measles-encephalitis in West Germany was reckoned to be 1:14500. The latest figures available are 1:1000 to 1:2000. We believe that this increased frequency may well result from the routine use of antipyretics. Considering the important part played by fever in combating the virus that causes the illness, this possibility cannot be overlooked.

6.2 German measles *(Rubella)*

In children, German measles is a harmless illness. Although not related to ordinary measles and not as infectious, German measles are spread in the same way by minute airborne droplets containing the virus. Children of any age can be affected.

Symptoms of German measles

Two to three weeks after infection a rash appears, sometimes followed by a fever. A characteristic symptom is that the lymph nodes around the neck and throat and at the back of the head become swollen. At first sight, the rash is similar to that of measles proper but here the spots are more evenly distributed over the body, though concentrating on the trunk, and tend not to merge. The fever can be high but fairly uncomplicated.

Exposure to German measles

German measles are infectious from one week before until ten days after the rash. The principal risk is to expectant mothers. If a woman without immunity is in contact with German measles in the first four months of pregnancy, her child may be born with malformations, or die in the womb causing a miscarriage or stillbirth.

If German measles is suspected, do not take the child to the doctor but let your doctor know first.

About twenty per cent of the adult population is still susceptible to the illness. Without immunization, eighty to ninety per cent of children catch the disease before the age of twenty and thus acquire immunity, or else they become immune through subclinical infection (meaning that the body has overcome exposure to the infection without becoming overtly ill). Whether or not a child has acquired immunity can be ascertained by a blood-test. In many countries, immunization is recommended before puberty for all girls who have not had German measles (see Chapter 7.4).

Treatment for German measles

Keep the child in bed and provide plenty of liquids as long as the fever lasts (for management of a fever see Chapter 1.2).

6.3 Scarlet fever

Symptoms of scarlet fever

After an incubation period of between two and five days, the child
breaks out in a fever rising sharply to
39°–40°C (102°–104°F), feels very unwell, vomits and is shivery. The tongue has a heavy white coating and the
back of the throat and tonsils turn
red. The child may complain of a sore
throat. The nasal membranes may be
affected, but there is no great amount
of phlegm as with measles. Diagnosis
may be confirmed by taking a throat
swab to test for the streptococcus
bacteria which cause the illness.

In typical cases, the cheeks are
dark red, but with a characteristic
pale triangle round the mouth. The
scarlet fever rash normally appears
on the trunk, but it may show only at
the groin, on the lower belly and
thighs. From a distance, the rash
appears to be a uniformly reddened
area gradually diminishing towards
the edges. Close up, the fine single
spots look like goose-flesh (Figure
22). Whereas the face with measles is
swollen and wet, with scarlet-fever it
is more clear-cut and dry.

After two to three days the coating
on the tongue peels off and leaves a
raspberry tongue, the fine papules
becoming visible on the bright red
membrane of the tongue (Figure 23).
After another one to three days, the
fever dies down. The last sign of
scarlet fever is peeling skin on hands
and feet after about two weeks.

Treatment of scarlet fever

Treatment of scarlet fever should
normally be supervised by a doctor.
To prevent spread of infection, the
child will have to be kept in quarantine for a period (see below). Keep
the child in bed for at least three
weeks and provide plenty of liquids
(for management of a fever see Chapter 1.2). At the end of the quarantine
period, the patient should be given a
thorough bath.

Nowadays the course of the illness
is nearly always harmless even without antibiotic treatment and, generally speaking, we prescribe only those
medicines which strengthen the
organism, rather than those which
merely suppress the symptoms.

Occasionally the illness may leave
pus-pimples with scabs around the
mouth or an inflammation of the
middle ear, both of which should be
treated by a doctor. More serious
complications which were once so
feared, such as inflammation of the
heart and kidneys *(nephritis)* and
rheumatic fever, have become very
rare in recent years. Even so, scarlet
fever in its classic form must be
regarded as a catabolic illness (breaking down substances of the body)
which affects, and even damages the

vital organs. Hence it is strongly recommended that the illness is followed by at least three weeks of strict convalescence during which time the child must be spared any exertion. During this period, the doctor will continue various checks and tests.

Exposure to scarlet fever
In Britain, North America and Australia, an outbreak of scarlet fever will be notified by the doctor to the Health Authorities. The patient will then be isolated for seven days and a throat swab is taken at the end of that period.

After being with someone in quarantine, visitors from outside should wash their hands thoroughly and dry them on a clean towel or paper towel. Thorough gargling is also recommended.

Unlike measles, recurrences of scarlet fever can occur. In our experience, this happens much more frequently after cases where antibiotics have been prescribed.

Effects of scarlet fever
After a good convalescence, with both measles and scarlet fever, parents can often observe a positive change in their children: a more individual facial expression, new abilities, new interests and a greater stability in general health.

To illustrate the effect these illnesses can have on children, a nine-year-old girl exclaimed in surprise after a severe attack of scarlet fever: "The whole world looks freshly washed!" She now saw all the colours much more intensely than before. She herself felt new-born.

6.4 Three-day fever *(Roseola infantum)*

In all the children's illnesses described so far — measles, German measles and scarlet fever — the rash appeared when the illness was in full course. With **"three-day fever"** however, the finely spotted extensive rash (similar to a German measles rash) appears only after the other symptoms of the illness have disappeared. Three-day fever occurs mainly in babies under the age of three.

Symptoms of three-day fever
The illness starts with the child getting a sudden fever reaching 40°C (104°F). This high temperature continues for three days without much change. Then the temperature drops as quickly as it rose and immediately the rash appears. Other symptoms are not marked or dramatic. Because of the sudden rise in temperature, febrile convulsion may occur (see Chapter 1.3), but it usually passes off

harmlessly. Antipyretics have only a limited success for some hours and burden the child, making it find fresh strength to renew the high temperature.

Treatment of three-day fever
No special treatment is necessary. For management of a fever, see Chapter 1.2.

6.5 Other infections with rashes

With a number of other illnesses, such as flu-infections, a slight patchy rash may appear towards the end of the illness. A typical phone call to the doctor goes like this: "Two days ago my daughter had a fever and a cold. Yesterday she was a bit better, today she's got a rash but no fever." Generally, the rash indicates the end of the illness and the parents do not need to bring the child to the doctor.

The sequence of these symptoms is the very opposite to that of German measles and scarlet fever where the rash appears with high fever and marks the beginning of the peak of the illness.

6.6 Diphtheria

Diphtheria, a highly infectious disease, is now very rare in western countries and had even started to decline before immunization against it was widespread. But even at the beginning of this century, it was still regarded as the children's angel of death.

Symptoms of diphtheria
Two to five days after catching the infection, the patient develops a sore throat and hoarseness, sometimes with fever. A dirty white coating extends over and beyond the tonsils. The symptoms are quite distinct from other upper respiratory illnesses. The patient is most likely to be pale, without high fever, has a quick soft pulse and tends to have low blood-pressure, swollen lymph nodes, inflammation of the mucous membranes and a characteristic sweetish smell in the mouth. The symptoms

reflect a toxic state which affects in particular the circulation and nervous system, and can lead to weakening of the heart muscles, collapse, and paralysis.

Treatment of diphtheria
Treatment of diphtheria nearly always has to be in the hospital. Diphtheria serum is used as well as antibiotics.

6.7 Glandular fever *(Infectious mononucleosis)*

Glandular fever is on the increase with pre-school and school-children. The incubation period up to the start of the fever varies, but is usually about a week. It is not known how long glandular fever is infectious after the onset of the fever. Fortunately no isolation is required, but when visiting the patient, avoid kissing!

Symptoms of glandular fever
Transmitted by a virus, the illness typically produces high fever, tonsillitis with widespread white coating, and characteristically thick lymph node swellings around the neck and other parts of the body. A swollen spleen and liver are also symptomatic. A skin-rash is less common.

Individual patients show a wide range of symptoms and the illness is usually diagnosed by blood tests. The fever generally lasts longer than with the illnesses described above and can recur. Although the patient may appear to be very ill and the internal organs are affected as with diphtheria, the fever does not leave permanent damage though there may be recurrent bouts of weakness afterwards, especially in older people.

Treatment of glandular fever
No special treatment is required (see Chapter 1.2 for management of a fever). Archangelica ointment may be used externally for easing the swelling of the lymph nodes.

6.8 Chicken-pox

This airborne illness is extremely infectious and mostly affects children under the age of ten. The incubation period is thirteen to twenty-one days.

Symptoms of chicken-pox
Over a few days, small spots appear irregularly over the body. These quickly grow into watery blisters ab-

out 2–4 mm (⅛″) across which become covered with crusts. Because the spots are at different stages of development, the skin looks like a star-map with different-sized "stars" (Figure 19). The blisters appear under the hair of the head, on the hands, in the mouth and genitals. Pains in the stomach indicate that the intestinal membranes have been affected. On the outer skin, the blisters are not painful but they are itchy and the patient is inclined to scratch them. There may be fever but it is usually of short duration. During the fever the child should be kept in bed, but if there is no fever, bed rest is not necessary.

Treatment of chicken-pox
Treatment is usually limited to whatever can be done to try to reduce the itching. Telling your children to stop scratching will usually have the opposite effect! Powder with an anti-itch ingredient can be applied. A lukewarm bath with camomile infusion or pine bath lotion is also soothing. If pus has formed in the blisters, pock-scars may remain afterwards, but the smaller ones usually disappear in the course of time.

Exposure to chicken-pox
Chicken-pox is infectious from two days before the appearance and crusting over of the blisters to one week after. As the disease is much more infectious than measles, children may be kept off school until the skin has completely cleared.

Chicken-pox can be carried not only through open doors, but even through an open window to another window. For this reason, children's hospitals and clinics take great care to keep it out, for once it has got in, the disease is very difficult to eliminate. Although the illness is relatively harmless, inside the hospital it can be a serious threat to patients undergoing special treatment and to others with low resistance.

Chicken-pox can be dangerous for new-born babies if they have not acquired immunity through their mothers. If you suspect that your baby may have been exposed to chicken-pox, consult your doctor without delay.

Chicken-pox and shingles
After getting chicken-pox, a few people may be inclined in later life to get shingles *(herpes zoster),* a related illness caused by the same virus. Children can be infected by adults suffering from shingles but then get chicken-pox. In shingles, blisters like little grooves appear on one side of the face, trunk or limbs. The blisters are often accompanied by pain and a high continuous fever.

6.9 Mouth ulcers *(Herpes simplex stomatitis)*

Children between one and four years old often get rough ulcers (aphthae) and reddening inside the whole mouth. There can be a high fever over a period of days. The aphthae are crater-like formations in the mucous membrane of the mouth which are flat, greyish and lentil-sized (Figure 20). They are also very painful and give off a bad smell from the mouth. Affected children often refuse all food and only with difficulty can be persuaded to drink. The illness usually lasts from seven to nine days. Weight lost will soon be regained.

A child who has suffered from the herpes virus is likely to get cold sores around the mouth and nose afterwards (see Chapter 5.15). An attack will usually last about a week and there is no effective treatment other than drying the blisters and reducing the discomfort with ointment. This is an infectious condition which is most often contracted from adults in the same family.

Treatment of mouth ulcers
Diluted tincture of rhatany and myrrh will sooth the complaint if the child can already rinse his mouth or will allow the inside of his mouth to be painted. Pure honey also helps the child to swallow a little liquid afterwards.

Particularly bad cases, where all food is rejected, will require hospital treatment.

6.10 Mumps *(Epidemic parotitis)*

Exposure to mumps
Children usually catch mumps over the age of five. The incubation period is about two to three weeks before symptoms show. Though mumps is not highly infectious, a sufferer can pass the disease on for about one week before the swelling shows and two weeks afterwards.

Symptoms and complications
Not all children become recognizably ill with mumps. Some are not susceptible, others are immune because of subclinical infection, and those that do become ill suffer in varying degrees. In one case, usually with a high fever, a child might have very swollen cheeks like a hamster (Figure 21) and feel very ill. But in another

patient, perhaps without a fever, the cheeks are swollen only for a few days. In yet another case, where the pancreatic gland has been the main target of the infection, a child will vomit and have colicky pains. In a case with complications, a child may get continuous severe headaches and will not sit up in bed. Here, the cerebral membrane has probably been infected and the child has **mumps-meningitis** (for recognition of this complication see Chapter 1). This condition is often not recognized and usually, in children, has no after-effects. It is often possible to avoid sending the child to hospital and nearly always possible to avoid a lumbar puncture. Antibiotic treatment in this case would be useless because it is a virus infection.

If a boy or man gets mumps after puberty, there is a risk of getting an inflamed testicle. Apart from being very painful, the inflammation *may* cause this testicle to lose its function. In rare cases where both testicles are affected, infertility can result. In girls and women, however, an inflammation of the ovaries usually does not have any serious consequences.

Deafness after mumps only occurs in one in 15,000 cases and true **encephalitis** even more rarely, though all such statistics should be viewed with caution.

Treatment of mumps
For treatment at home apply Archangelica ointment (Weleda) or warm lavender-oil compresses to the swollen cheeks. For abdominal pains, use a damp compress with camomile or milfoil infusion on the abdomen. In the latter case, the diet should be free of fats.

In general, high fever should not be brought down, but consult your doctor on this. As we have already said, fever weakens the activity of the virus and consequently tends to prevent possible complications.

For a discussion of immunization against mumps, see Chapter 7.4.

6.11 Whooping-cough *(Pertussis)*

With whooping-cough, there is no immunity from the mother and *all* babies, even those who are breast-fed, are vulnerable to the illness. However, the question of immunization against whooping-cough has been somewhat controversial in recent years (see Chapter 7.4).

Symptoms of whooping-cough
The incubation period lasts from ten to fifteen days and then the first sign of the illness is a harmless cough. This stage lasts from ten to fifteen days before the child develops the characteristic "whoop" or crowing noise as the child tries to draw breath. The

whoop continues for twenty to thirty days, so that the whole course of the illness from the first coughing to the final abatement can run for four to six weeks.

The first stage is known as the catarrhal stage, in which there is often a slight rise in temperature and the child is likely to have cold symptoms with a runny nose.

The next stage with the characteristic whoop is known as the paroxysmal (also spasmodic) stage. Mucous slowly collecting in the bronchial tubes brings on the loud and staccato cough which clears the mucous. The paroxysms wake the child during the night at intervals as frequent as half an hour to an hour. Between each cough, the child cannot catch breath, with the result that the face swells up and turns bluish. After some seconds, there comes a long whooping inbreathing through the constricted glottis. This is repeated once or twice. Finally the child coughs up the mucous and possibly some recently eaten food as well, and then falls asleep again, exhausted.

After each paroxysm, you can offer the child some liquid nourishment which will be absorbed by the gut before the next paroxysm starts.

The paroxysms themselves do not last longer than half a minute. It is important for parents to handle the situation calmly and gently. Slapping or thumping the child, or pulling the child up out of bed, will only make matters worse and will not help to ease the coughing-fit. Younger children may simply lie on their stomachs, push themselves up, cough away and then lie down again.

At the beginning of each bout, the child will feel very vulnerable. To help ease the breathing, talk the child through the crisis calmly and encouragingly: "Cough it all up. Now breathe in and cough again." In this way, the child will feel that things have just got to be as they are and does not panic. Often the calm presence of the grown-up is enough and so it is a good idea for one parent to spend the night in the same room as the child.

If there is fever at this stage, this is abnormal and the doctor should be called.

Your child will have lost weight during the illness but do not worry. It is quite common for children to develop an extremely good appetite afterwards.

Exposure to whooping-cough
Whooping-cough transmitted by bacteria and is infectious from the start of the coughing till about four weeks later, and in rare cases, six weeks. The infection is airborne, carried by water droplets breathed out. As a safe distance from infection is only five to ten feet (two to three metres), it is not advisable for susceptible children to be in the same room.

Whooping-cough in babies less than three months old is a matter for concern because at this young age babies cannot really manage the coughing fits and there is a high risk of brain complications. Therefore every precaution should be taken with young babies to avoid contact. In practice this means that mothers with babies whose older brothers and sisters have not had whooping-cough should be warned if whooping-cough is going about. The doctor can then, if the action is taken in time, arrest the infection in babies by giving an antibiotic.

Three to six month old babies can still suffer the illness badly but usually they are able to cope better with the coughing. Whooping-cough in healthy babies over three months old has often been treated successfully by us without recourse to antibiotics.

With proper treatment, complications are rare in children over one year old, so there is no need to be so cautious as in the first year.

Treatment of whooping-cough
Wrap the child up warmly in bed and give a hot lime-blossom tea so that the child sweats for a time. Then change the bed-sheets and change the child into dry clothes, and put a lemon compress on the neck and throat or chest (see Appendix).

Sedatives and cough-suppressants only increase the dangers of whooping-cough both in babies and in older children. With their use, the cough becomes more infrequent and less strong so that mucous remains in the lungs; pneumonia and lack of oxygen to the brain can result from this. A more sensible and less dangerous treatment is with medicines of anthroposophical and homoeopathic origin. In the case of a delicate child with pneumonia, treatment with antibiotics can be considered. In normal cases, antibiotics can be used to stop the infection spreading further, but have no influence on the actual course of the whooping-cough, other than prevention if administered early enough.

With rickets or lack of calcium in the diet, whooping-cough is much more dangerous. So we always recommend that babies under one year with whooping-cough should be medically examined.

Babies admitted to the hospital make much better progress if the mothers are admitted with them. While this is true generally speaking, we have found it especially noticeable in cases of whooping-cough.

6.12 Hepatitis A

Of the various forms of liver infection, hepatitis A is the most frequent and least harmful among children. It practically never causes permanent damage to the liver *(cirrhosis)*. Infection is usually caused by faecal contamination of the fingers and can be reduced by good toilet hygiene. The incubation period of the illness is from fifteen to fifty days. The virus, however, is excreted one or two weeks before the onset of jaundice, so that the child can already pass on the infection to others at that stage.

Symptoms of hepatitis
In about one third of cases, the condition is recognizable by jaundice. In these cases, the stool loses colour, the urine is abnormally dark and the child often complains of stomachaches and lethargy. The majority of cases, however, show no jaundice and only unspecific or no abdominal pain.

Treatment of hepatitis
Treatment is plenty of bed rest, warm liver compresses, as well as a light diet. The illness is usually over after two weeks. Consult the doctor to confirm if the illness is hepatitis A or another form of jaundice.

For preventive measures see Chapter 7.4.

6.13 The home medicine chest

We have often been asked why in this book there is no list of medicines for the medicine chest in the home. By giving specific remedies in every case we should infringe upon the doctor's freedom of prescription and we would encourage an uncritical use of the medicines. This would be quite contrary to our aims.

We do recognize however that there are parts of the world where there may be no doctor nearby with knowledge of homoeopathic, anthroposophical or herbal remedies. Parents in this situation may find it useful to refer to *Caring for the Sick at Home* (Bentheim).

6.14 The meaning and purpose of illness

Now and then the sort of question crops up in the consulting-room which really needs more time for a proper answer because of its wider context. One question of this kind surrounds the "meaning" of illness in children. Parents

frequently raise this topic, perhaps realizing that there are insights to be
gained from an anthroposophical understanding of the issue. We shall try to
respond in more detail here.

The gathering of experience through suffering is specifically a human
phenomenon. Since humans undergo a continuing personal development it is
possible in their case to ask what the purpose of any given illness might be.
Each illness affects different areas and processes within the human organism
and involves the soul and spirit.

To familiarize the reader with a number of terms that we shall use in this
discussion, it will be useful to sketch out an anthroposophical view of the
human being (see also the Introduction). A fourfold view can be seen as
follows: firstly, the physical body; secondly, the life body (sometimes called
the etheric body) which works on the physical body bringing about growth,
reproduction and aging; thirdly, the soul (sometimes called the astral body)
which is the seat of feeling and psychic experience; and fourthly, the eternal
spirit which is the essential self or personal being. It is the spirit in us which
says "I" and for this reason the spirit is often referred to as the "I."

The human body in its complex entirety is subject to the same physical laws
as determine the behaviour of solids, liquids and gases (mechanics, hydraulics,
aerodynamics and thermodynamics) and which operate in nature at large. In
the human body, however, their inter-relationship enables these different
physical elements to be the bearers of life processes and to express soul and
spirit. How our body is formed determines exactly how we can express our
soul and spirit potential.

The preceding description can be presented schematically as follows:

THE ORGANIZATION OF SOLIDS:
is the vehicle for form and shape (physical body).
The human being in space.

THE ORGANIZATION OF FLUIDS:
is the vehicle for time processes and life (life body).
The human being in time (human development).

THE ORGANIZATION OF AIR:
is the vehicle for soul activity and the ability to move (soul body).
Expression of the soul.

THE ORGANIZATION OF WARMTH:
is the vehicle for the individual will (the "I" organization or spirit).
Expression of the spirit.

The organization of warmth and air are described in more detail elsewhere (see Chapter 1.4 and 3.6). To add to the picture, let us here look at the fluid organism (the sum of fluid movement). We know that elementary life processes take place within the body fluids. Without water, life is impossible. For this reason Rudolf Steiner refers to the life processes within the organism as the life body. This life body is reflected in the movement of fluids in the body just as the soul is reflected in air and the "I" in warmth.

How the life body actually functions will be seen in more detail when we turn our attention to the connection between life forces and the capacity for thinking (see Chapter 13.9). A disorder in this area manifests itself in an illness such as mumps, for example, where there are changes in the circulation of the blood and in the secretions of the salivary gland leading to a swelling; similarly in the case of measles when there is a swelling of the tissues; or in German measles with the characteristic swelling of the lymph nodes.

An understanding of the four principles of organization outlined above makes it possible to gain insight into human pathology. Disorders such as swellings, shortness of breath, or fever may be seen not merely as unpleasant symptoms but also as an attempt by the human being to bring about a change in self. Illnesses make such a task possible. They come and go like independently regulating processes with a life of their own, bringing about a crisis in the human being out of which he will only be able to emerge by some effort or activity.

Seen from this point of view each disease has its beginning, its climax and its end. The illness infiltrates the organism with its own rules which are foreign to the organism and exerts an influence on both body and soul. As a result, when it goes, it leaves behind a change in the way the four members interact, a change determined by the nature of the struggle with the illness. The resulting experience is deeply unconscious in the physical body and more or less conscious in the soul.

Illnesses are vast configurations in time which are initially hostile to human development and bring into question the human being's own form and individual existence. Where there used to be a well regulated exchange of air there is the rattle of phlegm during the emergence of the illness. The skin which used to be delicate and pink now swells and may become fiery red. When the illness begins to pass, however, this means a victory for the child, a strengthening. The child has wrestled with the illness in the same way that it might have wrestled with a problem whilst learning something at school. The focus of this struggle will have been different according to each disease. With illnesses involving a high temperature, it is above all the "I" and its surrounding of warmth which forcefully involves itself in the life processes and exerts an abnormal influence on the metabolic processes. With whooping-cough on the other hand, it is primarily the breathing system which has to be reconquered. Illnesses that are accompanied by swellings of the lymph glands bring about a new taking-hold of the life processes. Concealed within the water-filled blisters of chicken-pox are substances belonging to the body which have to be removed from the life processes. This results in changes in the physical form visible not only in the blisters but also in the light scarring which is left behind. We can thus see from the form taken by each illness whether its tendency is to "come out" giving rise to symptoms on the skin, or to "go in," in which case the symptoms become apparent more in the blood or in the organs.

This distinction is most clearly evident when we compare diphtheria with the now almost extinct disease of smallpox. With smallpox, a short bout of severe illness with a high fever is rapidly followed by the spread of pus-filled blisters from the head right down to the soles of the feet. Combined with the resultant bleeding this soon leads to the total destruction of the organism, that is to say, death. Opposite in character but equally dangerous is the fully developed form of diphtheria. The skin is rather pale and the relatively low fever indicates that the body's resistance is at a low ebb. The throat is swollen from the inside and on looking into the mouth one can see a redness and the membraneous secretions developing on the tonsils. The pulse is accelerated and weak. The functioning of the heart and blood circulation is impaired. The overall impression is of a severe poisoning. Set against these two contrasting types of illness, measles seems to tend more towards the pox since it affects the bronchial passages and the skin most, that is to say, they have more of an outer manifestation. Fully developed scarlet fever on the other hand is more like diphtheria since it tends to affect the inner organs more. In the case of German measles, the symptoms are confined to the lymph nodes and a patchy rash rather like the measles. With glandular fever, the emphasis is again more on the internal organs although it tends to be less severe than the fully developed forms of scarlet fever or diphtheria.

In contrast to smallpox, chicken-pox is a harmless illness. Both are characterized, however, by the breaking up of the outer form of the body. This is also the case with herpes simplex (although normally confined to the inside of the mouth) with an enduring after-effect in the form of a harmless but unpleasant recurrence of herpes blistering on the lips. Where the patient suffers from eczema this illness can take on a more dramatic form so that something more like the pox is the result.

Every encounter with such illnesses reveals an imbalance which causes the "I" activity to adjust the equilibrium between the four members of a person's being. If one looks only at the source of the infection and treats its presence as the cause of the illness and its disappearance as a sign of the cure, then a number of questions remain unanswered: How does the illness relate to the being of this individual person? Why is this person affected in just this way where others are affected differently? What relationship does the source of infection have to the nature of the illness? No one can tell from any given cause of illness how the illness will develop or which individual will become ill. If one takes a careful look at the case histories of different people one will find that no two are the same. One person may have the measles quite severely and the scarlet fever lightly and the other the opposite. One person may avoid whooping-cough altogether and the other avoid mumps and so on. It is just in this grasping or not grasping of an opportunity for illness that something of the individual nature of each person is revealed, only we do not normally pay attention to it. The only question is how one develops a specific susceptibility to any given disease. This is a question that Rudolf Steiner researched by means of spiritual science. The results of his research throw light on the examples of smallpox and diphtheria as polar opposite forms of illness.

Steiner describes how when the "I" lays aside its physical body in death, the life body is gradually released from the corpse over a period of three days and nights (during which in many places it is still customary to hold a wake). Since the life-body carries within it as a kind of time picture the person's whole biography from the womb to the last breath, the "I" experiences its gradual release as a grand panorama of its entire life on earth. It stands, as it were, before an unbroken recollection that displays all the details of a lifetime.

This gradual release of the life body is complete after the three days and nights and it then rejoins the thought content of the whole world just as the elements of which the physical body is composed go back into the material earth. Then follows the gradual release of the soul-body which has been at work in the air organism during life on earth. This is a longer process which covers a period of about a third of the earthly life of the person concerned — corresponding roughly to the time spent asleep. This phase of life after death is referred to in religion, literature and art as the time of purification or purgatory. Here the "I" is able to relive everything that its soul experienced during its past life. However, all is now experienced differently from on earth. The individual now sees himself as others did. Someone, for instance, who exposed another person publicly out of righteous indignation will after death not re-experience his satisfaction or the "rightness" of his anger but rather will feel intimately what the other person concerned felt during this episode.

What is experienced during this purification serves not only to make what the soul has felt in the past life more objective but is also the basis of destiny for the subsequent earth life. If one has committed an injustice through ignorance of all the circumstances then this is the moment when the "I" will resolve to put it right in the next life. In planning its future destiny, the "I" will provide for the possibility of meeting the person concerned and making amends.

This formation of destiny has its implications for a person's future disposition towards illness. A life spent with a predominantly unloving attitude towards people and things would be experienced after death as a lack. It becomes possible to experience how this attitude affected and hurt others. On earth a person may have had good reasons for keeping himself to himself. Now he sees these reasons in a different light. He gets an objective view of them and sees the inadequacy and limitations of his self-centred earthly point of view. In religious traditions this process is also referred to as a judgment in the sense of adjusting one's point of view.

It is this new understanding which, during the passage from death to a new birth, can lead to a certain disposition towards illness in the next life on earth. In the case of an unloving attitude the person concerned would be predisposed to infection by a variety of the pox. The illness would then appear in life as a battle to overcome the previous imbalance, with the process of physical disillusionment related to an attack of the pox representing, as it were, a desire to come out of oneself. The earlier unloving attitude is thus overcome at a physical level and the "I" now receives the strength to stand in a new relationship with its surroundings. If the person concerned dies during the course of this struggle then the forces resulting from it will be available for the next life. The healing lies in living and suffering through the illness itself and in liberating the "I" from the imbalances which would have made further development impossible. The resulting gain is not affected by the length of one's life.

In the case of diphtheria, Rudolf Steiner explains how a life that was powerfully affected by emotions will dispose a person towards an illness which is wrestled with entirely on the inside of the body. It is as if the forces which previously expressed themselves in explosive outbursts are now compressed within and have to be overcome there. Here too, there is a healing at the end even if the resulting new possibilities may only be realized in a future life. In this way serious illnesses which affect destiny can be seen as the product of decisions concerning rebirth taken by oneself.

Thoughts such as these help parents to support their child in a different way through encounters with illness. This understanding of illness also corresponds to what we find in the many stories of healing in the New Testament.

We have described health in a human being as the ability to be open to and interested in the phenomena of the world around; furthermore, to be in a position to share in the world's problems and to do all in one's human power to set them right. There are different ways in which one can stray from this path. Some people withdraw more and more from the world and eventually brood on the feeling that the truth which can save the world is to be found only in themselves. Others let themselves be completely carried away by the demands of everyday life, increasingly denying their own being and are driven by events like a leaf before the wind. Those who are inclined to make themselves the yardstick for all that is around will lose their connection with their social surroundings. Those, on the other hand, who are too strongly influenced by social influences will lose their sense of judgment and inner security.

The capacity for devotion on one side and integrity on the other which are the positive characteristics of the "I" have clearly become unbalanced in both extremes described here. Human health requires that the "I" is able to make use of its capacities freely and in a manner that is appropriate to any situation. Schiller described this flexible use by the "I" of its capacities as "play". We can thus only speak of illness when the "I" loses its grip on itself or gets into such a "cramp" that it is no longer in a position to right itself of its own accord. To put it another way, both the "I" which gives itself up entirely and the "I" which withholds itself selfishly have lost the capacity to love. It is on our very capacity to love that the health of the "I" is founded: on the one hand to be involved in the world and allow other people and events to live in one's own soul; on the other hand to hold oneself back and leave others free. Such a loving relationship to one's surroundings is not only a sign of health in body and soul but also a goal towards which humanity as a whole is striving.

Christianity describes this very same goal as its "new commandment" (John 13:34). How difficult it is to achieve and how far we still have to go can be seen from the many forms of illness and error that humankind is still subject to. In its search for true humanity the soul swings constantly between the twin dangers of egotism and self-abnegation. One might be tempted to see this as a kind of unavoidable human fate and then question just how far we can be made responsible for our errors: "Surely we are the way we are? Who can be any different?" Once more the question of human freedom becomes of critical importance. We have every incentive to blame our inadequacies or problems on our physical circumstances or on other people but never on ourselves.

A good deal of courage is required to take full responsibility for our actions, for our whole way of being even beyond death. Such a resolve can only be taken by each individual for himself. No one can take this away — in this respect we are all completely free. The stories of healing in the New Testament make it quite clear that the struggle to make this resolve plays a decisive role in each one. Jesus asks: "Do you wish to be healed?" or "What would you that I do for you?" It is not simply a matter of Jesus seeing the illness and then conjuring it away but rather of the person concerned being willing to contribute something to the change in their condition. The impulse to do this comes from a realization that we ourselves are co-responsible for our condition and thus that real healing can only come about through our own active willingness to change. Herein lies the answer to the apparent contradiction between freedom and destiny — which is always experienced as necessity or fate. The recognition of our own personal involvement with our destiny is a central concern of Christianity with its twin ideals of freedom and love.

7 Prevention of illness

Nowadays immunization is the first thing parents think of in connection with the prevention of illness. We would like to draw attention to some other measures first and then look at immunization in detail.

7.1 On the psychological level

The psychological prevention of illness is a complex and fascinating area which we can only touch on superficially here by presenting a few general suggestions. Building up your own preventive psychological attitude to illness is something that relates principally to adult life. It applies to children only indirectly, through the example set by parents and other adults.

The first and most effective psychological measure in the prevention of illness is the enjoyment of your work. Love of work produces warmth of being which keeps the organism healthy. It is important therefore to arrange one's daily work in such a way that it can be enjoyed.

If your work is hectic or overtaxing, set aside a few minutes two or three times a day in order to look at things quietly. In that short period, try to introduce an element of calmness and order to your work attitude which will help you to tackle the day's tasks more effectively. Of course where the work is tedious and repetitive with no breaks, this advice may seem extremely difficult or almost impossible to follow. Even so, you should remember that reinforcing your negative attitudes to work of this kind will only increase its harmful effects. There is an unhealthy influence in being irritated, under pressure and always in a rush and panic. If we take these influences into sleep with us over a long period, sleep will lose its refreshing effect. We then become more susceptible to infections and become "run down." This phenomenon is increasingly recognized by scientists; blood-tests have shown that people who are happy in their work and not under stress have stronger immune systems.

We can all find this fundamental relationship with work reflected in people that we know. We are attracted to people who are fully engaged in what they are doing, not out of ambition but because they are involved and interested in their surroundings. Such people set us an example. They appear content, healthy and somehow refreshing. For children, too, it is of great benefit to be in the company of contented, hard-working adults. By contrast, there is something off-putting about those who work to rule with only their own advantage or profit in mind.

It is easier perhaps to see this relationship of attitudes and health in connection with minor ailments such as coughs and colds, but how about more serious and infectious diseases, such as diphtheria? Does this kind of preventive attitude offer enough protection? Even if I possess a positive attitude to life, will this be enough to protect my child? Will the child's power of imitation extend as far as this?

It is clear where our vulnerability to disease actually stems from: fear lies at the root of it. The very fact that we want immunization shows that we are afraid of disease. Only rarely do we meet someone without immunization facing an infectious disease with no fear at all. Occasionally, perhaps, you meet an old missionary nurse who has dedicated a lifetime to caring for extremely ill and infectious patients, without ever catching their infections.

Love for humanity and trust in destiny provide us with unshakable supports through most of life's difficulties. Even if these attitudes do not always prevent illness, they nevertheless help us to overcome it better. We have often seen very ill children admitted into hospital along with their mothers, and witnessed how the mothers have been able to help the children by their faith and love. Not all of us can act in this way. Each of us has our own individual fears which we have to live with and master in our own way.

Meditative and related exercises, if they are repeated regularly, can have a strengthening effect. But what is important here is the attitude of mind in which such exercises are performed. The danger of this type of exercise is that it can encourage a fanatical and egotistical obsession with fitness. There are people who cannot take a walk without thinking about the benefits of fresh air and physical exercise. While constantly thinking of getting fitter, they fail to notice the weather or the flowers blooming in the park, or whether the duck with her chicks is still there.

We suggest that many present-day attitudes to health and fitness should be examined carefully, for not only is a kind of health-egoism involved but also, in the case of some spiritually-oriented sects, even group egoism. While these sects undoubtedly promote psychological and physical well-being, there is often the danger that this is at the expense of inner independence and strength of character. Genuine personal development is achieved not through mindless adherence to a group, thereby surrendering our willingness to learn or to face inner conflicts, but only by overcoming our own crises and problems courageously.

If physical and spiritual exercises are used to help us become stronger and more responsible, they will at the same time help to build up and maintain health. People who live in this way will then be less dependent on sleep and food, less preoccupied with their own state of health, and consequently open to showing a genuine warmth and interest in others.

In addition to regular exercise, every kind of rhythm in the child's day has a strengthening effect so long as the right balance is achieved between activity and rest (see Chapter 12.1 on daily routine).

In modern biological research, there is growing recognition of the importance of rhythm in life. All life from the single-cell organism right up to the most complex mammal is dependent on rhythms which are finely tuned into each other. If the balance of these life-supporting rhythms is disturbed, the result in humans is illness, and in nature destruction and death.

7.2 Hygiene

The prevention of illness also requires us to know how infection is spread and how illnesses develop, knowledge that is particularly effective in preventing diseases such as whooping-cough in babies, and rickets, or caries.

Bacteriological hygiene must be carried out with a fair degree of thoroughness and care. It includes the isolation of infectious patients, disinfection of rooms and of objects used by the patients, and the use of protective clothing: gloves, mouth-mask or goggles. Modern surgery owes much of its success to thorough hygiene, and without it the high rate of mortality in childbirth during the last century would never have been reduced.

However, there is a transition that must be made from the carefully washed baby to the toddler crawling on the dirty floor. So what is the best approach? Should the child be kept away from all sources of possible infection or should it be exposed and learn how to resist? The same basic dilemma presents itself again and again in questions of treatment: for instance, should antibiotics be used for every bacterial infection, or only for those which the child cannot otherwise cope with?

As a rule the first child in a family is seldom ill, except perhaps when the parents catch something, because the child grows up alone. But as soon as it enters kindergarten, we can expect infections for the next two winters.

Every "bug" is brought home and all winter the child is more at home than at school.

With the second child things are much the same, but with the third child things change. Even as a baby, the third child is constantly exposed to the infections of the older children and catches the general run of children's illnesses at an early age, and often gets them unpleasantly severely so that it is quite a burden for the parents. As a rule, however, this third child becomes the healthiest and strongest of the lot.

7.3 Toughening-up

Many believe that increasing resistance to illness is largely a question of toughening-up the body and so are inclined to bring up their children under a hardy regime. The results of this are not always as straightforward as might be supposed. Traditionally, country children were always considered to be healthier, but in fact their good health was not due to cold washing every morning but because they were always warmly dressed against the cold. There is no doubt that a general disposition to infection can be reduced by a daily cold bath or shower and of course a certain robustness is developed by frequent exposure to rough weather. But we must distinguish clearly between immediate effects and long-term consequences. Regular washing in cold water can lead to a predisposition to rheumatism in later life. This is not to say that the use of cold water may not be the right thing in certain cases, but a general policy of "toughening up" children by this and other methods is definitely not to be encouraged because of the possibility of harmful effects in later life. Overexposure can even seriously affect the structure of the child's organism. Instead having cold showers, the child can wash with a diluted emulsion of rosemary (Weleda) which should only be as cool as is pleasant for the child, and this in the long run will have a strengthening and stabilizing effect.

Running barefoot through snow or an ice-cold stream as a test of courage is not a bad thing as long as the parents do not expect too much or accuse the child of cowardice if it refuses. Taken in a spirit of play, such "dares" are in order but have nothing to do with a course of toughening up.

Taking children to the sauna or hot-tub once or twice a week is good for toning up an organism that lacks activity and which has grown soft in air-conditioned rooms, but a child that is active from morning till night and plays a lot out of doors needs no such additional stimulus.

Finally we should stress that, in choosing any course of treatment or cure for a child, the character, physique and disposition of the individual child must always be taken fully into account.

7.4 Immunization

Artificial immunization is carried out for two main reasons: first, to protect individuals from the danger of certain infectious diseases; and second, because mankind feels threatened by epidemic diseases.

The reader may be surprised to find the whole question of immunization approached here quite differently from what is common practice. We prefer parents to decide for themselves which immunizations their children shall have and, with this aim in mind, we try to provide parents with the most important facts and considerations both for and against each type of immunization. In this way we hope that the parents' decisions will be based on knowledge of the individual child and not merely on the debatable results of statistical research. Complete freedom of decision does not of course exist where local regulations make immunization obligatory. However, even then, where immunizations are contraindicated because of underlying conditions in the child, this must also be taken into account.

The principles of artificial immunization are easy to understand. The object is to prevent certain infectious diseases. This is achieved by increasing the amount of antibodies which are similar to (or the same as) the antibodies produced by the organism when overcoming the disease. The two main methods are passive and active immunization. With *passive immunization,* specific antibodies from other humans are injected as a vaccine. These immunizing substances are soon broken down in the organism so that immunization lasts for about two months.

With *active immunization,* the body is stimulated (by an injection or other means) to produce its own antibodies. Active immunization affords protection against the illness for an indefinite length of time which varies with each individual but can last for several years.

Vaccines which are capable of multiplying, are known as *live vaccines.* Those made from material or metabolites of the infecting agent are known as *dead vaccines.* Both types are used in active immunization.

Immunization reduces the death-rate of an infectious disease very considerably, and also reduces at the same time the general likelihood of infection within a population. Unlike other preventive measures such as a holiday by the sea or in the mountains, immunization does not improve the general health of an individual.

Immunization is worthwhile when it can avert the risk of disease but it is only justifiable when no fresh major dangers follow from it. The value of immunization can be assessed by weighing up the following considerations.

On the one hand, the degree of danger of the disease must be understood. By this we mean, how prevalent is the disease, how grave are the possible complications, is the disease epidemic, how high is the death-rate?

On the other hand, the degree and quality of immunization should be considered: that is, how long will it last, how effective is it, what is the likelihood of complications, and what are the known side-effects?

Immunization can be regarded as worthwhile when the disease in question is liable to run a dangerous course, and when the immunization is good and lasts a long time. Complications resulting from immunization are an acceptable risk only when the illness itself is highly dangerous.

It must be stressed that the following discussions on specific immunizations are based on current knowledge (as at 1990) of the situation in the western world. Conditions elsewhere and as time progresses will vary considerably. Changes in recommenda-tions appear to be inevitable as there is constant research into the risks and effectiveness of vaccines.

Above all, we wish to emphasize that the decision to immunize or not, when taken by parents or doctors, should be based in every case on all the available knowledge about the individual child.

Antitetanus immunization

It is worldwide medical practice to treat dirty wounds by giving passive immunization against tetanus (lock-jaw). This involves giving an injection of concentrated immune globulins obtained from highly immunized human donors. The relatively danger-ous vaccine from horses and cows is no longer used. Because the body breaks down the immune globulins within a few weeks, passive im-munization of this kind is only worth doing in cases of severe wounds. In cases where tetanus is contracted the human vaccine in large doses has often saved a life.

Better protection is given by active immunization which stimulates the organism to produce its own anti-bodies. For a first series of immuniza-tions to last ten years, three injections are required, usually with an interval of one or two months between the first and second and up to one year between the second and third.

In the case of wounds which occur more than five years after the last immunization, a "booster" injection is given. But where there are very dirty wounds or severe injuries such as burns, the booster is given sooner. Where this booster has already been given more than once or twice, further immunization against tetanus during the next five to ten years will almost certainly not be needed.

Antitetanus immunization is one of the most harmless immunizations in existence. The protection rate is good although an immunized person may occasionally suffer a slight tetanus infection. The unmitigated illness is one of the most serious we know, with a mortality rate of between a third and a half.

It is worth noting that a person who has recovered from an attack of tetanus is not immune against a second infection. For this reason, even parents who would normally be against it, will allow their child to be immunized if they have actually experienced a tetanus infection.

In the developed world the risk of contracting tetanus in the first year of life is extremely slight. For this reason we suggest that immunization is given not at two or three months but only after the first year. At this age the child's constitution is much more stable and reactions can be more accurately observed.*

* Current practice in the UK is to immunize at the time of the triple vaccine at three, five and nine months. In future this timetable is expected to change to two, three and four months.

Immunization against diphtheria

In Britain and North America, immunization against diphtheria consists of three injections at prescribed intervals, together with tetanus (lockjaw) immunization and usually with immunization against whooping-cough (pertussis). This triple immunization is known as DPT, the first injection being given at around the age of three months (see footnote).

Immunization against diphtheria may cause a fever which, in itself, is not so serious. Other complications are rare but may occur if the immunization was given when the child was already incubating or suffering from another disease. The complications are then like those of diphtheria itself. Altogether the immunization is not quite as harmless as the antitetanus one. Protection by immunization should last for about five years, and can then be renewed with a booster injection. For the same reasons as those given for antitetanus, we suggest that unless there is an epidemic or local conditions dictate otherwise, parents who wish immunization wait until the child is one year old.

We cannot say anything with certainty about the effectiveness of active immunization against diphtheria. Though there have been fatal cases in recent years, it would appear that in none of these cases had the patients been fully immunized. Adults and children were equally affected.

In a case of suspected diphtheria, passive immunization is currently the required practice. This is a drastic measure as the vaccine is taken from a horse or cow which involves the risk of an allergic reaction to the foreign protein. It is also difficult to prove in less serious cases that the course of the illness is in any way improved by the passive immunization.

Immunization against whooping-cough

There is more controversy surrounding the whooping-cough immunization than there is with the previous two immunizations. In particular, it has long been known that if by chance the child was immunized when whooping-cough was just beginning, the illness can be very severe and lead to brain damage.

There is also the question of timing. If the first whooping-cough injection is given when the child is three months old, and is followed by two more at monthly intervals, the child will be six months old before full immunity is acquired and by that time whooping-cough itself is no longer such a danger (see footnote under Antitetanus immunization). The susceptibility to whooping-cough among babies under three months is very high even when they are breastfed.

A child with suspected whooping-cough should not be allowed into the same room with a baby under six months old. If a child with whooping-cough has been seen within three yards of a baby, the doctor should be informed within two days, as the infection can be contained by preven-

tive antibiotic treatment (see Chapter 6.11). If this moment has been missed and the baby has started to cough, these measures will no longer be effective. Generally it will be necessary to admit babies under six months to the hospital, preferably with their mother.

Vaccination against polio (poliomyelitis)

It is worth studying the background of polio epidemics which were becoming more and more serious until immunization was introduced. It was discovered that as the standard of living of a country rose so did the danger of an epidemic.

In more recent times, the pattern was that an epidemic would last for two years, followed by an interval of about sixteen years. This periodic phenomenon was explained as follows: during the epidemic those who were not struck down by the disease acquired immunity by being exposed to it and so the disease died down under the prevailing hygienic conditions. But this very hygiene prevented the new generation from coming into contact with the disease, with the result that it then had no immunity. After sixteen years, then, there were enough vulnerable young people and children for a fresh epidemic to take hold.

There are a lot of exaggerated ideas about the risk of catching polio during an epidemic. We should remember that an outbreak was considered serious if in one summer 40 people in a town of 600,000 caught polio. Most of the population would have acquired immunity by being exposed to the infection (subclinical infection). Therefore it was the insidiousness of the disease, its serious effects and the fear which it aroused, rather than its frequency or virulence, that led to the attempt by developed nations to stamp out the disease by means of immunization.

At first an injectable dead vaccine was developed, followed by a live oral vaccine which is now used in most countries.* A disadvantage is that in very rare cases (one in a million), paralysis occurs with the oral vaccine, as well as one case in a million where paralysis affects someone of the same household as the vaccinated person. We do not have this problem with the dead vaccine. After improvements of the dead vaccine its effects are as safe as with the oral vaccine. However, it is harder to use the dead vaccine among the adult population. The debate on the respective merits will no doubt last for some years yet.

In tropical parts there are still sporadic cases of endemic polio, even in vaccinated areas. We have to be aware that polio will be imported from developing nations into developed countries in which case large groups of unvaccinated people could under certain circumstances be affected. This begs the question as to

what conditions favour the appearance of polio. Dr Zur Linden's great contribution to our knowledge of the disease was to discover that a general susceptibility to polio results when people's senses are overstimulated. In the modern world, such effects are induced by sun, radio, television, traffic and industrial noise, background music in supermarkets and shops and so on, causing the whole nervous system to be weakened. It is further overstimulated and weakened by a high level of sugar consumption. To be aware of this and to take the necessary countermeasures is just as important as the immunization undertaken for social reasons.

We generally recommend this vaccination because, in the absence of it, there is the danger one day of an epidemic of sizeable proportions.

Immunization against German measles (rubella)

In the UK, immunization is now administered together with immunization for mumps and measles to all children between the ages of fifteen and twenty-four months.

Immunization is recommended in some countries for girls between the ages of ten and fifteen to provide them with antibodies to German measles. This is done because, in later life, exposure to German measles in early pregnancy may damage an unborn child. As repeated calls to the doctor show, it can be very worrying for a pregnant woman

---

* Current practice in the UK is to administer the oral drops at the same time as the triple DPT vaccine.

exposed to German measles to discover that she has no antibodies to the disease. The single immunization given between age ten and fifteen is hoped to give immunity for the whole span of a woman's child-bearing life. It is possible to be tested for antibodies to see whether immunization is really necessary but in some programmes immunization is given regardless of the test result.

German measles is only one of many possible causes of damage to the child in the womb, but it is one of the best known causes of malformation. There is a high occurrence of malformation when the infection takes place before the twelfth week of pregnancy, with actual malformation of new-born babies varying between eight and sixty per cent.

From the epidemiological standpoint, it would be best to give the immunization as late as possible and only to girls, as then the immunizing effect of the natural contamination of the population would not be affected. Where early immunization is practised generally for all children, including boys, at eighteen months, the result is likely to be that those not immunized will have less chance of acquiring immunity by subclinical infection (see Chapter 6.2) or by catching the disease at a later age. This means that for a woman who has not been immunized, the risk of getting German measles in early pregnancy would be greatly increased.

The live vaccine in use has been in existence for a number of years now, but how successful it will be, we shall not be able to say for another twenty or thirty years. In the meantime, the epidemiology of German measles will have changed; more people will have been immunized and there will be less chance of being exposed to the natural virus.

Immunization against mumps

There is a live vaccine against mumps which is administered by injection. Its only real justification can be to prevent permanent damage arising from mumps. As with whooping-cough, one of the arguments in favour quotes the heavy burden on families disturbed at night for weeks on end. Such arguments can be countered by asking whether it is right for a child's organism to be manipulated in such a way that it causes as little disturbance to others as possible.

Even the danger of meningitis with mumps cannot really be used to justify immunization because in the present-day course of the illness in children, the infection clears up in most cases without any after-effects (see Chapter 6.10). Immunization can only be justified as a protection against permanent damage such as infertility resulting from inflammation of the testes *(orchitis),* or serious deafness, which is rare. However, it is quite difficult to assess the actual risk of an inflammation of the testis with or without immunization.

The following considerations, based on our current knowledge, should be taken into account when deciding whether or not to immunize an eighteen-month-old boy. Most children will catch mumps before the age of fifteen; as a result, 70-90% of adults in West Germany have antibodies and continue to be immune without ever having been immunized. Let us assume, though, that the child in question does not fall into this majority group and so retains his susceptibility into adulthood. The question then arises: will he catch the illness during a wild (that is, natural) virus infection and become ill, or will he become immune through subclinical infection? If he caught the illness in its full form, there would be a ten to fourteen per cent chance of one testicle becoming inflamed. One third of inflamed testicles lead to loss of function. With our present knowledge, the physician cannot say anything more definite. Parents should be aware of these facts when deciding for or against immunization because the simple statement "mumps can cause an inflammation of the testicle leading to permanent sterility" says nothing about the actual risk.

Where permanent damage to the inner ear results from mumps, it is generally only on one side. Statistics relating to frequency are unreliable because the complication is often only diagnosed very late. In twenty years of practice, we have come across only one case. It is generally reckoned that there is one complication in fifteen thousand cases.

If immunization becomes more general, more people will contract mumps in later life. This means that we shall have more complications in future, caused not by an increasing susceptibility to infection but solely by immunization measures. With polio, the opposite occurs: if 70% of the population are immunized early, this makes the risk of infection slight for the remaining 30%. With mumps, however, the risk of complications in the non-immunized increases for the very reason that the rest of the population has been immunized.

Encephalitis, a rare inflammation of the brain which is not to be confused with the more common and often harmless meningitis, can develop from mumps with after-effects in the form of permanent nerve and brain damage. The course and outcome, however, are not as bad as in the case of measles. We have never yet come across such a complication with mumps.

How long the immunization against mumps lasts we cannot at this stage say with certainty although it is thought to be for life. Whether this expectation will be fulfilled, given the diminishing frequency of contact with the mumps virus, has still to be seen.

Immunization against measles

Now that smallpox has been eliminated by worldwide immunization, the declared aim of the World Health Organization is to stamp out measles as well. With this end in view, a programme of immunization, covering also mumps and German measles, has been going on for some years in western Europe. The live vaccine recommended at present, is usually not given until the child is twelve to eighteen months old because up to that age the child may have immune globulins from his mother in his blood which would slightly diminish the effect of the immunization.

The main reason given for the immunization programme in developed countries is the danger of measles-encephalitis. In undeveloped countries, there are risks of other complications.

The immunization is considered harmless if carried out correctly and it is hoped that the currently used method provides lifelong protection. However, the best immunization is obtained from just getting proper measles! This immunity is weaker if the illness was only very mild, as for instance in the case of a five-month-old baby catching measles from her brothers and sisters. The child may not show any symptoms on this occasion (because of immune globulins acquired from the mother) and it may get only a mild bout of measles if infected for a second time at the age of seven. The unanswered question is what will happen at, say, forty if the person comes into contact again with measles, after not having been in contact with the disease for thirty-three years? Will the individual then be likely to suffer a severe bout of the disease?

The present epidemiological balance is maintained only because measles are generally caught in childhood and people then have a good chance in the course of their lives to renew their immunity by casual contact with measles. Following the extensive immunization programme, uncertainty now arises concerning new-born babies which have hitherto been completely protected with antibodies acquired from their mothers. It has been discovered that, by the time they reach school age, immunized children already have a reduced amount of antibodies. Therefore, without casual exposure to the disease, will the antibodies of a thirty-year-old woman be sufficient to give her new-born child enough protection during its first years of life? It is certainly not the object of the immunization programme to create a severe illness for new-born babies or adults which, though not so common, will run a much more dramatic and dangerous course. Already we have to reckon with a number of illnesses which are severe in children for the very reason that the infection tends to occur in later life. Unlike the oral polio immunization, therefore, the measles immunization is "anti-social" and will only fulfil the aim of its promoters if the World Health Organization succeeds in stamping out this illness in a few years. If not, quite unforeseen problems will arise. That the problem has not yet been overcome in the USA is shown by the fact that epidemics still occur involving people who were apparently immunized.* In the meantime, the experts are bemoaning the fact that natural immunization is declining because there are fewer natural viruses in circulation. In addition, a second strain of measles has recently been discovered, thus calling the entire immunization programme into question.

One further illustration may show how difficult it is to judge the value of immunization for a particular individual and the ensuing effect on health. Let us suppose that there are two children who have suffered the same brain-damage. One has had measles and the other was immunized. Here it will be the parents of the immunized child who are left with more anxiety in case their child gets another encephalitis after, say, chicken-pox or flu.

In tropical countries and in third world regions, infant mortality from measles is higher and this factor must be taken into account when assessing an individual case. But even here the

* Between January and March 1990, two thousand cases of measles were reported in California, with twelve fatalities. We do not know whether those affected were not vaccinated at all or were unsuccessfully vaccinated. The health authorities have reacted by introducing a new immunization programme. It is worth pointing out that epidemics of such severity were not known before the implementation of general immunization programmes (except in isolated communities where there had been no measles for one or two generations).

long-term effects of immunization need to be considered, and it is questionable whether infant mortality would be much affected by programmes of immunization in those countries.

Given all these considerations, it can be seen that there is no general answer to the question whether to immunize or not. Each individual, by reason of his or her particular destiny, is affected differently either by the disease itself or by immunization.

Finally, the disease itself should be judged not only by its negative but also by its positive aspects. On the negative side, serious complications can, though rarely, follow the illness. On the positive side, the illness has a strengthening effect and the child emerges from the illness healthier and more robust. Indeed the whole family often feels closer and stronger after passing through the ordeal together.

Immunization against tuberculosis (TB)

This immunization is mainly a protection in the first year of life against severe complications of tuberculosis. In later life it has only a minor role in the general prevention of tuberculosis. More important in this respect is the treatment and observation of tuberculosis patients, the vaccination of cattle and the pasteurization of milk from herds which are not guaranteed free of tuberculosis. If the environment is free of this disease the immunization is only effective for a few years because the imperceptible boosts through slight infection are lacking. On the other hand under severe exposure even immunized people have become infected.

A tuberculosis test shows positive both for immunized and for naturally infected people, so that it is hard to establish whether a child has an infection over and above the vaccination. We recommend immunization for new-born babies only when a patient with confirmed tuberculosis (where the patient coughs up TB bacilli) is in the same household. In this case it is essential, too, that the baby is kept away from the source of infection. In addition, in countries where there is a high local incidence of TB, immunization may be appropriate.

Hepatitis A immunization

Nowadays if children contract jaundice, it is sometimes recommended that those not yet affected at home or in school should be protected by a (painful) injection of gamma-globulin into the muscle.*

It is better first to establish what kind of hepatitis the sick children have got, and if it is hepatitis A, to leave the other children for the following reasons. Hepatitis A is usually a harmless illness for children and

runs its course in most cases without severe symptoms. Additionally the immunization is often too late and protection would only last for a few months at most. The child is probably already protected by subclinical infection which could only be ascertained by a blood-test. An early infection with hepatitis A has the advantage that the child will not catch it again for the rest of its life. Finally, gamma-globulin is not effective against other forms of hepatitis.

In every case we recommend careful toilet hygiene and that the parents should decide individually whether the child is to be immunized in this way. The same applies to preventive vaccination before travelling to hot climates.

Immunization against flu (influenza)

The development of anti-flu vaccine raises interesting problems, as every year a new vaccine is required to meet the characteristics of a new flu virus, often originating somewhere in the Far East. This makes it difficult for immunization to be widely accepted. One strain of flu can quickly follow another, and a person already immunized against the first strain falls victim to the second. Immunization against flu is not generally recommended for children.* It

* In the UK, if there were several cases, a school would probably be closed and investigated. In an individual case, the child might be isolated. Elsewhere closure of the school is not usual practice but an individual case may be isolated. In the USA, injections for home contacts are recommended.

* In some countries, the vaccine is officially recommended for groups at risk such as children with cystic fibrosis, congenital heart-disease, and so on.

has no place in our consulting-room. Research into flu immunization absorbs much medical time and resources, and the question still remains whether even if a totally effective immunization could be developed, might not some other virus take the place of the flu virus?

7.5 Deciding whether to immunize

On the basis of the above, we deal with immunization in our clinic in the following ways:

We never press parents who do not wish immunization.

We try to explain to parents the arguments for and against each kind of immunization as set out above.

If the parents cannot decide for themselves, we advise immunization for tetanus for one-year-olds and, at present, oral immunization for polio at about the same time. In addition, we give immunization for diphtheria if the parents wish it after consultation.

We recommend vaccination against tuberculosis if there is tuberculosis in the family or if there is danger of infection in the immediate surroundings. In addition we give it if desired after consultation.

We have never recommended immunization against whooping-cough and we do not give it.

If desired we give adolescent girls immunization against German measles.

Except in special cases we do not give live vaccine against measles, mumps and German measles to eighteen-month-old babies.

We advise against immunization for flu.

We do immunize new-born babies of mothers with hepatitis B with the recently developed vaccine for this disease.

We use immunization with specific human vaccine in the following cases: with non-immunized children where there is danger of tetanus (lockjaw) after soiled wounds; wherever there is a suspected threat of diphtheria; with new-born infants in danger of chicken-pox where the mother has not previously contracted the disease. In certain cases we use gamma globulin where there is a definite threat of hepatitis A.

After all that we have said, we hope that readers will not be surprised if they come across doctors who are more reserved about the use of immunization as well as others who use it unreservedly. The views expressed here should not be taken in a dogmatic sense. It will also be clear that the more information is available the harder it is to make a definite decision.

Finally we should like to touch on a problem which constantly crops up in connection with immunization. Parents may learn about the importance of illness for a child's development only after their own child has been immunized. As a result, they sometimes worry that their child may be "missing out" on something. What can they do to make up for having immunized the child? The answer is straightforward. These children need simply to be brought up in such a way that their inner life develops as it should. Rudolf Steiner said of smallpox immunization, "Vaccination will not harm anyone who later receives a spiritual education." What he meant by spiritual education was that the individual is encouraged to develop his own spiritual activity without obstacles to spiritual awareness being placed in his path by a purely materialistic upbringing. The antidote to immunization, then, is found in an upbringing and education consciously directed at developing individual character and abilities through all stages of childhood and adolescence.

Here again we touch on the fundamental issue: to understand the interconnection between physical and spiritual development. We would maintain that just as courage and love of work are good preventives against illness, so illness can counteract spiritual underdevelopment. If we artificially prevent illness from occurring, we reinforce the body without having helped the soul in its development. Where the body is always fit and healthy, the soul may become less active and more shallow than in another person who has to harness forces to battle with illness.

We hope that this discussion makes it clear that really the parents themselves must make the final decision for or against immunization. As long as the state has only laid down recommendations and not regulations, the responsibility for decisions affecting their children remains with the parents. Where immunization is concerned, the doctor is not healing a sickness but is dealing with preventive measures. These measures must be determined by attitudes to health and sickness, attitudes which can be helped by discussion and should not be adopted blindly. The doctor can never give any absolute assurance that a child will be left undamaged by either the illness or the immunization, and the doctor's task is simply to co-operate with the parents in seeking the solution most suitable for each individual.

This leads us finally to a question which we are often asked: seeing that you regard illness as such a positive and necessary factor in the destiny of the child, why do you give treatment at all? The answer to this question lies in what we have already said about the place of therapy and medicine in our lives. The doctor is called upon to help and guide the patient through the crises of illness which destiny has presented. This the doctor does in the light of personal knowledge and conscience, acting in what he or she considers to be the most helpful and constructive way. How this is done will depend not only on the individual doctor's medical knowledge but also upon personal philosophy and view of life. A materialistic philosophy will seek to rid mankind of illness by any means, whereas a philosophy and knowledge which take the spiritual side of humankind fully into account will be more aware of the complex order of creation and will see both the positive and the negative effects of illness.

8 AIDS (Acquired Immune Deficiency Syndrome)

AIDS (Acquired Immune Deficiency Syndrome) is a phenomenon which is now receiving increasing attention and publicity. After a long search to identify the virus, AIDS has now been confirmed as a complex viral illness. A number of different causes were ascribed to the disease in earlier medical and paediatric textbooks but the actual virus was discovered in 1983. As yet (1990) no effective immunization or treatment has been found.

8.1 The characteristics of AIDS

The spread of AIDS

In the way AIDS has spread it resembles the great plagues of the Middle Ages. But the transmission of the AIDS virus (the human immunodeficiency virus, HIV) is quite different from that of epidemic illnesses which are spread through breathing and food. Preventive measures against AIDS are closer in kind to those of sexually transmitted diseases like syphilis or gonorrhoea, for AIDS is passed on predominantly by blood and semen. As a high concentration of the viruses can be found in seminal fluid, sexual intercourse in particular is a source of infection. Furthermore seminal fluid has a temporary weakening effect on the immune system and this is an important contribution to the physiological process for fertilization. The greatest risk of infection comes with homosexual intercourse where seminal fluid is absorbed into an organ (colon) which is not equipped to deal with it. The seminal fluid then passes into the rest of the body through the mucous membrane of the intestine, where it can develop its general weakening effect on the immune system.

Before the virus was identified, it was not known that stored blood (in blood banks) could contain the virus. Consequently many people were affected as a result of blood-transfusions given during an operation or after an accident. As the virus was also contained in the blood clotting factor administered to people suffering from haemophilia, some of these people are HIV positive. Also a great number of children have been born with the disease where the mother is affected and the baby has come into contact with her blood.

Course of the illness

The course of the illness is chronic and the outcome unpredictable. Many people who have contracted AIDS carry not only the antibodies but the virus itself in their blood without any visible signs of illness. Others become acutely ill only a few weeks after coming into contact. It is clear that individual and constitutional factors play an important part here and many researchers believe that the cause of the illness is not the virus itself but the immune system of the person affected which has already been impaired by other unspecified causes.

The acute stage of the illness develops intermittently, intermingled with changing symptoms of various infections (for instance, pneumonia, severe influenza, ear infections, gastro-intestinal infections and fevers of unknown origin). In addition central nervous disorders can appear as well as tumours of the skin and of the mucous membrane.

It is particularly distressing that very little can be done therapeutically. All that medicine can do at present is to try to contain the virus with anti-viral drugs as well as treating bacterial infections with antibiotics and applying general strengthening measures such as good food, rest or change of lifestyle. In addition anthroposophical medicine offers measures aimed at strengthening the immune system.

8.2 Prevention and cure

The best prevention of AIDS is of course to avoid possible sources of infection. This, however, is more of a shielding kind of prevention, related to the fear of infection. It can protect the individual but it cannot in any way help society to change its egoistic attitude to life. From what has been said, it is clear that our society requires quite a different kind of preventive measure: namely a strengthening of the body's resistance through acquiring a positive attitude to life that takes into account the well-being of our whole environment. Education which acknowledges the dignity of man will help to achieve this end (see Chapter 16.6).

The wide differences in the course of AIDS and the fact that many people have been infected for years without being visibly ill, show that

individual responses vary enormously. In terms of prevention, then, there
is room for manoeuvre not only
physically on the level of the individual's constitution but also on the
spiritual level. An individual who
practises self-discipline, who has developed a healthy idealism and who
cultivates a cheerful and confident
attitude to life will not be very susceptible to this illness. Should the
illness overtake someone with a temperament of this kind, the chances of
recovery, because of these attitudes,
will be better than those of a fearful,
doubting individual who has to con-
tend with great inner emptiness.

Anthroposophical medicine has a
whole series of constitutional remedies which support the "I" actively
working in the body (see Chapter
6.14) and this includes immunizing
activities. Any effort on the part of
the individual towards self-
knowledge and self-discipline will be
strongly supported by treatment of
this kind.

8.3 The challenge of AIDS

AIDS is somehow characteristic of
our times. We owe the identification
of the virus to modern biological
research techniques which have been
brought to bear on searching for a
possible vaccine or treatment. Without the electron-microscope and the
technique of protein analysis, it
would not have been possible to
discover the structure of this virus.
Also the infection is involved with the
sexual side of human relationships,
an area of social activity which has
these days become the focus of attention more than any other.

What kind of a picture is presented
by AIDS? The immune system is
attacked. The immune system sus-
tains the individual's physical integrity. It can be seen as a kind of
"biological ego." Once the immune
system grows weak, the organism
begins to lose its biological identity;
and in the symptoms of inflammation, tumours and nervous disorders
we see the structure of the body
slowly disintegrating. The personality
can no longer express itself fully in
this body. AIDS as an illness presents
a picture of physical dissolution, of
the disintegration of one's self. In this
the disease is a sign of our times, for
never has humanity as a whole been
so consciously ego-centred. Economic policies are promoted with a total
disregard for the environment or for
the customs of other peoples, and
personal prosperity is the prime consideration. Sexual behaviour, too,
reflects this egoism. Self-gratification
is paramount in sexual relations and
often leads to promiscuity instead of a

loving devotion to the other person. These egoistic tendencies are found everywhere in individual lives and in our social life. We may regard AIDS, then, almost as a vicarious illness: a group of people manifest the symptoms of the "dis-ease" affecting our whole society.

In this context we may look upon the healthy human body as being made in the "image of God" as expressed in Genesis. There is a perfection in the healthy human form but this perfection is diminished by illness which is like an impediment on the path towards perfection. Every illness, then, is the image of a task which the organism must fulfil in order to achieve wholeness. A severe illness can be experienced almost as a personal lesson set for the individual by God, and in this individual experience something is learned which cannot be obtained in any other way. Every sick or handicapped person values health much more consciously than healthy people. Wrestling with illness allows abilities to grow which make a human being more mature and more whole.

We conclude that our love and care should be devoted to AIDS sufferers. AIDS is an illness of our society with which we should all identify. The victims of AIDS show the symptoms of our common illness: they stand as our representatives. We should communicate this through, for example, taking affected children into the kindergarten and school, caring for them with special love and attention, and behaving towards affected adults in such a way that they feel that what they are suffering physically is something we must all experience spiritually. Our task is to overcome our selfish desires and to be more open to the needs of our time. If we can do this, AIDS can help our culture to become more Christian and more human, for Christianity teaches transformation of the soul and spiritual dedication to the great tasks of evolution.

9 Handicapped and chronically ill children

Some children are born blind or lose their sight through accident or disease. The world of their experience is reduced by one whole dimension. The pictorial way of imagining the world through light and colour is closed to them. But as a result, their remaining senses are all the more refined; they can hear more sharply and touch more alertly than those who can see. These children are much more sensitive to tone of voice and inflection of speech. They can tune into moods, attitudes and atmospheres much more acutely than those with sight who often, in the truest sense of the word, "overlook" these more subtle aspects of reality.

Other children cannot hear. It was once commonly thought that the deaf-mute were half-witted, until it was discovered that their limited ability to express themselves in speech was because they could not learn to think through speaking. But with the invention of sign language, these children have been able to develop their natural intelligence. Even so, the inner world of the deaf is full of silence. They cannot penetrate the surface of things to their deeper nature. They are inclined to become suspicious because they feel that an area of perceptions is closed to them and they cannot easily develop a trusting nature.

Other children are born with or develop damaged internal organs. Where a child has a congenital disorder of the kidneys which will eventually cease to function altogether, this means either a kidney-transplant or a lifetime on dialysis. What is the meaning of such an illness in a child's life?

What is the world like for children who cannot smell or who are colour-blind? How does a child confined to a wheelchair see reality? How is the world experienced by the lame, by the crippled, by a child with a stump and fingers instead of an arm? It is hard for us to know what dimensions of experience are hidden from all these or what special qualities they have developed to compensate. But we often find that children with limited mobility have above average mental energy. It is as if what cannot be translated into physical activity is made available as psychic potential. This phenomenon is also observed in children with a cleft palate. Whatever has been prevented from operating in the body becomes available as psychic activity. Such children are often not easy to rear. They do not always know what to do with their potential. They are inclined to excess, to undirected bursts of energy.

How does one act towards such children, or towards child diabetics, or towards those with heart-trouble, rheumatism, asthma, psoriasis or cancer? Our answer must be to invoke a fundamental premise: education and the overcoming of sickness are connected. Every illness presents a unique but hidden task, a unique opportunity for development. To discover this hidden task is the first step towards overcoming the difficulty. This discovery is always an individual experience and no generalizations can be made, but it may be possible to point to directions in which personal solutions may be found.

First of all, fear, anxiety and worry must be overcome. We should ask calmly: in what way does a sick or handicapped child experience the world differently and perhaps uniquely? How can I help the child to learn from this experience? If we wholeheartedly adopt such an approach, we shall be more likely to find the right way to tackle the situation.

We should realize that pre-school children feel their handicap only to the extent that adults let them feel it. Indeed they may only become aware of it because of unwarranted cosseting or because the disability is spoken about in their presence, or because they are unnecessarily indulged and spoilt as well as being subjected to expressions of pity. If, by contrast, we go about caring for them objectively, treating them — apart from their disability — just the same as other children, they will feel themselves to be "normal." Children can then identify with their situation, accommodating themselves within it, and will not have the feeling that they should be any different from what they are. The foundation is thus laid for that inner assurance which will be required later on.

When shocks come — as for instance when a squinting or limping child is teased, or when people in the street go out of their way to avoid a child with eczema because they think it is contagious — parents can still reassure the child. In the case of a two- or four-year-old, you can distract the child with a story or game, or by pointing out something. Later on you can say: "That boy didn't know you properly — if he had known who you are, he would not have done that." Or, "Well, you know, everyone has something which others can laugh at, or which they don't like, but we're not going to mind that." Older children can be told the story of the Ugly Duckling (Andersen) or Bearskin (Grimm). These stories tell how, after unsightliness or ugliness has been borne patiently for a time, it is changed into something beautiful and worthwhile. There is also the analogy of the pain the pearl oyster feels when a foreign body penetrates it and how it exudes mother of pearl to render the intrusive body harmless and smooth, resulting in the shining rose-white pearl.

With school-age children, it is possible to speak openly about a handicap. We should also discuss with other children how they can respect the handicapped person's self-control and self-discipline in keeping to a pre-scribed treatment or in managing the disability. In these discussions the question of divine justice often crops up. Why do some people have everything and can enjoy themselves fully, while others are deprived in various ways? But there again, you can ask, why can some people travel to far countries and see so much of the world, while others are prevented by circumstances from doing so? The question of individual destiny applies to everyone (see also Chapter 6.14 on the meaning of children's illnesses).

Finally, we must turn to a question asked by every severely handicapped child: how are we to understand and accept a destiny which prevents a person from learning a trade or profession, from having children or even from having self-control? If the answer was: "There is no sense in being severely handicapped for no real development can take place, and indeed children handicapped like that should not be allowed to be born," then everything we have said so far about the human personality is negated.

Rather than give such an answer, let us try to understand the meaning of a handicapped child's destiny. Here the idea of reincarnation can help. We have already mentioned this idea and we believe some children sense these things quite naturally in the same way that many people can feel the presence of those who have died.

From our experience we have found that children live with the idea of reincarnation quite naturally even though they have never heard adults speak about it. For instance, an eight-year-old girl dying of leukaemia comforted her mother with the words: "Don't be so sad — I shall come back again." In another instance, a four-year-old girl was heard talking to her baby cousin whose elder brother had died a few months previously. The little girl was overheard saying to the younger child: "How you've grown! When your brother comes down to earth again, he'll be pleased to see how big you are."

Some parents, seeing the enormous differences in the characters and abilities of their children, feel that they must have acquired them in former lives. Of course the reader may disagree, but it seems to us that any individual can test the possibility of reincarnation against his own life experience and so come to have a deeper insight into it. He may even be able to see reincarnation as a reality and discern its workings, for example, in the destiny of the gravely handicapped.

Let us take the case of a child who can neither speak nor walk. She lies or sits in her wheelchair utterly dependent upon those around her. During her whole life she is receiving, only making contented or discontented noises, but "does" nothing. Another child can manage physical work quite well under direction. His head is long and narrow, his body massive, his speech clumsy, his look is open and friendly. In the home where he lives, he does the same things every day helping with the housework and in the garden, and these simple tasks he performs with a zest often lacking in a normal healthy person.

What is the meaning of destinies like these? What can a person learn in such a life? What abilities are being prepared for a future life on earth? Such questions can lead to much fruitful thought. In the first instance, the child in the wheelchair spends a whole life in the experience of receiving, in the knowledge that in life we do not only give but also receive, that for all our opportunities and talents we are indebted to other people and to the world. If that child could only receive such an education from its handicapped life, in its next life the same child would not fall into a false independence from others. Being purged of egotism, the child would not cling only to things serving its own needs and desires, ignoring all else. Its life would now be based on gratitude, humility and respect for others.

The second child, working all his life happily and with regularity, has undergone a tremendous schooling, for nothing strengthens the will more than whole-hearted regular activity. Just as muscles are developed by regular exercise so the will requires constant practice in order to become strong (see Chapter 16.6). Having undergone this sort of training, the individual will bring energy and determination to the tasks of a next life.

Teachers, remedial helpers, doctors and therapists who believe in reincarnation have much a much wider philosophical basis for helping handicapped and chronically ill children and their parents than those who do not have this view.

Reincarnation is not concerned with being punished or rewarded but rather enables us to recognize and correct our own errors and failings and thus to work at our own development and that of the world. Michael Bauer once formulated a Christian aspect to the idea of reincarnation as follows: "To accomplish deeds of love, one life will not suffice, thus reincarnation is a necessity of love."

Generally it is the sick person who senses all this much more than the healthy person. We have always found that people afflicted with a chronic illness or handicap do not seem to suffer so much from it. It is as if they feel that this suffering is part of them and the very expression of their personality. Indeed it may even be the sick who bring comfort to those around them. Such a victory over illness is a sign of the instinctive understanding that every individual subconsciously brings to the impositions of destiny.

On the other hand, we have also seen how rebellion and resentment against sickness increase suffering. This is more obvious in people whose whole upbringing has conditioned them to the view that illness and suffering are only senseless by-products of life and should be eliminated. We regard it as an essential task of education to help the individual to attain an attitude that makes all life a meaningful source of experience.

10 Family planning

10.1 The relationship between parents and children

Growing up in a family of many brothers and sisters provides quite a different start to life from being an only child. There are certain experiences which belong specifically to the first-born, while the younger members of the family experience things differently according to their birth order. The oldest is judged against the highest standards in everything and is brought up to responsibility; the one in the middle is always remarkable for being "completely different" and then there is the youngest who is allowed to break all the rules. As they grow up, each child can look back with varying degrees of pleasure on the "ups and downs" of their particular place in the family.

On top of birth order, there is the varying relationship of the parents towards boys and girls and the relationship between boys and girls themselves. Parents may have a particular preference for boys or girls and preferences have very great influence on the development of the growing child. A girl brought up to be a wife and mother, or a boy brought up to become the "head of the family," will have to shoulder quite different burdens from those of a child who has been spared these roles. If however we learn as parents to regard the personality of a child as more important than his or her sex, our dealings with our children will be more open and less rigid.

All these factors which have a bearing on growing up in a family have themselves been subject to vast changes in recent times. Nowadays, to a much greater degree we can determine by choice how or whether a family is planned. Formerly the decision to start a family was based on economic realities and faced the prospect of an unknown number of children. Pregnancy of the unmarried was not accepted, abortion was a crime. To have a lot of children was a sure guarantee of care in old age. Questions of population growth and the medical and social aspects of having a family, were not matters of public debate.

Today all that has changed. Political, social, economic and even purely personal and medical reasons now determine family planning. Decisions about these matters are much more in the hands of the responsible individuals in the family itself. Formerly such things were regulated by the social norms. It is lack of awareness of this personal responsibility which is one of the underlying causes of increasing brutality in our social relationships. No longer feeling themselves constrained in any way, many people simply follow their own inclinations instead of acting responsibly towards society. Only a new attitude towards education and self-discipline can take us out of this crisis. The way in which individuals decide how to live with the consequences of family planning, whether in fact they "plan" at all, will depend on how they think and feel about their own development, about the existence of the not-yet-born and on how they view their social surroundings.

To all the various thoughts which govern family planning, we should like to add three which are not so often discussed:

The child needs rearing

Will the prospective parents enjoy rearing children? Are they prepared psychologically and economically to take on the task of bringing up a human being, whom at first they do not know and, then, all too easily come to feel is "theirs"? Even though it is quite natural for a would-be mother to feel that she wants to "have" a child, perhaps even to have someone who is her very "own," nonetheless this attitude can lead her to mismanage completely the upbringing of the child (spoiling, not allowing a certain freedom and, later, reproaching with ingratitude, and so on). No human being can belong entirely to another but sometimes that is only recognized when the desire for personal freedom and independence makes itself felt in the other person.

The child needs a broader perspective on life

Nowadays the fact that parents are generally still trying to solve the problems of their own lives is a decisive element in the atmosphere of the home. What attitude to their surroundings do the parents adopt? This is just as important for family life as the willingness to make the innumerable sacrifices, great and small, that are demanded of parents daily. In order to have some sense of inner security in our complex and changing world, it is important for parents to see modern life within some sort of historical perspective. This critical time in our civilization, with its extreme materialism and striving for technical perfection, can be seen as a necessary stage in the evolution of human consciousness.

The unborn child is a human being

What view do the parents have of life before birth? Do they think that the child comes as a "blank page" into the world, or begins its earth-life with expectations and abilities which stem from experiences in former lives? (See also Chapter 6.14 on the meaning of children's illnesses). Through the centuries, students of philosophy and theology have devoted a great deal of thought to the question of life after death. Far less has the question of pre-existence been raised and debated. But those who have a feeling for pre-existence will come to consider the whole question of family planning in a very different light.

10.2 Birth control

Today we know enough about the processes of conception and birth to be able to control them. Legislation in many countries has given women much greater freedom of decision and responsibility in this area. While we are a long way from seeing everything run exactly according to our plans and wishes, the results of research into *in vitro* fertilization (test-tube babies), sterility, abortion, prenatal diagnosis of inherent malformation, and contraceptive methods have all vastly increased the individual's scope for decision and action. We can expect even greater possibilities in the future.

Here, we do not intend to present new guidelines or doctrines on what may be ethical or permissible, but rather to suggest some viewpoints which take account of life before birth and life after death. These are based on the spiritual insights of Rudolf Steiner.

Steiner describes how life after death is divided into two major periods (see Bibliography). The first period is concerned with working over the experiences of the life just lived, beginning with a process of purification of the spirit. The second period is concerned with the preparation of a new life on earth. Many generations before birth, the individual is drawn towards a particular part of the earth, and towards a particular nation and ancestry. Thus Johann Sebastian Bach was born into a family of generations of musicians. There he found the preconditions necessary for the development and realization of his abilities. In this way, every individual seeks out the most fitting hereditary stream and waits for the right moment for incarnation.

It is not easy in our time for an incarnating individual to find either a suitable body or the right moment. Sensitive parents may distinctly feel something of the child who intends to incarnate with them. Dreams, inklings, a quite definite feeling that someone is there who belongs can all provide intimations. Often the moment of conception is consciously experienced by one or both parents even to the extent that the girl or boy appears to the mind's eye, and later grows to be exactly as seen.

Rudolf Steiner's research shows that the child's desire to be born and to accomplish a certain mission, mingles with the physical love between the parents. Only when the child's resolve to incarnate matures and the parents are ready to receive the child can conception take place. It is not until the third week of pregnancy that the spirit of the child (the "I") can completely unite with the embryo. Then the "I" uses its own life-body, or etheric body (see Chapter 6.14), to work at the embryo's process of growth and differentiation. All this usually takes place before the mother-to-be has missed her period and so confirmed her pregnancy.

If we look at contraception and abortion from the viewpoint of the unborn, we get a completely fresh picture. The connection between sexuality and love and between sexuality and egotism becomes a question that affects not only the couple and their respective wishes and needs, but also the wishes and needs of the child-to-be. The child has sought out a particular couple for its incarnation, and has also chosen a particular time and a group of contemporaries. If the chosen couple are using contraception, this will prevent the child-to-be from being born into that family. It will be forced after a time to look for another, similar, pair of parents. This will have consequences of destiny for the first pair, as indeed all our deeds affecting other people or things have consequences which will eventually come back to us to be requited.

Incidentally, from the point of view of the unborn, we should take into account the difference between hormonal and barrier contraception on the one hand and contraception by means of the coil on the other. In the case of hormonal and barrier contraception, fertilization is nearly always prevented, whereas with the coil fertilization does occur quite frequently but the coil then prevents the fertilized ovum from implanting in the uterus. It can be seen that there is a difference of effect upon the incarnating process of the unconceived child, a difference in degree of approach to earth and of disappointment at being refused admittance.

Contraception, however, does not make such a deep incision into the life of the mother as does abortion. After an abortion many women experience deeply their break with the being of the unborn child and can give expression to this experience. They often say that they had the feeling that they have lost a good force or power. They feel themselves somehow empty and hollowed out. Some even say: "If I had known beforehand what it would be like, I should never have had the pregnancy terminated." Not all will express themselves as strongly as this. Much depends on the motives which led to the termination of the pregnancy. A woman who was in a desperate situation or who for health reasons had her pregnancy terminated will look back upon this event differently from one who did it from a personal whim. The first of these women will require quite different counselling and psychological assistance to come to terms with her situation.

The motives of the parents are also important where a pregnancy is achieved by fertilization outside the womb with subsequent embryo implantation (commonly known as a test-tube baby). Here, too, the parental attitudes will have a marked effect upon the destinies of mother and child. Prospective parents should examine carefully their own motives. They should ask themselves whether their motives are purely a selfish desire for children. Looking at the question from the viewpoint of the child-to-be, we should ask whether this method of conception is right for the human child, which will be forced to begin life and development outside the womb. This is normal and natural for fish which release their eggs and sperm into water for fertilization to take place; but procreation in this manner is quite unnatural for human beings. The process can become an experiment with unforeseeable consequences for the child. What will be the lasting effect upon the child of having been deprived of the spiritual warmth of his mother's organism?

The more methods of contraception, abortion and artificial insemination that become available, the more imperative it becomes to examine the inner motives that impel us to use them. The methods in themselves are neither moral or immoral. It is the motives which bear the moral value of our actions. And the motives are a personal matter. Each of us bears the responsibility for our acts, for our own development and for the development of those entrusted to us, and it is up to us to choose our motives in freedom, unhampered by the customs of society. More and more people are coming to see that morality arises where the individual changes motives from being predominantly self-centred to serving the good of humanity.

Finally there is, of course, voluntary sexual abstention. If there is no sexual activity, then no particular attraction is exerted on the unconceived, whereas attraction *is* exerted when coition takes place with contraception.

The points of view which we have advanced here only touch briefly on what is a complicated subject. Nevertheless we hope that they will contribute towards a realistic appraisal of a subject where personal wishes and ideological standpoints stand in the forefront. Our discussion here is intended to widen the scope of the reader's awareness of all that is involved in decision-making and to show how much our own actions are interwoven with the deeds and sufferings of other people.

10.3 Genetics and prenatal diagnosis

Today there is a whole series of hereditary illnesses and inherent malformations which can already be diagnosed during the first half of pregnancy. By means of amniocentesis (the examination of the amniotic fluid), cell culture and chromosomal analysis carried out in the sixteenth to eighteenth week of pregnancy, it can be ascertained whether the foetus has been affected by a genetic disease. If the foetus is affected, the law in some countries allows a pregnancy to be terminated. Of course many people have ethical objections to this practice and even to prenatal diagnosis.

Objections to amniocentesis are usually countered by arguments like the following:- many parents can now accept pregnancy knowing that modern prenatal examination will tell them whether their child will be normal or not; furthermore they know that only 3% of children concerned will be born with a serious handicap and these children can be eliminated by termination of pregnancy; and again only about 1% of the healthy foetuses subjected to amniocentesis are physically damaged by this test.

Arguments of this kind are founded upon a concept of the human being which has been reduced to the purely materialistic. It is not untrue but it is one-sided, for a human life cannot be understood statistically (after all very few people die exactly at the end of their statistically calculated life expectancy). Each individual life and destiny can only be weighed and evaluated according to its own determining factors. If we take into account the lives of the 1% of children damaged by the test, we would certainly not quote statistics in defence of amniocentesis.

When prenatal diagnosis is recommended in order to prevent children being born with a hereditary disease, or malformed or otherwise severely handicapped, the underlying assumption is that the future life of these children is of no human worth. This view can only be maintained from a completely materialistic viewpoint. If, on the other hand, we acknowledge the reality of life before conception and birth, and the meaning of life as lived by a severely handicapped or ill person (see Chapter 9), then the decision to terminate a life that has already begun in the womb will not be so easy. This does not mean to say that we condemn prenatal diagnosis on ethical grounds but, because it expands our room for action, we require a greater sense of responsibility; and with responsibility must come the readiness to accept the full consequences of our actions.

When a mother decides against giving birth to a child which she knows will be a Down's syndrome baby, four people enter into a relationship with the incarnating individual and this relationship will remain and carry consequences. The four people are the mother herself, the father, the paediatrician or the specialist giving counsel, and the gynaecologist who terminates the pregnancy. If we take the full picture into account when decisions of such a nature are made, our conscience and our sense of responsibility are thereby sharpened. As a result, we shall take more seriously into account the individual who has sought such a hard destiny and who, when denied the opportunity through abortion, must find other ways of realizing that destiny.

At this point, we should not gloss over the fact that more and more families are adopting handicapped children. Many mothers now continue their pregnancy to full term even though the geneticist has diagnosed Down's syndrome. These mothers have felt deeply that they are already joined to their child's being and destiny, and have acted accordingly. Our destiny is formed by our past deeds, deeds not only in this life but in former lives, and we are bound to one another in multifarious ways, in all that we owe to other people and they to us. Insight like this can reconcile parents to the handicap of their child and can lead them to ask their child: "Why do you need *me,* why am I bound to you, what can I do to help you bear your destiny, how has your suffering deepened my own experience and knowledge?" In this way the handicap and destiny of the child can be accepted by parents who might otherwise have resented their fate and cried: "Why does it have to be *me* of all people who has been landed with a handicapped or malformed child?"

We live in a time where the relationship between knowledge and technical know-how on the one hand and morality on the other is out of balance. Precise research into the laws of destiny and into the soul and spiritual being of man can help to restore the right balance (see Chapter 6.14). In the same way, our attitude to experiments on animals which we conduct for the "benefit of humanity" will change when we know more about the animal's being. Then we shall feel more responsible towards them and towards the earth which we share with them.

Our view is that these are questions not only for the experts but also for each one of us. It is not necessary to have studied in order to think about pre-existence, the destiny of the earth and the meaning of life. Nonetheless there is a widespread inclination to leave important decisions in areas such as prenatal diagnosis, artificial insemination, breeding experiments or genetic experiments to specialists, church or state. We consider that it is important for everyone coming into contact with these questions to work at them actively. A new morality can only come about when the individual's sense of responsibility is founded on personal insight. Such a morality will emanate from the individual and will not be the result of collective norms that restrict the freedom of the individual.

Working towards greater knowledge of our own actions will lay the foundation of this sense of responsibility. Certainly many mistakes will be made through lack of knowledge and misjudgment about what can or should be done. Because of this, it is all the more important that individuals should have the courage to face the consequences of their actions even though at first they may have only a vague idea of what the real consequences are.

Part II

Foundations for Healthy Development

All education is really self-education. As teachers we are only a part of the surroundings of the child which is educating itself. We must be the best possible surroundings so that the child can educate itself in tune with its destiny.

Rudolf Steiner

11 The first months

Every new-born child brings with it the plea: "Help me to become a true human being." So every adult involved with the child should be asking: "What is needed for a healthy human development?" But in nearly all adults, a lot of educational attitudes, preferences and notions stem from a person's own childhood with all its memories, both pleasant and unpleasant. Parents who, in their own childhood, suffered a strict upbringing, will perhaps allow their children more freedom. Those who wish they had been governed with greater strictness will hold the reins more tightly.

In contrast to this, our suggestions for education and upbringing will be based on the child itself. Whatever style of child-rearing is adopted, it can be measured against the questions: What stage has the child reached? What is the next step in its development? The child is not burdened with our experience and its only desire is to become a human being. It has no desire to be a guinea-pig for this or that pet idea. It is on the way to learning to adjust itself to light, sound, food, warmth and cold. It is becoming familiar with the room, with the house in which it lives, with its immediate surroundings and with the people and conditions around. The child does not want everything at once nor, on the other hand, wants to be denied its due.

In order to develop the right feeling for what the child needs, we must examine the different stages of a child's development. Then it will be easier for us to see where exactly each individual child stands. Often parents ask us: "How can I do the right thing? — everyone I ask tells me something different." It is important, then, for parents to develop their own judgment. No one lives as close to the child and with as much responsibility towards it as the parents do. In the end it is they alone who can decide what is right for the child. The role of others is to express points of view and give advice based on their own experience which can help parents to observe their child and its surroundings more closely and to develop their own individual judgment.

11.1 Impressions after birth

The pregnancy and birth are over. "Who are you?" the mother's eyes ask the unknown being who has just been put into her arms. During the next days every little movement of the baby is watched with anxious care and delight: the sucking motions in his sleep, the yawning, the delicate play of the fingers. The breathing, sometimes scarcely perceptible, is occasionally interrupted by a series of somewhat deeper breaths or a little grunt as the baby stretches itself. When the mother bends closely over the child, its breathing becomes deeper or faster for a moment, expressing happiness as her nearness is felt. If the baby is lying asleep beside her, the mother can sometimes see the eyeballs floating beneath the closed lids (this can also be seen in premature babies when their eyes are open). The transitions from sleeping to waking, and from waking to sleeping are still very fluctuating at this stage.

The child's gaze does not yet rest upon objects, but rather picks up and reflects the soul quality of its surroundings. And then to this is added the sensation of light. Instinctively we adults search for the baby's personality in the eyes, sensing that it is not yet present there. If the eyes are open, they seem to search for something near the mother on which they fix their gaze for a moment before they grow tired and close again. After a time they open again and once more try to reach that something. This rhythm of seeing and not seeing is an important part of the first experience of self. Here we realize that we owe the certainty of our earthly existence entirely to our sense perceptions. Through the activity of perception the child becomes more and more aware of itself over the following months. By the age of two or three, the child will come to perceive its own unique identity.

The desire to experience the surrounding world through the senses permeates all the activity of the newborn baby: it enjoys being replete, and when hungry it greedily seeks the breast and can suck in masterly fashion. The baby gives itself up to sleep or tries to absorb the light, sounds, noises, cold and warmth that are all around. Soul experience is entirely bound up with this opening and closing, desiring and being satisfied; and so the baby's sense of daily rhythm develops long before it is really aware of time. In the same way, the child's movements are quite reflex and uncontrolled. The mother spontaneously feels that she can soothe her child and ease away these jerky movements that often appear so helpless.

Hospital birth

If you are having your baby in hospital, it is a good idea for the child's father or grandmother — or at least someone closely connected to the mother — to be present during the birth, helping and sharing in the joy. After the birth, the mother should try to have her new baby beside her during the day: the first days after the birth are decisive for the relationship between mother and child.

Efforts are now being made in some western countries to make hospital births as warm and human as in the home. All the technical apparatus in a delivery ward does not really need to be so much in evidence as to destroy the right atmosphere. Experienced maternity staff will assist at the birth discreetly, the operating staff and the obstetrician being in the background but on call in case of emergency. All concerned should be aware of the significance of a birth and should share in the happy event.

It is increasingly the custom in some countries to lay the baby on the mother's tummy immediately after birth. In the excitement, it is often forgotten to keep the baby warmly covered. Because the baby is wet, it quickly becomes too cold. The skin of the new-born baby is well protected by the *vernix caseosa,* a cheesy coating all over the body. When washing the child after birth, care should be taken to leave as much of this vernix on the skin as possible.

11.2 The first feeding times

These days, we often hear a young mother say that she wants to share feeding the baby with her husband, and for this reason does not want to breast-feed. The new baby, too, has something to say on this subject, something which the mother will only "hear" when she holds her baby to the breast for the first time (see Chapter 14.1).

Whether breast-feeding or bottle-feeding, it is important in the beginning that the sixth feed during the night is not missed out. In order for the mother to cope with the extra burden if breast-feeding, the father, grandmother or other helpers should try to spare the mother and child as much as possible during the day. A breast-feeding mother should rarely have to give up the night feed for health reasons, leaving the child to be given a milk or herb-tea feed by someone else.

Babies are sometimes laid to the breast too often because mothers are uncertain or perhaps believe in the principle of "demand-feeding." Not every smacking of the lips and stretching means hunger, and if mother and child become accustomed to constant little feeds an unnecessary dependence will arise, even to the extent that the ensuing difficulties may need the doctor's help.

We often hear views such as, "Just leave the baby, he'll let you know when he's hungry," or "Don't spoil the baby, she's got to have a fixed rhythm." In fact the new-born baby does live in a rhythm, but it is a living breathing one. It has been discovered with free feeding times that the average interval between feeds often lasts for rather more than four hours with the result that the corresponding feeding time next day has been retarded by about an hour as if the baby had a daily rhythm of around twenty-five hours instead of twenty-four. After six to ten weeks the baby adjusts automatically, sleeping through the night and taking regular four-hourly feeds during the day. Usually this slight difference in the rhythms can be ignored and baby can be put to the breast every four hours, but it is pointless and indeed unconducive to the flow of milk to wake the baby out of a deep sleep and force it to drink simply in order to keep to the correct rhythm.

11.3 The first sense-perceptions

Sound and noise

On entering a room with a baby in it, people automatically alter their behaviour. If not the slightest sound is coming from the baby, even the noisiest person will grow quiet and tiptoe up to the cradle. On the other hand, if the baby is yelling its head off, it will get everyone around moving at the double. Between these two extremes the baby's life develops. In this the mother usually plays the chief part. The mother's happy voice full of warmth, and her words of endearment intermingle gently with all the little noises that the baby makes in her presence.

All noises which are not human are at first alien and disruptive. Very often the baby's reaction is noticeable in its breathing as it sleeps or in its quickened pulse and heart-beat. Not just the pneumatic drill in the street, but also the sewing-machine or the washing-machine two rooms away can be heard by the child. We must assess the noises in the baby's surroundings not simply by their effect when the child is awake but rather by whether they are suitable for the child's age. Acoustically human life develops between the extremes of absolute peace and the plethora of human, instrumental and technical noises. The more carefully we can control the sounds coming to the child from its surroundings, the keener and more sensitive will the child's hearing be later on. To cite from personal experience, we have more than once been telephoned for advice by a mother whose baby was feverish, and in order to hear the mother speaking on the telephone, we have had first to ask her to turn off the radio blaring in the background.

Before it has learnt to speak and think, the child cannot in any way distance itself from surrounding impressions, and especially from aural perceptions. Our ability to distance ourselves is only slowly developed as a result of learning to name and recognize things. This means that during the first year of life, the child is quite incapable of "switching off" and is totally exposed to every impression with its whole highly sensitive body. What the child experiences in this way is delicately registered by variations in pulse and breathing. Of course a house full of musical talents should not be completely silenced but the instruments should be practised or played at a certain distance from the baby and pieces selected as much as possible with the child in mind. All technical sounds and the continuous droning of radio, television, video and cassettes should be kept away from babies as much as possible.

The effect which sounds and noises have on babies can be observed in their play. If you give a baby a rattle or something attached to an elastic for it to make a noise with, you can see the sort of movements which the child makes. Its wriggling and kicking tend to become quivering and jerky. It is quite different when you provide a simple wooden clapper for it to play with. Then the child's movements harmonize with the sounds and become noticeably orderly. In both cases, the noises give the child great pleasure, but only in the case of the clapper, do we have the impression that the child adopts a more restful attitude and has come to terms better with the sense impressions.

Again, different effects are produced on a child by the parent singing or humming quietly nearby. The baby is lost in wonder, its movements are more relaxed and, if tired, it soon falls asleep because it has opened itself to the music and can abandon itself more easily to sleep.

Air, humidity and smells

All are agreed that fresh air is good. But in the city when we open the window we have to take what comes in. For the baby, it does not matter if the air is cool but there should not be a draught from an open door or window. For this reason it is useful to have a veil over the baby's bed. Whether the window should be opened just a little, or left closed for the most part and only opened now and again, depends not only on the temperature but also on the humidity or dryness indoors, and on the amount of noise outside. The question of heat conservation has also to be taken into account. A good solution is to open the window wide to change the air when the baby is not in the room and then close it completely. Avoid at all costs that the baby is continuously breathing in cooking smells and cigarette smoke. That is bad even for adults who are not so engulfed by their sense impressions as babies.

As far as humidity is concerned most of our modern heating systems are unsuitable for babies, primarily because they do not leave the air humid enough. Even humidifiers fitted to the heaters do not completely solve the problem. In order to maintain sufficient humidity in the home, several quarts of water need to be vaporized each day. This can only be done with electrical humidifiers which have their own disadvantages (noise, bacterial growth and the like). But if it is necessary to use such a device for health reasons (if for instance the family are prone to catarrh), be careful to get one that operates quietly and that works with normal tap water and without filter paper. The kind we recommend brings the water to the boil by means of two electrode plates. They are cheap but hard to find. If you do not have such a thing the best solution is to air the room briefly but frequently. Another way is to put a pot on to simmer away at low heat out of reach of the baby. If the baby's air passages become infected, the surrounding atmosphere can be improved by adding a few drops of eucalyptus oil to the boiling water. Chronic colds, coughs and hoarseness are generally exacerbated by modern heating methods.

Sunlight

The new-born baby opens its eyes in the half-dark and seems to be looking for something. If we let light fall on its face, the child's eyes will shut again immediately. This changes after a few weeks, and the baby when awake will look around even when there is plenty of light in the room. Now it is time to let the baby sleep outside, sheltered from direct sunlight and from the wind. Begin with fifteen to thirty minutes daily according to the weather and slowly increase to two hours or longer. Of course have a look at the child from time to time. Some people do not like the idea of putting a three or four week old child out into the open even though it is warmly wrapped up and has a bonnet on his head. But exposure to daylight is most important for a baby in our latitudes. The particular quality of light directly overhead in a blue sky has a valuable formative effect on the human body. After mother's milk, this light is the most important factor in promoting the formation of a healthy bone structure.

Sunlight from blue sky, when enjoyed in the right amounts, contributes towards preventing rickets and promotes general strengthening of the body (see Chapter 15.2). If the baby has its face and forehead exposed to the blue sky overhead (but protected from direct sunlight) for up to two hours daily, with the hood of the pram down, the child will benefit and it will be impossible for rickets to develop. Hazy light from the horizon does not have the same properties as the blue sky overhead which is not always obvious in a city landscape.

Warmth and cold

The new-born baby's regulation of warmth is undeveloped and easily upset. If a baby is born in too cold surroundings, it will tend to have too low a temperature for hours afterwards even if wrapped up immediately after the birth. It is therefore most important, and one cannot do enough, to keep the new-born baby evenly warm. Paediatrics in Germany is currently learning a lot in this area: premature babies in the incubator are now dressed or at least on a warmth-retaining sheepskin. Formerly they lay naked on a cotton sheet under the warm fan of the incubator, but with this practice, the babies lost far more warmth than now when dressed.

At home, too, parents should watch that their babies do not get cold. When bathing the baby, it is far better to have a radiator in the room rather than a fan heater. The difference can be seen in the baby's mottled skin. Outside in the fresh air, cool cheeks and cool hands are quite normal even in a warmly dressed baby, but when in bed the baby's hands and feet should always be cosily warm. As a lot of heat is lost through the head, a woolly hat should be worn outside, and inside a thinner cotton cap or bonnet (unnecessary of course in hot climates).

If for no special reason a baby is prone to have cold hands, a pure woollen vest with long sleeves usually helps, and the vest can be left on during nappy changes even if it is a little damp at the bottom. The particular qualities of wool are discussed in greater detail below, as this is a topic which is often disregarded.

During the baby's first weeks, it may still be necessary to put a covered hot-water bottle in the bed (be careful not to make it too hot). In a cooler room, or if you do not care for a downy or eiderdown, the baby, once wrapped up, can be put into a woolly sleeping-bag or wrapped in a blanket.

Using sheep's wool
Unbleached sheep's wool can absorb up to thirty per cent of its own weight in humidity without feeling damp. Because of its good insulating properties, humidity can evaporate through the wool without any chilling effect on the skin. No other textile has this property. Perspiration is also absorbed and the excess body heat is not prevented from escaping as is the case with synthetic textures. That is why the bedouin in the desert wear woollen or sheepskin clothing.

Some mothers do not like wool because they feel that it irritates their own skin, but such soft quality vests are available for babies that they can be worn even by babies with the most sensitive skin. The garments must however be hand-washed in a very mild soap solution so that they retain their softness. The objection that wool cannot be boiled is hardly valid, for unbleached wool only needs to be washed in a warm solution of 30°C (86°F) to become clean and not smell. Furthermore wool lasts; a thick knitted woollen pair of nappy-trousers (see Appendix for knitting hints) will still do for a second child if it has always been washed in the right way. It is important that the wool is 100% pure fleece wool, unbleached. Ready-made articles of clothing are of course expensive. But because fewer are required and need to be changed less often that balances out, while the advantage to health cannot be measured in money terms. If you are able to knit, then of course there is less of a cost problem.

For very sensitive skins, vests and bonnets of pure silk may be the solution. This textile has almost the same warmth-regulating properties as wool and is very pleasant to wear.

Cotton underwear is only suitable in very warm weather when there is not much variation in temperature. Synthetic materials are unsuitable in any case as they retain humidity and keep in the body heat.

Far too often we have to examine children in our consulting-room who are not warmly enough dressed. But we occasionally come across the opposite extreme: an overheated child under endless layers of wool, with a thick cap pulled right down to the eyes, not even allowing the forehead to cool off. The ideal is therefore to find the right mean between the two extremes of overheating and underheating. Too much warmth cossets the organism and hinders the development of the body's regulating mechanisms. Too little warmth or even deliberate exposure to cold gives rise to reflexes and regulatory adjustments in the body which go

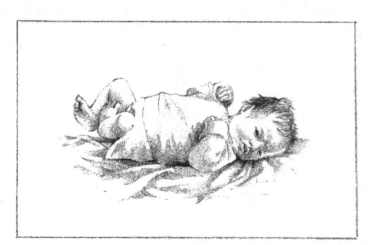

Figure 26. A young baby's limbs are loosely bent (gradually straightening out in the first 3 months)

beyond normal conditions and provoke extreme reactions. In both cases, the development in the child of flexible and sensitive reactions to warmth and cold will be impaired (see Chapter 7.3).

11.4 Laying the baby down

We know from the way we carry a young baby that it cannot hold up its head and body. Only when lying on its tummy can the baby raise its head for a moment (Figure 27). But it is not generally known that gravity can have a directly deforming effect on the body of the child during the first months. A baby that is always turning its head the same way because light and people are coming to its bed from that direction will develop a flattening of the skull on that side. This deformity can extend along the trunk right down to the pelvis. If not recognized in time, usually by the end of the third month, the damage cannot be fully rectified. In rare cases a wry-neck (torticollis), a broken collar-bone during birth, or a swelling on the head (haematoma) can be the reason for the baby lying on one side only. The baby should therefore be laid alternately on each side.

Once the baby is able to turn itself and prefers the light side, the head of the cot should be turned round so that the light comes from the other side. In the case of a wry-neck or haematoma, the baby will need a support made of nappies rolled together to prevent it turning back on

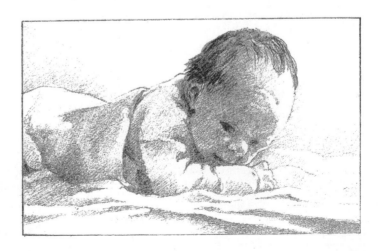

Figure 27. Lying on its tummy a baby can stretch its neck and move its head sideways. Even a newborn baby can lift its nose clear of the ground (birth to about 6 weeks).

to the "forbidden" side, at least temporarily. Consultation with the doctor will be necessary in a case like this.

As for whether the baby should be laid to sleep on its back or tummy, laying the baby down on its tummy was widely recommended in Germany twenty years ago, following American influence. The idea was that the children developed their motor-functions better, the back became stronger, the pelvis was relieved of pressure and could develop better. Since then, however, deformities due to laying the baby on its tummy have

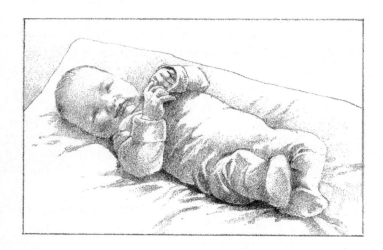

Figure 28. Finger-play starts when the baby lies on its back.

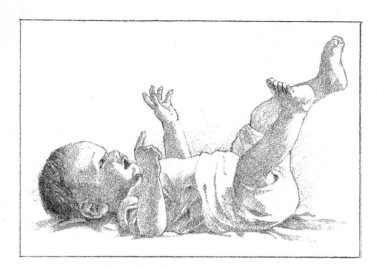

Figure 29. The baby lying on its back open to the surroundings. In warm weather expose only the face and forehead to the blue light of the sky in order to prevent rickets. The baby should not be exposed to direct sunshine for more than a short time.

become known, for example, the outward splaying Charlie Chaplin feet or a flat chest.

If we follow the development of the respective children (those laid on their tummies, and those laid on their backs), we notice that the "tummy babies" are ahead of the others with their movements to begin with, but the "back babies" are more peaceful and develop more varied finger-play (Figure 28). Observing individual children, we note that the "tummy babies" learn to stand earlier, but "back babies" soon overtake them in alertness and agility.

So we recommend not being dogmatic about how to lay the child down. In the first weeks the best policy is to lay the child on each side alternately. If the baby settles only when laid on its tummy, it should be left to sleep that way. When awake, put the child to play on its back so it can study faces, objects and the play of its own hands. If the baby only sleeps on its back, lay the child on its tummy for short periods when it is awake.

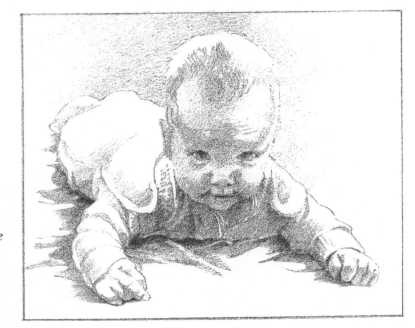

Figure 30. The child learns to raise itself from the ground. The elbows begin to take the weight. The fingers are still bent (3–4 months).

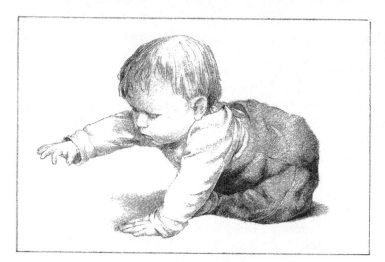

Figure 31. The first movements forward have been discovered because the child wants to reach something. This is the start of crawling (10 months).

11.5 Nappies (diapers)

During the baby's first weeks, we recommend that cotton nappies (diapers) are used, and that the baby is wrapped in a shawl. It is preferable not to put on leggings or a stretch-suit. Plastic or rubber nappies are also undesirable; they do not allow the wetness to evaporate, which is bad for the skin.

Children born by breech-delivery have a tendency towards hip weakness. This can be counteracted by using a cotton nappy with an extra roll of cloth between the legs, which bends the knees out and up. Breech births are very rare in the UK and USA nowadays.

After a few weeks, the baby will begin to kick off its nappies if they are put on too loosely. To prevent this you can put on a pair of woollen leggings and then wrap the child in a shawl which will also prevent kicking too freely.

We do not recommend that babies are allowed to kick too freely all the time, as was formerly thought good. During the first months, a baby carries out a great number of reflex movements. If we watch the child's eyes we can see how the child is endeavouring to gain control over these movements, and here we shall want to help, if possible. By "swaddling" the baby correctly, the wild kicking movements are restrained and the baby is given support in its efforts to control movement. The

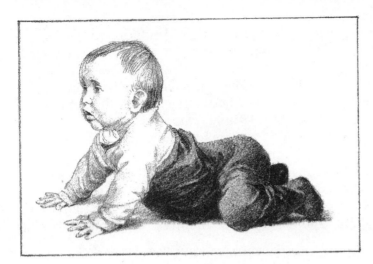

Figure 32. At about six months the child spreads out its hands, straightening arms and legs, looking rather like an "egg figure." Movements, gaze and baby-noises are now much more expressive.

baby's gaze will become calmer and more alert and it can now concentrate on learning to use its hands.

During the first eight weeks, however, allow the child some free kicking time during nappy-changing which should occur at least five times in the twenty-four hours. In addition, do not swaddle so tightly that the baby cannot move his hips at all; this could hinder the development of the acetabulum (hip-joint socket). This is especially important in cases of congenital dislocation of the hip.

Congenital dislocation of the hip should be attended to as early as possible by the doctor. If it is overlooked and the dislocation is only recognized when the child begins to walk, an operation will be necessary, and this usually entails further corrective measures as well. Chronic bad posture and bad weight distribution will lead to early arthritis, which can be a painful and troublesome handicap.

11.6 Washing, bathing and general care

The baby's skin, like the adult's, has a fine film of fat for which there is no real substitute. There is no sense in washing this film away with a daily bath and then rubbing in a skin cream instead. In most cases it is sufficient to give baby a quick bath twice a week and to wash the face, folds of skin and nappy area daily. Sputum, urine or excreta need only to be washed off gently with plain water without soap. Do not rub hard. Remains of skin cream or excreta should be cleaned off with oil. Ordinary sunflower-seed oil is quite adequate for cleaning, and a lot cheaper than proprietary baby oils. The folds of the skin at the neck, the armpits, behind

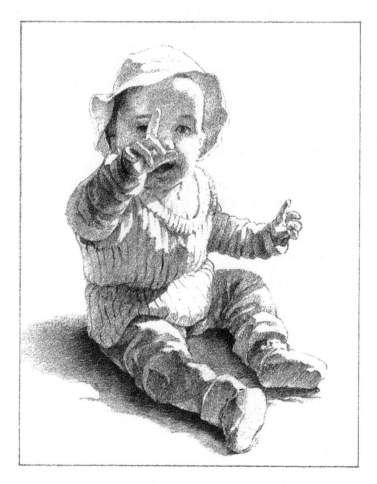

Figure 33. Sitting straight up, the child now has got its hands free for playing (10 months).

the ears and in the nappy (diaper) area should be cleaned with a thin application of oil. Too much powder in these parts easily becomes crusty when it gets wet and can then be a cause of irritation. A little powder can be used if there is chafing or heat rash. Too much powder, raising clouds, can cause the child to cough and is dangerous for the lungs.

11.7 The baby's bed

We recommend a basket cradle, with padding all round in one colour and a pale pink-violet veil. This gives protection against irritating air movements and allows a pleasant subdued light to shine through in which the child can sleep peacefully. It also protects against direct sunshine by an open window and of course does not allow any ultra-violet rays through. This must be taken into consideration when using sunlight to prevent rickets. In this case the veil is drawn aside in such a way that the sun is still shaded, but the baby's head is exposed to the blue light of the sky.

Whether you use a cradle, pram or cot it is important to keep it next to the mother's bed. This is often not done with the consequence that the parents have to get up repeatedly during the night. The mattress for the baby's bed should be of one piece, smooth and firm. There should be no pillow except perhaps a thin homemade one filled with grain such as millet which can be renewed from time to time. It fits the roundness of the head and does not interfere with breathing like a soft pillow filled with down.

11.8 Getting about

As with cars, the appearance and construction of prams are dependent on fashion. Prams are not all well-sprung and ideal for their purpose, and hardly any have pneumatic tyres, which are best. Although most people take great care to push their babies gently, it is surprising how

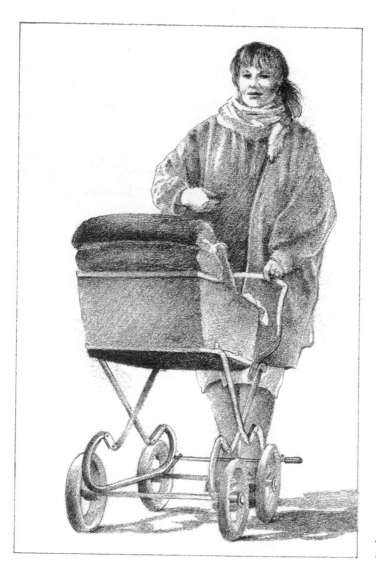

Figure 34. The baby should be facing you in its pram.

many are unaware how much their babies are exposed to jolting and vibration in a pram. Because of their design, most prams have to keep to the pavements and babies in them are exposed to the exhaust fumes of traffic. But with a well-sprung pram on pneumatic tyres, you can go for a walk on country footpaths and lanes. Whatever kind of pram you have, the baby should be facing the adult. If the child has its back to you and is facing right into the traffic and bustle of the street, you are exposing it to a whole lot of unrelated impressions which cannot be assimilated. If your pram has transparent sides, we suggest you cover them with a single coloured cloth.

Carry-cots are the best for the first weeks and baby-carriers (papoose-bags) are fine once the baby can hold its head up, that is after four months. Make sure that the baby is dressed warmly enough when being carried in this way.

The disadvantage of all these ways of transporting the baby is that the parents are tempted to take the baby with them everywhere, even into the really unsuitable atmosphere of supermarkets and other places with harsh lights, music and noise, not to mention the possibilities of infection. Even car journeys should be carefully weighed up as to how necessary they really are.

The most suitable surroundings for the baby are those where its faculties can best cope. Before it reaches the stage of crawling and exploring the room, a baby feels happiest in its mother's arms or in its bed. Anything else is an unfortunate necessity which may be forced upon us by circumstances, but we should realize that these experiences are only a hindrance to the development of the child. The fact that babies will tolerate an enormous amount and seem to put up with all sorts of things is something that we should never take advantage of.

12 From babyhood to childhood

12.1 Daily routine

The transition from baby to toddler comes when the baby learns to walk. Now the child is no longer a quadruped and its hands are free to get hold of all sorts of things, pull them down, and inspect them. The daily routine now starts to take on different aspects. The child toddles from one room to another and follows the mother around. It begins to sit properly at table with the rest of the family — who now have to learn not to make the child the centre of attention, but let it take its proper place without

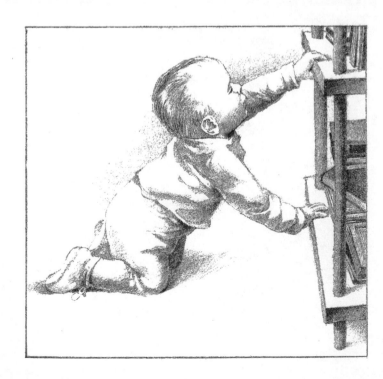

Figure 35. Something is attracting the child upwards. Hands are already skilful and strong (1 year old).

disrupting the lives of the older children.

Sleeping habits will also change. During their first year, babies sleep both in the morning and in the afternoon — outside or by the open window. But in their second year, they sleep only in the afternoon. Many of them can no longer go to sleep by an open window or in the open air, and have to take their afternoon sleep in their room. It is important then for them to get some sunshine before or after their afternoon nap and not to sleep through the best part of the day. The earlier their afternoon rest, the better they will sleep at night. The more punctually and regularly meal-times and bed-times are kept, the less the child will react with tempers, grumps, tiresomeness and boredom. Children love solid habits best. A regular routine not only helps the child to become aware (see Chapter 13.4) but is the best foundation for the training of the will (see Chapter 16.6).

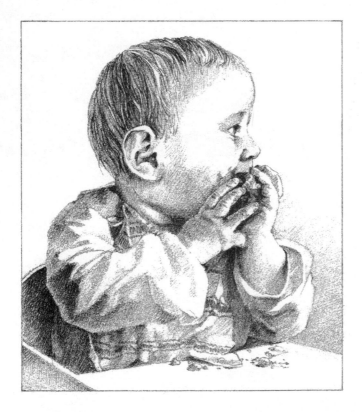

Figure 36. Learning to eat in a high chair (second year).

12.2 Nappy (diaper) and potty

Once the baby starts to toddle about, waterproof pants over the nappy (diaper) can be used. Disposable nappies are useful when you are visiting or on a journey. As children at this age do not wet their nappies as often as little babies but wet them thoroughly when they do, they see to it themselves that they do not stay wet too long, and the problems of getting chilled or of chafing the skin are no longer so great. Besides the "critical moment" is generally known in advance and the nappy can be changed immediately after the event.

Potty training is not important at this stage. Do not make a fuss about whether the baby performs successfully or not. Potty habits develop most naturally if you have a wooden high chair with a hole in the seat for a potty under it. A useful type is the sort of high chair which can be folded down and used on the floor between meals (Figure 38). After meals, the nappies can easily be removed while

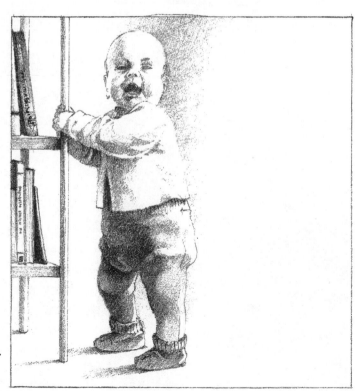

Figure 37. The feet have now learnt their function. Soon the hands will be quite free (1 year old).

the child continues to sit in its chair for ten minutes. Then if you are lucky, the baby will have moved its bowels and in this way will grow used to regular times. The same times can be kept up when the child starts using the toilet.

12.3 Clothing and footwear

Young children have a great fascination for shoes. They love putting them on and taking them off. Later they identify people by their shoes and play at being the people whose shoes they are "wearing." Of course

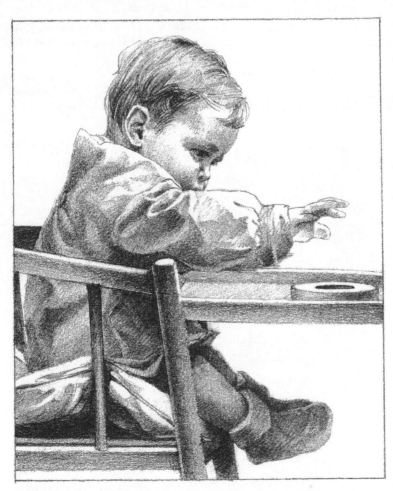

Figure 38. The high chair is also a place for playing.

Figure 39. Grand-parents and grand-children are always fond of each other.

the mother must play the game, too, and recognize who the "person" is supposed to be.

But in the beginning it is hard for children to get shoes on. They curl their feet up instead of stretching them out into the shoe. Shoes for beginners have to be well loosened or opened up before being put on.

For a time it was thought that shoes were a support for the feet of little children. That is just as wrong as the idea that you need shoes to learn to walk or that insoles can form the feet.

Feet develop best when the baby goes barefoot, or in stockings or slippers to prevent cold or to prevent sliding on a slippery floor.

Out of doors, a grassy lawn is good for the feet and indoors a mat or carpet of sisal bast, wool or bristle. All of these they give the feet something to feel and grip actively. Shoes pamper the feet and make them passive.

To have flat feet at this age is normal. The arch develops at the age of five as a result of proper exercise.

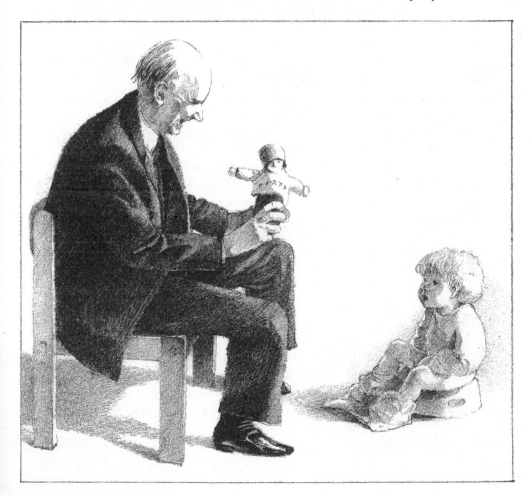

But if the child does not walk, it will not develop an arch. With persistent flat feet due to weak connective tissue, orthopaedists are almost unanimous in the opinion that insoles are only desirable in cases where the whole skeleton may be adversely affected by bad posture. Normally the best therapy is to encourage the child's own exercise. Going on tiptoe is very good for developing the arches. You can call it "flying like a bird" and get the child to run on tiptoe with raised fluttering hands. Exercising like this is much better than making formal demands on a child with which it will soon lose interest.

There is considerable divergence of views about the best kind of outdoor shoe. The ideal is usually far removed from what can be obtained in a shoe-shop or chain store. The most healthy kind of shoe is of unlined leather large enough to allow thick woollen socks to be worn in winter. The shoes should be tipped with rubber for grip and the heels should be flat. Synthetic and lambs-wool linings usually only cover the upper and back part of the shoe and are not nearly as warm as woollen socks which cover the whole foot. Moreover synthetic lining does not allow the moisture of the feet to disperse, and consequently the feet are more prone to getting sweaty and to suffer from athlete's foot.

It is often said that the soles of a baby shoe should be as soft as possible, but we cannot agree; after all, the whole purpose of a shoe is make it easier to walk on rough ground and in bad weather. For puddles, snow, or muddy ground, strong soles and heels are best. For pavements, soft soles are comfortable but they do not offer any protection against the jarring of the joints and backbone.

To sum up, the foot develops a healthy shape and function not through the shoe but through its own activity. Shoes are there only to protect the feet from harsh surroundings.

As far as clothing is concerned, the advantages of wool continue to outweigh all the alternatives (see Chapter 11.3). You can continue to dress your child in a woollen vest and you will try to avoid synthetics. At night a knitted woollen sleeping-bag is recommended, preferably made from unbleached sheep's wool. This bag can be used between the ages of one and four, and even until six because at this age children tend to throw off the bed-clothes at night without being able to cover themselves again. In this type of sleeping-bag they can move around and lie whichever way they want and still keep snug and warm.

Everyday clothes should be as practical as possible: that is, they should allow freedom of movement, they should stand up to wear and tear, be warm (or cool) and absorb moisture. Beyond that the child's liking for a particular article can help to determine choice. Sunday clothes should reflect the mood of Sunday.

As far as colour of clothing is concerned, Rudolf Steiner draws attention to this question, especially in his book *The Education of the Child*. He points out that it is not so much the colour which the child sees that is important but the effect of the complementary colour. If for instance you look at a red patch for some time and then quickly look at a white patch you will see the complementary colour green on the white. Similarly blue produces orange-yellow. These "opposite colours" are created while the eye sees the original colour. Complementary colours are much more intense in their effects in children than in adults, and indeed they can have a profound effect upon the child's physical condition. In the case of an overactive child, red clothing will produce the complementary green which has a soothing effect. In the opposite case of a more intro-verted child, whether slow of tem-perament or simply withdrawn, blue will be stimulating because it pro-duces the complementary orange-yellow, which is a stimulating colour.

A change in the perception of colour takes place when the child reaches the age of nine. Before then the child's "I" lives more in the surroundings; and from the age of nine onwards, it lives more within itself (see also Chapters 13 and 17).

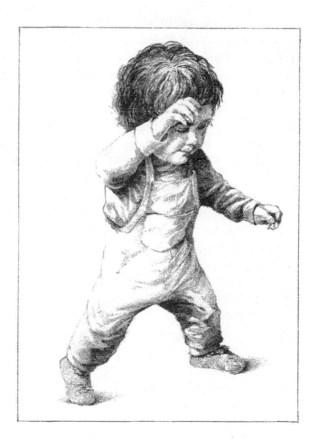

Figure 40. This child is
practising tirelessly.
Sight, touch and balance
are hard to coordinate.

12.4 Swimming and gymnastics for babies

A baby's activity is stimulated by certain events in the day such as bedtime, nappy-changing time or playpen time. These bursts of activity are all more or less spontaneous, whereas if we try to encourage a specific muscular activity or motor skill, this can amount to interference in the child's natural development. A healthy baby does not need extra stimulation. So we should ask whether swimming is really beneficial for a young baby.

With a handicapped child who requires special exercises, the whole art of therapy consists in applying the kind of exercise which corresponds most closely to a normal development. Swimming does not correspond at all to the phase of development that a healthy infant is going through. After all, the first year or two of life are taken up with trying to come to terms with gravity. This development reaches its peak when the baby has learnt to walk. Swimming with all four limbs is quite a different experience and unrelated to walking.

Furthermore, baby skin loses fat and other valuable substances in water and absorbs very little that is of value instead. What is lost has to be replaced, what is absorbed has to be assimilated, and the resultant cooling after the swim makes unnecessary demands upon the organism. We recommend, then, that babies are allowed to play in an environment like a swimming-pool only after the age of two.

The only advantage of letting babies swim, is that it gives pleasure to the parents and allows them to enjoy the company of others all busy with their children in a congenial group. There is no evidence that babies are braver people or better swimmers in later life just because they were introduced to the swimming-pool before the age of one. On the contrary an older child who has consciously overcome a fear of water will have developed more courage than the child who has been accustomed to swimming from a very young age. As a general principle, children should not be made to swim until they are ready.

12.5 The playpen

The playpen is an intermediary stage between the baby's bed and the room which is still too big for the child (Figure 41). The playpen should be made of wood, with bars and a floor at least 10 cm (4") above the floor of the room to raise it above the draughts. If the floor of the playpen is not raised, you can put a strip of material around the sides to keep the draught out. Make sure that the joints at the corners are padded to prevent the child from trapping its fingers.

Set the playpen up in a place from where the mother can be seen. At six months, the baby can be laid in the playpen as long as it is awake and playing so that it can see the mother

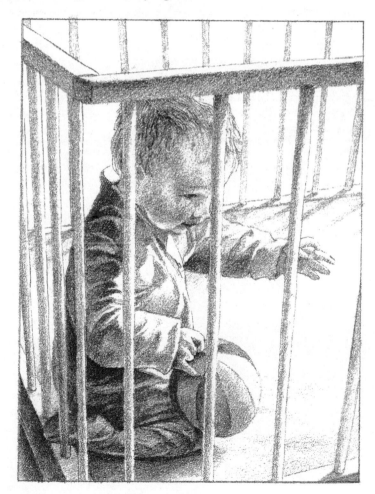

Figure 41. A sunny morning in the playpen. Not a prison but a protected space where the child can play.

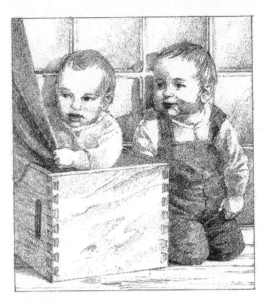

Figure 42. Even babies enjoy the company of a friend some mornings.

Figure 43. This 10–12 month-old enjoys watching his mother from the safety of the upturned stool.

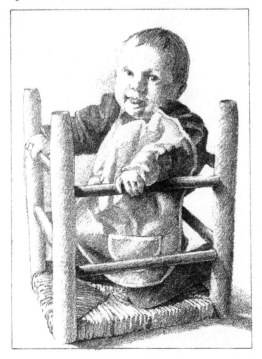

while she is doing her housework or just sitting nearby. In this way you will avoid the bad habit of just going to look at the child when it demands attention or is fretful. The child is now taking part in the mother's life and not the other way round, and its natural urge to imitate is stimulated when the mother is busy doing things. Very soon, the child makes its first attempts to stand up holding on to the bars of the playpen which are constructed for that purpose.

Most children are happy playing in the playpen during the morning. If the child grows tired and lies down, the mother can cover it or put the child to bed. Because the child has seen plenty of its mother during the morning, it will normally be quite satisfied to go down to sleep. In the afternoon, however, the child will want to get out and so a walk or a period outside fits in quite naturally.

Once the baby has found out how to crawl, the day will come when it feels the playpen is a restriction. Now the mother's attitude is all-important: if the child is put in the playpen at any time as a punishment, then the playpen has become a prison. But if the child is frequently popped in for a moment so that the mother can get on with her work then there is a limitation which has naturally arisen. The baby cannot develop its imitative powers properly if the mother is always interrupting what she is doing to run after the lively little creature crawling about everywhere and catch him before he pulls down this or that object.

If you do not like the idea of a playpen, you should at least have a moveable bed with bars and a solid head and foot, out of which the baby cannot climb before it is two years old. There are two good reasons for having a bed of this kind. First, it is useful during periods of disturbed sleep (see Chapter 17.1). Second, when the child is ill the bed can be wheeled about and kept near the mother. You cannot really expect a baby to stay alone in bed in its room while the mother goes about the rest of the house. But babies are usually quite happy in bed when they can see the mother through the bars (Figure 14). In addition, there is room in the bed for them to move and play while, at the same time, they are not exposed to draughts and dirt as they would be on the floor. When they get tired, they will lie down and drop off to sleep. In this way, the mother does not always have to be carrying her child about or keeping a close eye on it.

12.6 The playroom

Not every child can have its own room but if there is a playroom or nursery room in the home, it can be fitted out in such a way as to help the child's development. Here are descriptions of two very different rooms. Which one do you think is more suitable for a child?

—A room with a white ceiling, brightly coloured wallpaper with pictures of little puppets, balls and sailing boats, a practical floor covering of PVC and a synthetic carpet, curtains with strong contrasting colours, and on the wall a calender of a baby-food firm. The furniture is of washable orange-coloured plastic. You can see that the parents have had professional advice and have been to some expense.

—In the second room, ceiling and walls are painted with a light warm pastel colour. One corner and the sloping ceiling are panelled with cheap boarding. The linoleum floor is covered with a sisal carpet, on which a patchwork rug and sheepskin rug are lying. An old sandpapered wardrobe, un unpainted wooden table in the corner with children's chairs, a plain double bunk-bed, a stand with shelves for the toys, a couple of boxes to push about, sit on or to build with, a picture on the wall of which the mother is particularly fond and above the child's bed a Renaissance picture of an angel. The colour and material of the curtains are such that even during the afternoon sleep the room is enclosed in a cosy darkness, and

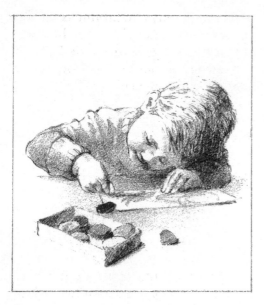

Figure 44. Starting to draw. Wax crayon blocks are easier to hold than sticks.

there is no glaring contrast with the wall colouring. Altogether the colour scheme is warm and welcoming.

In decorating a room, glaring colour contrasts only blunt feeling for the quality of individual colours. You can see this clearly by contrasting a car-park full of different coloured cars with a wood's delicate shades of green and brown. In the first case the colours thrust themselves upon us, while in the second they draw the soul out so that it becomes active in its perception. At an age when the impressions of the senses have such a powerful effect on development, it makes a vast difference whether the child is subjected constantly to caricatures, glaring colours and smooth shiny surfaces, or whether it can have all around carefully balanced gentle shades of colour which allow the soul to breath.

And wallpaper? A wall painted all of one colour becomes a unit of space and area, whereas wallpaper patterns impose a foreign element on to this space. Sadly, the common picture patterns try to be jolly and childlike. If we begin to take them seriously, however, what is in them? What distorted caricatures of life we are offered! And where in the real world do we find such an endless repetition of false images? Where are all these innumerable pussy-cats, balls and Little Red Riding-Hoods?

It does make a difference to a child in later life if it has grown up in rooms which are suitably equipped. If you are uncertain about what colour and furniture to choose, the following may help as a guiding principle: the object in question should express outwardly its intrinsic nature. Take, for example, a plain unvarnished table of solid wood. The proportions and thickness of the top and the legs, the run of the grain and the joinery of the parts all exhibit the very nature and purpose of the table. But a plywood table hides the brittle quality of the layers and shows outwardly something that it does not possess inwardly.

For keeping the place tidy, the chaos of toys can be swallowed up in a chest or hamper. If during the baby's first year, the mother starts to have her own quiet and peaceful routine of putting the toys back in their place once a day, and especially if she can arrange them with love and care, the child may well come to join in tidying up by imitation later.

Equally important for the child is whether the mother really likes being in its room or not. The child's room will remain only a bedroom as long as the mother carries on all her interesting activities elsewhere and never spends any of her working or resting time in the nursery.

12.7 Holidays

A lot of young parents want to get back as soon as possible to their favourite holiday places but these are hardly ever what suits the baby. Every change of surroundings means an uprooting for the child from the home in which it is much more firmly anchored than the parents. The child's sense of being is much more related to the familiarity of surroundings than is the case with adults. If, however, a regular change of air is necessary for health or other reasons, it is best to go with your child to the same place for several holidays in succession. The place and accommodation should be chosen for their suitability for the child. Going back to the same place the following year the child will acclimatize much more quickly and will derive a lot of satisfaction from recognizing everything again.

If the parents have to go away for any reason, the child should either be left in familiar surroundings and cared for at home by someone the child knows, or it should be taken with the parents. Only in extreme circumstances should a child be separated at the same time both from the people closest to it and from its home (see also Chapter 16.1).

12.8 Toys

The enormous choice of available toys nowadays represents quite a problem. Children are inundated with innumerable and ingenious products which are all thought to be suitable. If, however, you observe a child absorbed in play, you soon notice how little the play activity has to do with what the toy itself purports to be (Figure 43). Play reflects the urge of the child to be actively involved with its surroundings. The child does what it sees others doing. A two year old will stir away happily

Figure 45. Experiencing balance through play: in the body and outside it.

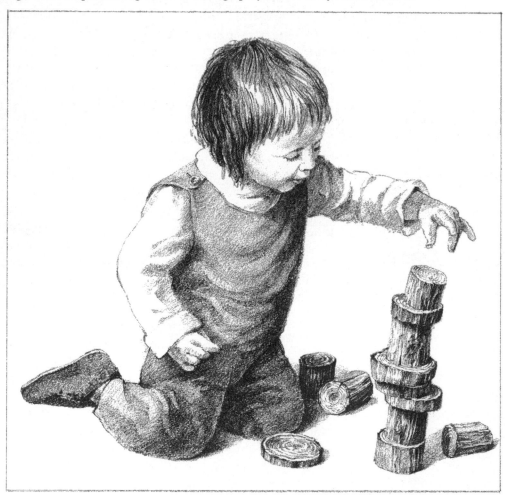

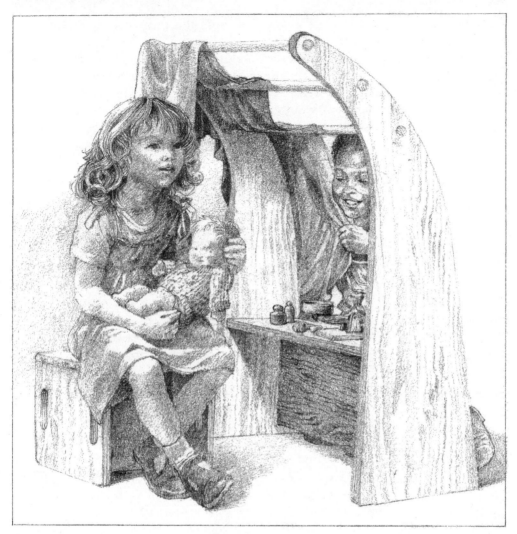

Figure 46. The best toys are simple and made of natural materials.

with a stick on the floor, cooking soup like its parents. It "turns on" the gas. It goes "click" just like one of the parents taking a photograph. The child examines the plates as they rattle cheerily when they are taken from the sideboard for a meal. It likes to be actively involved with everything the adults are doing. It experiences fulfilment in what it is doing — not in just looking at a perfect plastic doll. If the doll has not got a face, the child will invent one out of the imagination and so the doll cries, is angry, or grows tired. A doll's face that is always smiling, or a fixed caricature, is a false imitation that stifles the imagination.

What then is a suitable toy? Ideally, a doll should have a simple shape and construction suitable for the age of the child. To begin with, a little silk cloth stuffed with wool and tied at the top and corners to indicate head, hands and feet, is perfectly adequate. Later the child will enjoy a wooden doll that can stand, sit or lie. Later again, a doll can be made of cloth.

Any object which allows the child's imagination to work is suitable as a toy. A finger can be a toy, which the child watches and sees doing all sorts of things. The corner of a cushion can be a toy, which the child can fold over or push in. A plain box that can be opened and shut and things put in and taken out; or a bit of wood that can be tapped on the table and the noise investigated. Later on a bowl and a bottle top to scoop up water and make a lake; or a pot and lid; or a brightly coloured knitted ball stuffed with wood to be rolled, thrown, pushed and wrapped up; little bits of coloured cloth.

Why is it so important that the child does not get any of those perfectly designed clever toys as presents from father, mother, uncles and aunts? It is because toys like these do not allow the child any play of the imagination, and the material, colour and form used in them are absolutely at variance with the child's sense of reality and aesthetic sense. It is most important to allow the child to develop healthily through activity and free imagination. On this topic, Rudolf Steiner says: "The child, however, does not learn by instruction or admonition, but by imitation. The physical organs shape their forms through the influence of the physical environment. Good sight will be developed in the child if his environment has the right conditions of light and colour, while in the brain and blood-circulation the physical foundations will be laid for a healthy moral sense if the child sees moral actions in his environment. If before his seventh year the child sees only foolish actions in his surroundings, the brain will assume such forms as adapt it also to foolishness in later life ... If people could look into the brain as the spiritual investigator can, and see how it builds its forms, they would assuredly give their children only such toys as are fitted to stimulate and vivify its formative activity. Toys with dead mathematical forms alone, have a desolating and killing effect upon the formative forces of the child. On the other hand, everything that kindles the imagination of living things works in the right way." *(The Education of the Child,* pp. 25–6).

The link between bodily activity and brain formation has been well established scientifically; for example Bobath-gymnastics use movement-therapy to treat early brain damage. To counteract speech defects and dyslexia, agility training and balancing exercises are used. Everything which the child undertakes with interest and which seizes the imagination works on the fine structure of the brain which at birth is still very unformed.

The toys and playthings that are good for the child's development are, however, not necessarily the products most advertised by commercial interests forever seeking markets. If today's parents fail to realize what is good for their children, future generations will inherit or grow up with grave deficiencies, not even knowing why they suffer from emptiness and boredom, or why they lack imagination and a lively productive spirit.

13 The child's development and social environment

Is the human being the product of both heredity and environment? And which of the two is more influential in human development? These questions are constantly raised and discussed, and not just by specialists. Genetics, sociology, child-psychology, social-paediatrics and other branches of science keep the issues alive through endless new research.

In the chapter on children's diseases (see Chapter 6.14), we looked in some detail at the human "I" and how it goes about making the inherited body "fit" better. This approach enables us to see heredity and environment in a different light: they can now be understood as complementary fields of activity both of which are needed by the "I" in order to fulfil its development.

Seen from this point of view, characteristics latent in heredity no longer appear merely as the random result of genetic mutations. It is not by chance that the first child in a family has, say, curly hair, the second straight hair and the third the sparse hair of his grandfather. These characteristics are "planned" in advance: the "I" itself, active before birth, selects its parents and the inherited characteristics which will best suit the development of its personality.

It is the same with environment. This term is commonly taken to mean a set of external and often hostile circumstances with which the individual has to wrestle as part of the process of growth and development. But here again we must see things from the viewpoint of reincarnation. Environment is not alien to the child but the chosen surroundings for its particular destiny. Even more, our environment is a living extension of our own being as humans within the created world, a broader "life" with which we have both past and potential unity. Thus each child takes from its environment what is properly and rightfully "its own." One child takes everything which furthers a musical talent, while another leans towards everything technical. One child is actively and purposefully acquisitive of what it needs, while another is receptive to impressions and lets itself be moulded. Where do these very different tendencies come from? If we observe children developing, we notice clearly that none of them starts life with a blank page. Abilities and weaknesses, aims and proneness to certain illness are projected from former lives into this one.

The individual takes from heredity and environment what he or she has an affinity to. The task of education lies in guiding this process of assimilation, and in shielding the child from "too much," "too little," "too early" and "too late." On the other hand we also have to prevent the child from developing only those attributes towards which it is predisposed. The full outcome of a life on earth consists not just in developing those natural talents brought in at birth, but also in increasing, widening and further developing the total personality. There is an unlimited potential for learning within a single human being but, equally, there is the danger of total inertia and lack of development.

13.1 Learning to see

In an earlier chapter, we described the searching look of the new-born baby, a look that cannot maintain direction, let alone concentrate on anything (see Chapter 11.1). Over the following weeks, the baby's eyes will remain open for increasingly long periods. While being fed, the baby usually watches its mother. But it is frequently noticeable that the baby's eyes repeatedly seek out one direction even though there is nothing particular to be seen there: perhaps a bit of the wall or a piece of cloth some distance away. If we turn the baby's head away, the eyes will go on looking in the same direction for as long as possible. This reflex, which is called the "doll's eye" phenomenon, shows clearly how the baby is learning directional vision. Instead of the eyes floating freely in the way which is characteristic of the sleeping child or newly born baby, now the axis of vision is being directed. If we insert our own head into the direction of vision, the child will at first look right through us quite unaffected by the solidity blocking its view. Only gradually will the baby notice our head and react with its eyes, quickening its breathing and making movements. The child's eyes now begin to focus on our head and if we move slowly, it will follow with its eyes. If however we keep still (as mothers usually do because they feel that their babies are drinking them in with their eyes) we shall see our own reflection in the baby's pupils slightly below the centre. This means that the child is not looking at a sharply defined head, eyes, nose or mouth, but is looking past the outline of the head, either above it or a little to one side.

The extraordinary thing is that the child's soul takes part in what is seen through the eyes. With its mother, the baby reacts peacefully and happily watching her. With unsure, over-tired or harassed people, the child becomes restless or its mouth trembles in a timid wary way. Even though the baby has as yet no clear and definite sense-perception, it does "see" something: it "sees" the emotional condition of the adult. You can observe this, too, when a person goes to the cradle of a sleeping baby and a gentle little smile (on one side) flits suddenly over the child's face. Then you cannot help but feel that the child is aware of something even while asleep and with its eyes closed.

Directional vision and perception of emotional states appear at the same time long before proper objective vision is possible. So we may well ask whether the child cannot perceive to some extent purely spiritual or soul qualities which are hidden from our objective vision. We may call to mind how medieval painters painted halos round the heads of angels, madonnas and saints, to make visible their noble soul-character. Once a mother asked us in the consulting-room: "Why does my baby always look past me over my head?" She was surprised and delighted when we answered: "The baby is looking at your halo." In the same connection, a baby at that age is attracted by all that glitters brightly and shines red. Objects with these colours seem to irradiate something similar to what emanates to the child from a free and open person.

After some time, usually in the fifth week, the first conscious smile appears, the beaming smile of a baby who has found its mother's eyes. The child has now accomplished the transition from gazing into the surroundings to looking straight into the pupils of the eyes. This is the moment when, in the meeting of the eyes, soul meets soul, and thus a fundamental condition of human existence is fulfilled, namely the seeking and "recognizing" of other people. As the baby "recognizes" its mother, it smiles. From now on, the child seeks out the mother's gaze. Even in later life, the child is not happy unless it has felt, at least once a day, the interested and understanding gaze of its father or mother. Nor can the child develop properly in school unless there are teachers who bestow a look of real interest.

At the same time as the baby experiences this interplay between itself and other people, its attention now begins to be attracted to other things. When carried past the window, the baby sees "something bright" moving across its vision. When it is happy and lively, its hands and arms agitate spontaneously and this "something that moves" suddenly appears, disappearing again just as suddenly; then it slowly comes back again when the child is still, and a second "something that moves" joins the first, perhaps touching it; then the two tiny hands begin to play together (Figures 28 and 29). The baby learns to feel them, and as it learns to look at them the play becomes more directed and the baby becomes more aware of itself. This awareness of self is further strengthened by the baby's contact with other people: when for instance it feels its own mouth when drinking at the mother's breast, and when it feels the loving touch of the mother's hands and arms.

This quality of contact and touching is also in the baby's gaze, and consequently the objects that the child is given to look at are important. The things perceived should truly represent what they are. A silly round moon-face painted on a musical box has nothing to do with the chimes emitted, nor has the plastic material of a baby's rattle anything to do with the noise it makes; but a piece of wood preserves its integrity in the noise it makes when struck. Depending then on what is presented to its perceptions, the child will develop a sense of what is true or false. If the adults around have lost their appreciation of what is genuine and real, how can the child develop a sense for the integral value of sense-objects? All then becomes debased and spurious. Therefore it is of critical importance at this age when sense impressions work so deep that the parent should be very much aware of the nature of the objects presented to the child (see also Chapter 12.6).

Around the age of five months, the child begins to recognize faces and to make associations between individual features such as voices and spectacles or hair-styles. The child recognizes a familiar person, and knows when it is with a stranger. It starts to be shy. The stranger can then observe how the child's defensive reaction operates: first taking the form of uneasiness, then turning to the mother or starting to cry, depending on the distance from the stranger and from the mother. A baby on its mother's arm will tolerate a stranger at a distance of perhaps three feet but not when the stranger comes a few inches nearer. If the baby however is further away from the mother, then the stranger will only be tolerated at a greater distance. When the stranger sits down or the mother props the child up, the distance is reduced, as confidence is built up through activity.

If the mother should say: "Don't be afraid" then all is lost, for although the child may not understand the words, they will simply reinforce the feeling that the person is really a stranger.

The child's field of spatial awareness is highly flexible, expanding and contracting with the child's feelings and clearly influenced by the mother's own feelings. The limits of this visual field will expand with wakefulness and contract with tiredness. Visual awareness responds, too, to isolated and pronounced impressions of colour: for example, a child will recognize its father when he comes through the door alone, but it will not recognize him among a group of other people — only when he comes a bit nearer. We can see therefore that a child's alertness and interest are not trained by a multiplicity of impressions, but by the perception of single verifiable things.

Finally something which you can observe in every child at some time. Up to now we have talked about the seeking and finding gaze of the child; but there comes a time when the child consciously turns its gaze away. The child begins to enjoy playing at "hiding" or "peek-a-boo," shutting its own eyes or covering them to make someone vanish away, or getting the mother or someone else to shut their eyes or cover them and so disappear. Later in the child's life, of course, the moment comes when its gaze is turned aside because the child is ashamed. The appearance of an adult may remind the child that something has been done which was perhaps not quite right. The lowered gaze is an expression of shame, of the feeling of being excluded. This feeling represents a force which requires cherishing. It is the "I" itself which is ashamed of the consequences of its actions and would rectify its error. Similarly in later life the blush of shame is a sign that the "I" would conceal itself from another person's gaze and will not readily be seen as it is at present. Anyone who has had to do with children will know how adults can go far wrong in this area. On the one hand, there are parents or teachers who seem to want to relieve the child of all difficulties and obligations and, in extreme cases, even make a lack of shame into an educational aim. On the other hand, we find family or school situations where the child's personality is simply ground down by the moral strictures and judgments imposed by adults.

What we have described above relating to spatial awareness and the distance at which a stranger is tolerated, are aspects of a child's "soul space." The child consciously experiences self within this space which fluctuates, its "expansion" and "contraction" depending on the child's mood and alertness.

13.2 Learning to walk

From its early days in the womb, the child has been constantly moving. Even fertilization was an event where the slowly moving egg came into contact with the rapidly moving sperm-cell and together they became one. There followed a process of flowing and turning, a contracting and expanding from which the various organs emerged becoming separate and interconnected, differentiated yet growing towards an interrelated function. Even before birth, then, the organism is in motion as it grows and develops, and after birth this movement continues. The child goes on growing. As time passes, however, its scope for movement develops beyond what is dictated solely by the organs.

During the medical examination of a newly born child, we see that, when the baby is laid on its side, it will hold all its limbs loosely bent, so that the whole child looks as if it has been rolled up (Figure 26). Arms and legs are bent and the hands loosely closed. If you touch the baby's cheeks with your finger, its head will turn towards the stimulus and the child will try to suck the finger. If you lay the child on its back and turn its head to one side, it will be able to move the arm of that side sideways along the mattress and bend the other arm up to its head without being able to lift it from the mattress. If you let the child lie with its tummy on your hand, holding it up in the air, its head will hang below the horizontal line of the backbone. If you then turn the baby on to its side (still in the air), it will bend the upper leg more than the lower. If you let the soles of its feet touch the mattress or a wall, the baby will stretch out the forward foot and bend the hind leg so that when this is repeated on the other side it gives the impression of walking. If you lay the child on its tummy, it will free the nose by raising its head and turning it sideways (Figure 27). If you lay the child on its back and allow its head to loll backwards, the arms will spread-eagle themselves and come jerkily together again. If you beat the mattress near the child's head, the arms will shoot outwards on the mattress. If you lift the child up, its eyes will open in the half-light. If you put your finger into the child's hand, its fist will close over it and cannot let go. If you allow the child to lie naked in a warm room on his mattress, it will make kicking movements alternately by pushing out the arms and legs. These movements at first appear without rhythm or reason. On looking closer, however, you will see the basic rhythm of walking on all fours.

When the baby is two and a half months old, most of these inborn reflexes begin to disappear. Now the baby of its own accord begins to close its fist, to suck, to lift its head. It ceases to make reflex walking movements but moves one leg after the other continuously and no longer jerks out its arms and legs in an uncoordinated way. The loss of instinctual abilities signifies an important step towards becoming a human being, for animals are able to learn to walk from the reflex of stepping soon after birth. A foal can keep up with the herd only two hours after being born, but the human baby is still busy developing its brain and the rest of its body and goes through an arduous process of learning to stand and walk which fully occupies the child for a year. Then the child truly "stands on its own feet" and directs its steps wherever it wants, no longer blindly following the dictates of its body, no longer subject to animal urges. When we compare the rate of development of different animals, we discover that the faster an animal develops, the more its abilities are bound to its physical organs. The slower the development, the more these abilities can be extended by processes of learning. Because the human being has to learn everything that makes an individual into a human being, there is potential to extend all these attributes. A human's personal "freedom of action" increases with every new ability. That is why the human being in contrast to animals matures physically with singular slowness over a period of sixteen to twenty years. In this way the human person acquires the ability to keep learning all through life, that is to say to become freer. This also means that if the inborn reflexes continue for too long, then there is a disturbance in development which the doctor needs to recognize as early as possible.

At three months the baby can already hold its head up. It has got "control of the head." Lying on its tummy the child can raise its head and shoulders a bit above the ground (Figure 30). Month by month the child raises its head higher above the ground and uses forearms and then fists to prop itself up. Finally at six months the child spreads out its hands and straightens its arms and now stands on its hands, looking rather like the all-head-and-no-body figure which is the child's first drawing of the human form. This supporting function of the arms can be noticed by an adult when he himself is groping about in a dark room or playing at blind-man's-buff.

At three months when the baby is lying on its back and can see its hands in front, it learns to grasp. Then it brings everything moveable to its mouth to be tested. While its grasping is slowly developing from first closing its fist, then to a pincer grip and finally to a proper grasp using the thumb, the baby begins the conquest of space around. We can estimate how far the child has taken possession of its own body from the number of its defensive movements: a three-month-old baby no longer likes its head being touched, while a six-month-old baby will react by pushing away if you try to hold it by the chest. Similarly the tendency of the head to adopt an upright position works its way down into the body. This can clearly be seen in the way a mother carries her baby. She supports the new-born baby under the head, the three-month-old baby at the shoulders, the eight-month-old below the hips, and the eleven- to thirteen-month-old sitting on one arm while her other arm is free for other things. At about ten months babies learn to sit up straight (Figure 33) on their mattress, and are ready to sit properly, whereas before that they sat bent forward with their heads above the middle of the supporting triangle of feet and buttocks.

Before it is five or six months old, the baby readily adopts a curled position. This it now gradually gives up in favour of stretching out. It lies on its back stretching out arms and legs when kicking, and both its feet land simultaneously on the mattress. When it raises its head, it stays central and does not flop about. This inclination to stretch enables the child to open itself to its surroundings and is not to be confused with the urge to stand up. At this point the urge to stand up, as we have already described, has only reached down into the hands, the middle of the back and below the hips, whereas the stretching urge takes in the whole body. This can be recognized in that babies will stretch their legs against a blanket and apart from hopping impulses they show no readiness to stand.

Neither the curling up and shutting themselves out from the world, nor the stretching and opening to the world are impulses toward locomotion (in a free human sense). Locomotion is rooted in a third form of movement which becomes recognizable from the third month onwards, and joins with the urge to stand that is working its way down through the body. This third form of movement shows itself in the turning movements of the lower part of the body.

At ten months when the baby is sitting, the hands have become quite free for play. Now the predominant action of grasping alternates with conscious letting-go and later with throwing-away. Only the feet have not yet become "possession" and the baby does not object if they are touched. After the baby has learnt to kneel on one knee, it learns to haul itself up on the bars of its pen or cot or by some piece of furniture to a supported standing position (Figures 35 and 37). The few weeks in which it manages to stand up but not to sit down again appear rather agonizing.

It is at this age that the first important method of moving has been developed: rolling, wriggling and squirming along on the tummy, or sitting, or crawling (Figure 31). The method which the child chooses depends on which is first successful, and this is then retained. It also depends on the kind of flooring. The use of artificial walking aids disturbs the individual process of learning. We do not recommend them as they open up a means of movement which the child has not won for itself, thereby impairing its own activity. Furthermore the constant use of these appliances gives rise to problems such as the tendency to stand and walk on tiptoe, which can retard for months the development of normal standing and foot movements.

Some children learn to crawl after they have learnt to walk, others never seem to go through a wriggling stage while still others can walk at ten months as if they were eighteen months old. For learning to walk, any time between ten and eighteen months is quite normal.

The question is often put to us as to what is "best" in terms of a normal development. This we cannot answer in a general way even if we wished to, because all human beings, unlike animals, go through an individual personal development. This development, seen spiritually, always swings between a too early and a too late. To do the right thing at the right time is the highest art of living, and every human being inclines towards this ideal whether consciously or unconsciously. Early maturity in an individual is often linked to a lack of inner freedom. When this occurs, a person is then more strongly marked by innate talents and lives life accordingly without acquiring much that is new. By contrast, late developers acquire their abilities through a great deal of patience and hard work and can use their attributes more freely. They often show more understanding for the problems of others.

After learning to walk, the child faces a whole lot of other tasks: climbing stairs, hopping, jumping.

The achievement of walking itself goes through many stages: from the straddling waddle of the toddler (Figure 40) to the light, springy step of the nine-year-old. All these forms of movement are learnt through imitation. None of these arbitrary movements is instinctive. We can see, then, how the child's developing movements can be encouraged by good example. Whether we go about hurriedly or languidly, whether we walk noisily or softly — all is observed, taken in and imitated by the child. Not only that, but the child also perceives the inner attitude of the adult expressed in movement and so learns to express its own moods through movement (see Chapter 16.6).

13.3 Learning to speak

The first real signs of forming sounds appear as if by chance when the baby is eight to ten weeks old, soon after the first conscious smile. These sounds are delicate, produced with the outward breathing mixed with throaty sounds from the palate. The child itself notices them and tries to repeat them. These murmuring sounds only appear when the baby is in a good mood as when being fed or having its nappy (diaper) changed,

but never with children in a children's home. Mother is delighted and tries automatically to imitate this gurgling, which quite astonishes the baby, and a dialogue ensues which repeats itself daily with little variation. About the fourth month this kind of articulation ceases. Often a pause ensues in which the baby merely listens.

At about six months other strongly voiced sounds like "dada-baba-mama" are attempted. The child tends to trumpet them and make other labial sounds, now accompanying the baby's kicking in a rhythmical manner. These sounds alone do not however lead to the development of speech. For that it is necessary for there to be speech around the child. From the example of speech heard around it, the child begins to form more sounds and so gradually finds its way into speech. Right from the start, babies speak in "whole sentences" and utter a whole sequence of ideas together. When, for instance, a baby says the word "Mama" it means "Mummy come here," "Mummy where are you?" or, "Mummy I want to be carried" and so on. "Car," "dog," are similarly utterances of whole statements. More and more words are acquired and these can represent for the child a whole series of notions and attributes. Connected ideas are increasingly expressed in two and three word sentences such as "Daddy car," "Soup hot" or "Mummy home."

Here is an example. An eighteen-month old girl wanted to accompany her mother shopping in town but was told: "You can't come into town. It's noisy, crowded with people and cars and it's smelly." And so the child was left with her big sister, who later reported that the little girl had said: "Mummy, town, cwowdy, 'melly."

If adults copy these attempts at speech and start talking "baby language," they deprive the child of the correct model which is required and the child is left with simplified sounds. When adults speak to a child in a normal fashion, then the child has the opportunity to pick up all the nuances of its mother-tongue.

Usually in its second year the child utters its first words. It is noticeable that children of well-educated parents begin to speak comparatively late, and it would seem that they cannot find their way into the large vocabulary of their parents. After a few months however they have caught up and for the rest of their lives they retain a head start in the use of words and expressions. If, however, the parents have a limited vocabulary then the child has not much more to learn than the example presented. Children in this situation often start to speak earlier but their vocabulary remains limited, a disadvantage which can only be overcome once they go to school and receive the necessary stimulus. It is very difficult to correct the speech of children whose parents' manner of speaking is in any way artificial and has something officious, haughty, clipped, or affected and so rings false. The feeling that a facade is erected in this manner of speech impinges on the child's soul and undermines its finer sense of what is true or false in what is being expressed. It is the same with moods and feelings expressed in the speech of the adults around him, for the child absorbs these nuances instantly and picks up the attitude being expressed long before it understands the actual words. As a result, children experience directly, through the way that they are expressed, emotions and moods such as joy, seriousness, coldness, sharpness or mildness, and tend to imitate them even though they do not understand in detail what the mood or attitude is all about.

Normally no exercises are required for learning to speak. Also the correction of words wrongly pronounced should be avoided. Speech should always express something directly. If I interrupt the flow of language by a correction, I destroy its directness. The only thing that a child will learn from this habit is to interrupt their parents in the same way. Why should a child not say "squiddle" (for squirrel), "tolly" (for trolley), "programme" (for programme), "uptairs" (for upstairs)? The adult will take care to pronounce these words especially clearly and can be sure that the child will not make similar mistakes when it is fourteen years old.

Almost every child shows a temporary inclination to stammer when its urge to communicate is greater than its ability to speak. Patience and tolerance of this fault will help to overcome it. If, however, impediments of speech such as lisping, stammering and stuttering appear, it is of great importance that one-sided training or exercises should be avoided before the child goes to school because if speech formation is made conscious the whole process of imitation is disturbed. At this age the best remedy (which always helps) is for the adult to speak clearly and well, and above all slowly enough in the presence of the child. Nursery rhymes, children's songs and verses, reading aloud, or better still the

telling of fairy-tales all excite the child's enjoyment of the sound of the language and encourage its own self-expression.

In addition, it is a common error to believe that a speech defect can only be cured through speech-training. As we have seen, the development of movement precedes that of speech. Speech is a metamorphosis of bodily movement. The larynx carries out in miniature the same movements as the body. Therefore all defects of speech are accompanied by greater or lesser impairments of movement. If movement can be practised through games such as throwing a ball, walking on stilts, balancing, threading beads and similar skills, it is surprising how much better the problem sounds become articulated. In this connection we recommend collections of verses and finger-games. Infant-eurythmy is also particularly effective (see Chapter 16.6 and 16.8).

In the case of a child with defective speech, we can do only what is good for the normal development of speech, but more intensively. Only when the child is old enough to go to school, is it ready to work directly on any residual speech defects. At that stage a programme of speech exercises can be followed without harmful effects.

Finally we shall discuss the question of growing up with two languages. In Argentina, for example, many children grow up with one parent speaking English and the other Spanish. The child does not then grow into a single mother tongue but hears two right from the beginning. Such children start speaking later than the norm with a single tongue. At first they mix the words of both languages but then learn surprisingly quickly to express themselves in each separately. Later they are envied for their mastery of both languages and also often for their ability to learn other languages more easily. When they grow up, however, and are asked whether they would bring up their own children in the same way, they usually reply: "No, my child is going to have one mother tongue. It is going to grow up in the language of the country and learn the second language only when it is quite sure of the first." A person who grew up with two languages observed: "I don't feel absolutely at home in either language. I dream in Spanish, but I think in English and speak whichever language is required by the situation."

Because thinking is substantially based on language — as the following chapter will show — we do recommend that the child, at least to begin with (that is until it starts to call itself "I") should grow up with one language. Each language has its own kind of logic, dictated by the surface structure and grammar of the language in question, giving shape and order to thought. Identifying with this framework of logic is known to aid the development of thought and to contribute to the strengthening of the personality.

If the parents speak a language different from that of the country in which they are living, it is not easy for them to bring up their children in one language only. If, for instance, English-speaking parents living in South America wish their child to grow up speaking Spanish, how should they go about it? The main objective should be consistency, that is, an adult should always use the same language directly to the child regardless of what is used towards others when the child is only listening. Try to ensure that a particular language is always associated with particular people and situations. With both parents speaking English at home, the answer here would probably be to send the child to a Spanish-speaking school. By "compartmentalizing" in this way, children have been known to grow up managing even more than two languages without confusion.

Any bilingual upbringing has both advantages and disadvantages. The facility for language learning which is gained has to be set against the feeling of never being absolutely sure of any one of the languages spoken and, as we have already mentioned, every individual needs a deep familiarity and relationship with a native tongue as part of mental development. Parents from different linguistic backgrounds will therefore have to take a number of things into account when deciding what to do.

13.4 Learning to think

What is thinking? It is our ability to bring coherence, sense and order into everything we experience. Our thought-life is a network of relationships by means of which we are able to grasp realities, even those beyond our senses. For example, we experience that we can understand not only those things that we see and perceive, but also those that we can grasp only conceptually, as for example, mathematics. Thought is also bound up with our experiencing ourselves as an integral part of the world around us. When we act upon a thought, we feel that we are playing a part in shaping the reality in which we live and we are expressing the intimation of a wider and greater whole. Within the laws which govern this whole, our thought discovers the means to become ever more free and personally independent.

In the growing child, we can observe different stages in the development of the ability to think.

Intelligence tied to the body

Long before the child "knows" that it has something in its hand, it can work with it. A baby feels an object, looks at it, tastes it and listens to it and so experiences its quality and consistency — whether it can be grasped, whether it will topple over, whether it will roll. We often see how a child intentionally loses sight of something in order to find it again, never tiring of the game; and so in the activity of its hands and senses it happily experiences the constancy of things and, thus, by extension, its own continuity of existence.

If as adults we form a concept of the same object, we describe its position, shape and consistency, type, relation to its surroundings and to ourselves, and so on. We grasp in thought what the child experiences through its senses. For us the world is divided into "I" and "you," "mine" and "yours," but these are ideas which the child cannot yet differentiate because it feels itself actively involved in what is being experienced. The child experiences the worlds of sense and of thought as unseparated. Herein lies the key to understanding the infant's soul-life. Adults can think separately from the activity of our senses, but the young child experiences both together, and so for the child, the experience of sounds, smells and tastes is much more intense and filled with a more vivid reality than in later life. This quality we can sense in our childhood memories which are of a far greater intensity than those of later life.

The first step in the development of thought is direct perception of the sense and meaning of objects or activity in the child's surroundings. There is no "thinking through" an action for the child. As adults, we conform to habits of logic every time we put a lid on a pot or open a door to go out, whenever we put things back where they belong, when we close the window because it is too windy, clean something that has got dirty and so on. Because the child perceives actively, without the intervention of logic or reason, it feels directly involved in all that is happening and cannot distance itself like we coolly calculating adults do. And so the sense and meaning of the child's surroundings are reflected in its play. Imitation then comes about because of the very way a child observes and remembers the world. Its intelligence lives in its perception to such an extent that the thing perceived is remembered not as an abstract thought but as a physical reality. The child recalls by re-enacting the reality. Just as memory-thoughts arise in an adult's mind, spontaneous actions by the child evoke the thing or person remembered and of course this is done by means of imitation. What has once been imitated can be repeated. By repetition skill is acquired, the body training itself closer and closer to the ideal of the action or event perceived.

The power of imitation may, then, be understood as the working together of three elements: sense perception, thought, and "a physical memory." The high degree of similarity between the observed model and the child's imitation is not an indica-tion of motor intelligence. It is attributable to the fact that it is the same thought in both. Any imperfection or change in the imitation is most likely due to a limited or biased perception in the first place.

As the living intelligence begins to emerge from the body and work in the mind, the ability to imitate diminishes. Before that, however, the major achievements — learning to walk, speak and think — are already behind the child. Consider how it would be if children could think at birth and were able to judge in advance whether or not they were up to learning all that they had to. Obstructed and confused by thought, they would never be able to adapt their bodies consciously to walking and talking, nor would they make these skills their own as they do through instinct and intuition.

The influence of speech on thinking

A fresh step in the development of thinking is taken when the child begins to speak. It learns to speak in the same manner as it learns to walk, imitating intuitively without grasping the thought content. Only gradually does the thinking element separate itself from the speech element. Take the following instance: a child is gathering sticks in a park. Suddenly it stands still, seeing a "stick" moving on the ground. Thoughtfully it observes: "That not 'tick."

The inner life of thought is just beginning in this child, but it is sufficiently developed for the child to find a concept and a word to relate to the worm which it sees. Naming and distinguishing arise first of all from perception. Before conceptual thinking begins, names and simple statements appear. For the child, its whole surroundings appear to "speak." The lump of clay makes a rolling noise, the walking stick clicks, the door squeaks and bangs when the current of air blows it shut, the water gurgles down the drain and vanishes. Everything lives in its own way and has something to say. Even fingers can talk to each other and tell stories. This way of experiencing things as if they were speaking, endures for the next few years in that special imagination which belongs to childhood: grandfather's boots look like the wrinkled old man down the road; the stove can move ominously in the darkness: apples laugh happily and pears look at you with funny faces; slices of bread turn into hedgehogs or a house; the wooden block in the playroom is now a jug, now a car or a church tower going ding-dong. If you whisper everything becomes more mysterious and you can hear even better what things are saying.

At this time of life, words work magic in other ways, too: when the little ones after supper still linger at the table not wanting to go to bed for another five minutes, a whispered "Come on, we're going to play taxis," sometimes helps. In a moment, one of them is sitting on your shoulder ready to drive away from the table and off to the bath, while the second child can hardly wait to be the taxi driver too. In moments like this, we see time and time again how the child's thinking is still highly mobile and imaginative.

The first flash of pure thought

We have discussed how the development of thinking does not proceed in completely separate phases but rather through a continuous process through which the dominant elements change, succeeding one another but working on into the next. Each time a new element appears, it reduces somewhat the effect of the previous one which, as a result, does not operate so exclusively or so strongly as before.

The birth of memory is a sign of the first flash of pure thought activity. In its second year the child still feels itself a part of its surroundings. It calls itself by its own name just as if it saw itself from without. Should it bump into the corner of the table, the child will behave almost as if the table hit it and may even hit back. If the crying child is carried into another room where the table can no longer be seen, the tears will dry up quickly. If the child sees the "nasty table" again shortly after, it will often start crying again, for the memory is still bound to the perception of the object. The child's thinking is not yet aware of itself and is still living in the sense-perceptions (as we have already described). Thus we may speak of a "locative memory" at this age.

As the consciousness of self begins to dawn, memory begins to free itself from the sense perceptions and to become independent within the soul. This moment is often experienced as a joyful fright. It often comes when the child has suddenly been left alone, or with some intense experience, or with a sudden sense of loss in which the child's feeling of being separated from the world is sharpened. Here is an example: Christopher, aged two, comes into the kitchen where his mother is making a meal. He picks up the empty basket by the stove to carry it away. His mother says: "Leave it there, Daddy needs it right away." Christopher puts the basket back on the floor and answers standing straight up: "No, me — me take to Daddy." This first experiencing of the "I" marks the moment when the child begins to distinguish between self and surroundings. Now the child is no longer content to perceive and name everything, but will add its own thought activity to what is happening. The persistent "Why?" of this age emphasises this process. From now on, the child is always wanting to repeat in word and thought what has been perceived.

Thus we see how the experience of the interconnection of the sense world becomes inward possession in three stages. First actions are observed, instinctively imitated and so "understood." Then the meanings of words that name things, actions and events are grasped. Finally there comes the ability to comprehend inwardly: the child no longer calls itself by its own name but grasps the idea of its own identity. This the child does by its own thinking, for memory as such only begins with the child's first utterance of "I." From now on, the thought network increases from year to year and undergoes further development with the change of teeth (see 13.9 below) and with puberty until at last it reaches the point where the adult is able to think in abstract concepts (see Chapter 16.6). This thought network is a part of the "life-organization" (see Chapter 6.14) which is no longer required for bodily growth. This discovery by Rudolf Steiner is of momentous importance for education and medicine.

We can therefore see why thinking only becomes adult after the growing period is over. Furthermore we can understand why people who have learnt to be creative in thought go on increasing their spiritual capacity right into old age. This is possible because more and more forces are freed from growth and regeneration. At the moment of death, the whole network of life- and growth-forces is lifted clear of the body, exposing the complete picture of all memories both conscious and unconscious in great clarity. This experience of the whole life-organization freeing itself, and a whole lifetime being reviewed in pictures has been often described by people who were very close to death.

As we have seen, the child develops through first being active in perception, then through expressing itself in words, and only in the end through reviewing in its mind what it has experienced. In this pattern of development, thought retains its proper function, operating in proper sequence. Unwanted explanations and reasoning only disturb the child's natural urge to imitate and lead to abstraction and precociousness. For this reason, the child is best nurtured and stimulated not by being forced prematurely to absorb intellectual concepts and abstract reasoning, but through a medium like fairy-tales which appeal to the child's fantasy and imagination. The images in fairy-tales need no explanation for they reflect themes related to the inner development of the human being. The pictures speak for themselves and work on in the child's soul without adult intervention. They give wings to and activate the child's imagination but leave it truly free. For what child ever really saw "a golden palace east of the sun and west of the moon"? No bounds are set to the imagination. Those who have heard plenty of fairy-tales in childhood will find it much easier as adults to grasp concepts relating to personal development and fulfilment: the journey and adventures of the unrecognized prince past all obstacles to the wedding with the princess. In ourselves, this "way" is our own search for our higher being, union with which is the goal of our inner development.

We do not subscribe to the view that fairy-tales should not be told to children because of the cruelty in them. Whoever tells the same fairy-tale over and over again comes to see the truths concealed in it. The content appears cruel only as long as the underlying truths remain hidden. Young children are far more perceptive than adults in this respect and readily look on "the fight with the dragon" as an ordeal which has to be gone through on the path to goodness. Fear arises only if the stories are told theatrically. If they are told calmly, the child will feel at home in the events described, for they reflect realities of the life of the soul in which evil and the triumph over it play a considerable part. The soul's development is not helped either by ignoring or by overstating these realities, but it is helped by learning to face up to evil and master it. While cruelty and evil are to be confronted in fairy-tales, then, it is also important that children are exposed only to those (such as Grimm's Fairy Tales) in which good overcomes evil. Tragedy in human destiny can only be understood by the child when its soul life has reached a certain maturity. For this reason, many of Hans Christian Andersen's Fairy Tales are not really suitable for children.

13.5 From childhood to adulthood

It is absorbing and thought-provoking to watch the stages of a child's development through learning to walk, talk and think. Scene after scene passes before our eyes:

The child begins to stand up and to make its first steps. It starts to control its own movements.

The child begins to talk. Before it calls itself "I" (that is, before conscious thinking begins), the child is unable to tell a lie. Learning to talk means at first only speaking the truth.

The child begins to think. It begins to develop a conscious inner life and can now say "I" meaning self. This gives the child great joy; you can see this joy in the eyes of a toddler.

The way in which a child develops gives rise to a number of interesting questions. What happens in later life to these facets of early human growth? Do any of us in later life ever again have such a joyful awareness of self? Do any of us know ourselves as surely as the child seems to? Do we not rather feel invaded with things we cannot fully identify with? Do we really have a conscious inner life? Or do we mostly only react to external circumstances, content to "cope" with life? What happens to our sense of truth? How much untruthfulness is hidden in our stock phrases, polite-

ness and conventions? Which of us really wants to know how someone is when we ask, "How are you?" How many of us really stand on our *own* feet? How many of us feel we are forced to be something that is not truly us, that we are at odds with our destiny, that we cannot direct our lives as we should really like?

In the Gospel of John we find the words: "I am the way, and the truth and the life." (John 14:6). We witness the truth of these words as we watch a child developing towards the point of saying "I am." But at the very moment when this consciousness of self lights up, the first signs of a crisis to come are simultaneously revealed. This crisis can be expressed in terms such as: "I do not know my way. I do not know what I really want to do in life." Or "I know what I am not, but where is my true being to be found?"

Those who have lived through this crisis and emerged with a sense of self-discovery, often recognize in their experience the real birth of the I, the "second birth" as described in the Gospel of John (John 3:1-21). This second birth marks our conscious union with the power of Christ, power which already works in the child and gives the ability to learn to stand, walk, speak the truth and have an inner life. The child is not conscious of the power of Christ, but the adult who has consciously united self with it can at the same time discover three fundamental motives for inner life:

To accept destiny positively and to be ready to learn all that it offers for personal development.

To seek truth in our dealings with our fellow men. To make no compromises as regards our inner life, this being all the more important because our outer life often demands that we should be adaptable and ready to make compromises.

To watch over our inner life and development and to shoulder co-responsibility for it.

This threefold union with the power of the Higher Self, the Christ-I, that is associated with every human soul, can also be sought through the way of art, in movement, speech and voice as practised for example in eurythmy (see Chapter 16.8), or through discipline of thought.

It is an ancient piece of wisdom that even the wisest of us can learn from a child. In the development of the child, the highest ideals of human evolution are realized before our eyes in a parable of nature. What the child experiences and does unconsciously can become the highest moral force when practised consciously by the adult.

13.6 The playgroup

Many mothers with an only child feel they must try to overcome the isolation in which the child finds itself. How is an only child to learn about joining in socially and standing up for itself in a group? For this kind of problem, the playgroup seems to be at least a partial solution. The playgroup, apart from offering mothers short periods of freedom without their children, also gives them the chance to meet and discuss common problems and to help each other in overcoming them. On top of that, the children find friends to play with.

When the playgroup offers parents the opportunity to do something together at these times such as baking, weaving, singing or making music, this will create a busy and stimulating atmosphere for the children. It is not so stimulating when the parents merely sit and watch in the background drinking coffee and chatting.

There are certain needs in the child's social development which are not met by the playgroup, however. To make human contacts, children need a role-model which other babies and infants cannot provide them with. The ability to sustain an I-you relationship begins around the age of three when the child learns to identify self. Before that age it is best if the child lives in daily intimate contact with only a few people, and especially with one person in particular. For this, the home provides a better ground than the playgroup.

In another respect, however, mothers' and parents' gatherings can contribute to social education. Through such encounters, people come face to face with the more widespread isolation in which many find themselves today; for not only does the single mother with one child feel cut off, but also her neighbour with three children, the grandmother in the old folks' home, and many others who live on their own. Where these difficulties are aired in regular group-meetings, some progress is already being made towards their solution.

Added to these instances of isola-tion, there is the increasing problem of parents — especially single parents — feeling helpless or even alien towards their own children. As a result, the demand for professional advice and counselling in child-related problems or even for institu-tional care, is growing rapidly in the developed world. When we take into account the rapid decline in the over-all population of the number of children, together with the increase in the numbers of old people, and when we consider that more and more children are growing up in deprived circumstances without proper care and support, we feel grave concern about how in the future these children will develop the necessary social instincts and capacity. But there is also in this trend, an opportunity for caring adults to take on additional responsibility for children beyond their own family. In this way, perhaps, conditions will be created in which mutual sharing and caring can be offered to those most in need.

13.7 The kindergarten

In Britain, North America and elsewhere in the English-speaking world, children are admitted to kindergarten, the preparatory year before full school, at the age of four to five. In Germany, new legislation encourages the admission of children to the kindergarten once they have reached the age of three. Universally speaking, in many cases, parents start looking for a place before that where the child can be looked after.

It is never an ideal solution to put a child under three out to care, though of course there may be compelling reasons (such as work) for doing so. Possible alternatives for working parents are to take turns being at work and in the home, or for two mothers to join forces, or for a home-help to come in, look after the child and the household. Some parents may be able to find an adoptive family with other children or even a "day-mum" to whom the child is brought. These solutions are not always possible and then it will be necessary to find a nursery group or crèche.

Children who have not had a regular home background but have been brought up in one of the ways mentioned above make themselves noticeable to the kindergarten teacher. They are less controlled and not so self-contained. It may be necessary for the kindergarten to provide special curative measures and so compensate for much of what has been neglected or caused in the earlier years.

If the mother can be at home all day, the question is quite different: *when* should the child go to kindergarten? Does the child need to go at all? The answer must be given for each individual case. In a good situation with one parent at home and other children to play with, there is no real need. On the other hand, where there is a good case for sending the child to kindergarten, much will depend on what the kindergarten itself is like and on what sort of a teacher there is. A highly technical household will want the kind of place where they bake, wash and cook. But if the kindergarten is of the "do as you please" type or, at the other extreme, pursues a pre-school education programme, it is probably better to keep the child at home.

We usually recommend sending a child to kindergarten where, after consulting with parents, we find that the daily routine at home is pretty chaotic, or where perhaps there is tension or a "bossy" attitude towards the child. In such cases, a child guidance specialist or counsellor can often give helpful advice on how the home background can be made more conducive to the healthy upbringing of the child.

In our view, there is no reason why

a child suffering from a chronic illness or disability should not go to kindergarten; but of course it will be necessary for the parents and teacher to discuss the potential problems, possibly also with the doctor. From a social point of view the integration of a handicapped or sick child into the kindergarten is extremely important not only for the child himself but for its healthy companions who can thus learn consideration for others.

13.8 When is a child ready for kindergarten?

There are two principal signs to indicate when a child is ready to go to kindergarten:

—When the child can go off by itself: when for instance the child has deliberately run away from home and found its way back again, or wanted to go home with a friend without waiting to be picked up. This tendency is so pronounced in some children that they occasionally disappear — to the consternation of their nearest and dearest — and turn up in their own time to say where they have been. If a child still clings to its mother's skirts and does not dare to go any distance alone away from her, the time has not yet come for kindergarten. Of course, in such cases the mother should check whether it is her own attitude that is hindering the child from acquiring the necessary independence.

—When the child can listen to a story from beginning to end: this shows that the child's mental pictures can be guided by words, and consequently the child can meet the demands of the group.

In our experience these two stages usually occur about the age of three and a half. If they are not apparent by the time the child is four, it is advisable to have a word with the doctor.

(For organization of the kindergarten day, see Chapter 16.6).

13.9 When is a child ready for school?

The school entry age in most countries is between five and seven. Specialists who have done extensive research into children's maturity, recommend starting school between eight and eleven. We consider it crucial that, at whatever age it begins, education is adapted to the age in question. Then a suitable pre-schooling or a home education would achieve the same thing. Some children might then do better if they were removed from the home surroundings while others would benefit from being kept at home.

There are a number of signs when children are ready for school at about the age of six or seven. The main indications of maturity are as follows:

The body change
Compared with the toddler and kindergarten child, the six or seven-year-old shows a distinctive change in body shape. The trunk has lengthened, the angle of the ribs above the abdomen is no longer broad but narrows to an apex. The chubby hands have disappeared, the gaze no longer wanders about but can rest on one thing, is alert and ready to absorb. The limbs, head and trunk are in better proportion.

The appearance of second teeth
The appearance of the first permanent molar or front tooth shows that the enamel of these teeth, the body's hardest substance, has been fully developed. Education generally takes little account of this fact. In anthroposophical terms, once an organ has reached full development, the forces which developed it are then used for regeneration and maintenance of the organ (see 13.4 above and Chapter 6.14). But this does not apply to the enamel of the teeth, which is not regenerated. As a result, the formative forces thus released become available for sustained thought activity (see Chapter 16.6). In the child's mind, continuity of concept becomes possible, that is, concepts can now be retained in thought, or in other words remembered.

The thinking of the school-child
In the section on *Learning to think* (see 13.4 above), we saw that the little child has a "locative" memory at first. Then the child finds its way into the repetition of words and actions, and only then the kind of memory develops which is entirely inward and enables the child to remember things without external stimuli. This ability to remember is the first indication of abstract thinking. Now the child is able to direct its own thought, and

can answer specific questions: the child can, for example, repeat a story heard in the kindergarten.

With this stage, of course, the ability to imitate starts to decline. Up to now, the child could only "comprehend" by copying the action perceived. This mode of learning through imitation needs to be examined more closely. A complex activity, it can only be understood in depth when one regards thinking as a metamorphosis of growth activity. The more the growth forces are engaged in developing the body's organic structure, the better the child can imitate, because the body's ability to grasp and repeat an action directly through sense perception is due to the intelligence still working in the body.

For this reason, a marked lack of ability to imitate can be an early symptom of grave disabilities of soul and spirit, even indicating autism. This is also why the child's body up to and into the change of teeth is so exposed to the influences of its surroundings in so far as the development of its organs is concerned. If a child has to imitate much that is senseless and chaotic or if it has to experience interrupted and disconnected activities, this will have consequences for its physical development (see Chapter 17.9 and 18.3), for each organ develops properly only when it is influenced in the right way. This extremely flexible and malleable phase culminates in the decline of the imitative faculty when the child is ready for school. The metamorphosis of growth activity starts to take place with the change of teeth, when each individual enamel crown has been fully developed. Thereafter the intelligence acts more and more within the soul.

Social maturity in school
Once a child can fit into a larger group of children, social maturity has been attained. For this the child will have learnt to keep still for periods, not moving its arms and legs, and be "all ears". Usually social maturity comes later than the intellectual maturity required by a school-child. Social maturity in most cases is only attained in the course of the first or second year at school.

Skills and self-expression through speech
These abilities are often insufficiently developed if the earlier upbringing did not provide enough stimulus. If, however, the abilities have been properly developed, the school-child will be able to throw a ball into the air with one hand and catch it, hop on its left foot and right foot equally well, and do more dexterous exercises showing skill with its fingers. In speech, the child will be able to form complete grammatical sentences.

The absence of any one of these signs of maturity need not mean that you should postpone sending the child to school. In cases of doubt, consult the doctor or school advisers. One should take all the known factors into account, such as the age of the child relevant to the class; the oldest child in a group will experience school quite differently from the youngest. Partial disability or handicap should not, if possible, prevent a child from being admitted to a class of children of the same age.

We recommend that parents avoid preparing children for a school inter-view as this will only inhibit them and will often only result in a complete block at the critical moment. Admission to a school should not depend solely on the result of an intelligence test, as this can only show a small part of the spectrum of the child's total abilities.

14 Nutrition

14.1 Breast-feeding

In recent years, breast-feeding has come back into fashion in western society. It is to be hoped that this trend will continue and that, in Third World countries, too, where it has become a kind of status symbol not to suckle one's own babies, breast-feeding will regain its former importance.

We should like to run through the arguments in favour of breast-feeding with the hope that the important message that "breast is best" will be promoted even further by our readers:

Breast-feeding creates an elemental relationship between mother and child. It lays the foundation for the social feeling that we need each other and are there for each other. It is Nature's picture of giving and receiving.

Breast-feeding promotes the restoration of the womb after child-birth.

Breast-fed children are less prone to infection and overcome it better.

Breast-fed children are much more immune to digestive disorders and inflammation of the bowel, sepsis and meningitis.

Breast-feeding is simple, less time-consuming and it is cheap.

Practical questions about breast-feeding

How do you learn to breast-feed?
From the baby! That is apart from one or two tips from the midwife or from an experienced mother.

How often should the baby be put to the breast?
In the first weeks as often as the baby is hungry and cries. After that a four-hourly rhythm will be established.

For how long should the baby feed?
Five to ten minutes at each breast. There is no point in feeding for longer because after five minutes about three quarters of the milk will have flowed out. If at first the baby demands only one breast every six to eight hours do not be surprised if the flow of milk does not come properly. Give both breasts at each feed. Later when enough milk is there you can feed from alternate breasts.

How often should the baby be weighed?
Once a week (unclothed) in a warm room. Mothers can also check the amount of milk they produce by weighing the baby (clothed) before and after a feed, and noting the difference. This is especially recommended when the baby is not gaining weight properly. Also this should be done twenty-four hours before taking the baby to see the doctor.

How many motions should breast-fed babies have?
The answer is: one in ten days or ten in one day! The stools may vary in colour and even appear green. Breast-fed babies normally thrive whatever the frequency or consistency of the stools.

How long should I continue to breast-feed?
We advise feeding only from the breast for the first five months. Over the next four months, the baby should be gradually weaned to pap food. We find that to continue breast-feeding after nine to ten months causes mother and child to be too strongly attached to each other.

In their second year, some babies will cry noisily — often at night — for their mother's breast out of habit, even though they may not actually be drinking any more, and this quite frequently becomes a problem requiring the doctor's attention. This is a clear signal for the mother that it is now time for the child to become a little more independent.

What should I eat while breast-feeding?
Normal food that does not cause constipation or flatulence. She should drink plenty of milk, possibly also diluted almond purée from 7% almond purée, where available. Alcohol and nicotine must be strictly avoided. Mothers with low blood pressure may be allowed a cup of coffee, particularly in the morning. Fruit may also be eaten provided that the child does not react to it with increased wind or sore bottom. If reactions to certain fruits do become noticeable, avoid them for a period. The effects of particular foods vary considerably according to the age and general health of mother and child, so it is impossible to set a general rule about avoiding things like fruit or coffee altogether.

Problems with breast-feeding

If the mother's **milk has a slightly bluish colour**, this does not mean that it lacks enough nourishment.

Yellowness in a baby's skin and eyes is no reason to suspend breast-feeding (for jaundice see Chapter 5.2).

The only known **reasons for not breast-feeding** are if the mother has an active tuberculosis or an abscess of the mammary glands (see below), or is HIV positive.

In some rare cases, **a deficiency in Vitamin K** can affect fully breast-fed infants aged between two and sixteen weeks. Babies suffering from this deficiency may tend to have blood-clotting problems which can result in brain haemorrhage. This complication occurs in roughly one in 30 000 healthy infants. It is interesting to note that the problem has not so far been observed in babies fed on powdered milk who absorb a small amount of Vitamin K daily through this form of nourishment. This leads to the assumption that in rare cases the amount of Vitamin K occurring naturally in breast-milk is insufficient. In order to counter this possible danger nowadays, Vitamin K is given to all new-born breast-fed babies in amounts of 1–2 mg injected or taken orally three times in the first three months. In general practice this large dosage is recommended as the problem is almost impossible to foresee. However we do not recommend treatment in this way but keep to a lower dosage which is closer to natural conditions. Our recommendation is to give the child one to two teaspoons of carrot juice daily, which is equivalent to a dose of about five micrograms.

Cracked nipples can be treated with lanolin or a prescribed ointment. By rubbing the nipples with undiluted lemon juice not only during pregnancy but also when feeding, the nipples are hardened and undesirable bacteria eliminated. If the nipples are very sore, the milk may have to be pumped off for a time and fed to the baby either with a little spoon or with a bottle and teat with a very small hole.

Where there is **not enough breast-milk,** put the child to the breast more frequently and give him both sides. Do not let him suck too long (to prevent the nipples becoming sore). The mother should drink plenty and wear a warm upper garment with long sleeves; a cardigan which unbuttons in front is ideal. Get help where possible with the housework from grandmother, sister, neighbour, friend or father. Do not give the baby any additional food to begin with but if, after feeding at both breasts, the baby is still clearly unsatisfied, you can give a little fennel tea with 3% sugar to top the feed up. The baby will however be ready for the next feed all the sooner and that is good. This method is particularly suitable for the second and third week when the mother is back home. It does not matter if during this period the child does not put on any weight, but there should be no loss of weight. The most common mistake is to give supplementary food because you are afraid of not having enough milk. Only three mothers in a hundred have a genuine problem of not providing enough milk themselves. In these cases a transition to a supplementary milk feed will be made in the fourth week as a matter of course (see 14.2 below).

Where there is **a family history of allergy,** it is considered wrong to give a baby even the smallest amounts of feeds containing cows' milk as a *temporary* measure during the initial period after birth. In a baby that is slightly allergic, this can induce sensitivity to cows' milk. If the child is then fed only on mother's milk for quite a long period and subsequently is given a foodstuff containing cows' milk, the child can quite possibly show strong allergic symptoms.

If **a child refuses the breast,** the mother should consult another mother experienced in breast-feeding, or a midwife or doctor.

Retention of milk in the breast can be treated in a number of ways. Keep trying to give the baby the breast while gently massaging the breast to stimulate the flow. The use of a quark-compress as an external measure gives effective relief.

Even in the case of **an inflammation of the breasts** it may not be absolutely necessary to give up feeding immediately, but here the doctor should be consulted. Quark compresses are helpful. The earlier the treatment is started, the better the prospects·are for continuing breast-feeding.

In the case of the baby getting **an infection or digestive upset,** continue to feed. Flatulence and tummy-aches are unfortunately not so uncommon these days even with breast-fed babies (see Chapter 2.7).

If a mother has to undergo dental treatment requiring **a local anaesthetic,** she should avoid giving the baby one or two feeds after the treatment. If she has plenty of milk, she can draw off a supply beforehand. Whenever medication is required, the doctor should always be asked whether the drug will get into her milk and harm her baby.

Every woman who has **too much milk** should try to give her surplus to a needy child. In the UK this is organized within the local maternity hospital. There is no external system for the distribution of surplus mother's milk. In other places, the parents of a premature baby may be able to make their own arrangements to collect the milk once or twice a day and take it to the hospital. It is a precondition of course that the donor should be healthy. In these days of AIDS there is much more need for getting a clean bill of health as a donor. Parents can of course satisfy themselves as to the health of a donor and accept the risk between themselves. Where there is some doubt, the donor's milk can be pasteurized.

A serious problem is posed by **residues of pesticides and weed-killers** in our food chain. Pesticides are absorbed by plants and residues are passed on to animals and humans where they can accumulate and even affect mother's milk. Although this has been known for over thirty years, there has been no official opposition to the use of weed-killers and pesticides in agriculture. Although milk preparations contain residues in lower proportions, we still recommend breast-feeding as its advantages are incomparably greater. in addition, the mother can make efforts to obtain residue-free and naturally grown food. This should be done as early in life as possible.

14.2 Supplementary feeding

It becomes clear that a mother's milk is insufficient when the baby does not thrive properly. Of course, the more often you put the baby to the breast, the more your milk production will flow. But it sometimes becomes necessary to supplement mother's milk with milk of a different origin. This is known as supplementary feeding.

There are various ways of introducing supplementary feeding. In Tables 2 and 3 (see pages 243–44), we show two fairly typical examples. When the mother finds that her milk is running down for the evening feed, then she can give a "half-milk feed" (half cow's milk and half water) or a half-milk semolina pap. After the breast-feed give as much as the baby will take, usually about 50 g (1¾ oz) or about three tablespoonfuls. This amount is sufficient for healthy children and will not hinder the production of milk. The extra feed in the evening is also useful if the mother is in urgent need of a good night's sleep.

A baby will sleep longer afterwards — with luck, all night!

If your milk is not enough in the daytime, either, you will have to supplement the other feeds, too, though usually in the morning there is more milk.

As the intestinal flora changes markedly with supplementary feeding, you must take note carefully of the baby's stools. There should be a heap in the nappy (diaper) at least every other day. Diarrhoea — known as dyspepsia in babies — can occur more readily with this type of nourishment. In such cases continue to breast-feed and give the additional nourishment as described in Chapter 4.1.

Feeding with a spoon must be learnt. The action of sucking causes most of the food to flow out again and must be caught patiently with the spoon and shoved in again. You have to push, tilt and wipe the food in against the upper jaw.

14.3 Bottle-feeding and weaning

Any form of baby-feeding which is not with breast-milk is normally administered by bottle. This is always a substitute for the breast and, in primitive living conditions, can be dangerous.

If breast-feeding is not possible, we recommend that after the first three weeks one of the various feeds prepared from cow's milk is given as a substitute for mother's milk. Where possible untreated milk fresh from the cow should be the basis of the recipe. The directions for making up the feed are extremely simple (see below).

In the first two weeks, the baby has to be introduced to the selected food in gradually increasing amounts. Thereafter as a rule give a daily ration of ⅐ to ⅙ of the child's weight until it has reached 6 kg (13 lb). Then keep to this amount until the end of the baby's first year giving from 800–1000 g (1¾–2¼ lb) per day. Additional drinks are not necessary.

As can be seen from the nutrition table (see page 243), bottle-fed babies should be weaned to fruit and vegetable juice (starting at one to four teaspoonfuls daily, up to a maximum of ten) earlier than breast-fed babies, and also introduced earlier to a vegetable and/or fruit feed. This must however be done quite gradually. Watch that the baby is neither overfed with milk nor has too little

protein. Compared with mother's milk, every other kind of nourishment is unbalanced. Even the best conditioned and vitaminized brand of baby-milk can never equal the balance of mother's milk nor come anywhere near its freshness.

On average, cow's milk contains more than double the protein in mother's milk and mainly casein which is hardly present at all in breast-milk. Cow's milk has half the milk-sugar (lactose) content of mother's milk. Only the fat content is about the same. As for mineral content, cow's milk has four times as much with, in particular, relatively larger amounts of calcium and phosphorous. Even so, babies fed on cow's milk are more prone to rickets than breast-fed children. Iron can be more easily assimilated from mother's milk and therefore iron deficiency occurs more rarely.

Undiluted cow's milk would burden a baby's digestion because of the difference in concentration of proteins and minerals, and would cause illness after a short time. For this reason, cow's milk is normally diluted with water during the first nine months (for amounts see Recipes 1 to 3 below).

The dilution however leaves the milk with insufficient nutritional value. The deficiency must be made up by adding sugar and almond purée and later sugar and cereal-flour. We prefer making up your own mixture with fresh milk to using dried commercial products which try to adapt cow's milk to mother's milk. Dried milk can never come up to the quality of fresh milk, quite apart from the fact that, in a commercial dried product, you have no control over when, where and to what quality the ingredients were produced.

It is best, then, for the child to have fresh and untreated milk, best of all from an organic or bio-dynamic farm or a dairy where the cows are organically fed. If such milk is not available then use the freshest green-top or pasteurized milk.

Long-life (UHT) or sterilized milk is not recommended. Fresh cow's milk should be heated briefly to 80°C (176°F), especially in summer, as this will give some protection against bacterial contamination. Moreover, since cow's milk is an alien substance for the baby, heating it makes it more digestible.

Intolerance to milk is rare. Even what is sometimes known as "milk-crust" (a yellow seborrhoeal crust on the scalp) has in most cases nothing to do with milk, though it often gets better if the baby is given rather less nourishment. While genuine intolerances are rare, they can occur with any kind of food (see Chapter 4). If a genuine allergy to cow's milk is diagnosed, other baby-foods are available as alternatives, for example, preparations from soya beans.

Nearly all children have a very good tolerance of cereals and thrive splendidly on them but there is a known allergy to one of the constituents found in cereals. Wheat, barley, oats and rye contain gluten, a complex protein containing gliadin which in rare cases cannot be processed by the organism. The related condition, known as coeliac disease, affects one child in one thousand in Europe. It is recognized by three signs: failure to flourish, large amounts of soft stools — more than a cupful per day — and the baby being generally out of sorts. Coeliac disease requires specialist diagnosis. It is useful to know that rice contains no gliadin and is always tolerated.

The various cereal-flours used as additives to milk or diet for diarrhoea all have their advantages and disadvantages. Rice cereal (see Chapter 4.2) is easily digested, and the stools become firmer. It is much to be recommended for young babies, and for older ones with diarrhoea. Oatmeal makes somewhat thinner stools and easily causes bloating. Barleymeal is easily digested, but must be prepared at home by boiling down. Wheatmeal (the meal should be wholemeal if possible and sieved) is less common, semolina normally being used instead, and should be without added vanilla. We recommend organically or bio-dynamically grown produce.

In digestion, cereals are broken down by fermentation. The baby's stomach cannot activate this in the quantities required for each feed until the child is a few days old and sometimes not until a few weeks old.

For this reason the change-over to a cereal-supplement milk should be done only gradually, building up over several meals, otherwise there will be digestive upsets. Compared with mother's milk, cow's milk products remain much longer in the stomach, therefore there should be an interval of four hours between feeds.

Care of bottle and teat

The bottle and teat should be boiled once a day during the first months and laid out to dry on a clean dish towel.

After use clean thoroughly with a bottle-brush under running hot water. If washing-up liquid has to be used, it must be rinsed off afterwards under running hot water. The bottle-brush must be cleaned in the same way, and should put somewhere warm to dry quickly after that. The teat can be cleaned from time to time with cooking-salt. The use of disinfectants is not recommended.

Cow's milk

Bacterial decomposition
Bacteria causing decay grow in milk at temperatures over 5°C (41°F). It is important to chill the prepared feed in a bath of cold water before putting it in the fridge, otherwise it can remain lukewarm for too long. Further it is important to keep the feed in a temperature just above freezing. The temperature inside a fridge can rise above the optimum level for several hours when a whole lot of uncooled food is put into the fridge.

Pasteurization or boiling
By this method, most of the bacteria present including those of TB are destroyed. The milk is no longer so nourishing but it will not cause diarrhoea, which is a threat particularly in summer. Treating milk by quick heating and cooling is not so destructive. For household use, it is enough to heat the milk to 80°C (176°F).

Sterilization or ultra-heat treatment
Sterilization is effected by prolonged heating over 100°C (212°F), ultra-heat treatment by a brief heating over 140°C (284°F). Both treatments make the milk guaranteed sterile and so long-lasting, but at the same time rather dead, and are therefore not recommended. Furthermore it is often found that the treated milk contains a great number of dead bacteria.

Homogenization
Milk fat is broken down into smaller droplets, then the cream no longer rises to the top. This can be advantageous for commerce but not necessarily for the consumer.

Preparation of the baby's milk

There follow a number of different recipes for making up a baby's feed. Recipe 1 contains no cereal and may be used up to three months. Recipe 2 contains cereal and is suitable for babies over three months requiring more nourishment. Recipe 3 is a cereal recipe for use between three and ten months or until replaced by a full milk feed. Recipe 4 is a supplementary feed for temporary use.

Do not provide nutrition that contains cereal for the first months of the baby's life because (1) fats, carbohydrates and protein are in a very unbalanced proportion; and (2) cereals present too early a demand on the baby's digestive system before it is strong enough. For these reasons, our first recipe does not contain any cereal. Older babies can cope with cereal very well and it can be recommended for them without any hesitation.

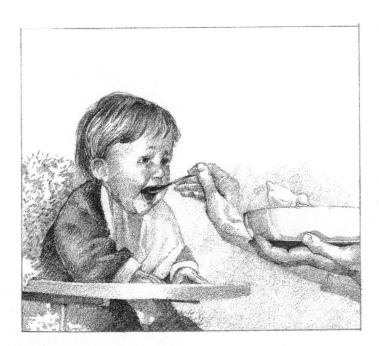

Figure 47. Learning to eat solids from a spoon.

Recipe 1 (for up to three months)

This is a complete feed based on cow's milk which is suitable for babies up to three months old. It can also be used for supplementary feeding but, if so, use as fine a hole as possible in the teat. With too large a hole, the baby may find the ease of feeding preferable to the breast. The composition corresponds to what is called adapted food and does not have the disadvantages of commercial ready-to-use preparations. Lactose (milk sugar) extracted from whey is obtainable from chemists (pharmacies) or health food shops. All cow's milk – preparations are lacking in Vitamin C and therefore this should be added no later than in the sixth week of the baby's life (see 14.4 below on fruit).

The total feeds for one day should not exceed ⅐ to ⅙ of the baby's weight. With very young babies, start with six feeds a day, reducing to five then four after about 4-8 weeks.

Many premature babies when they are three months old will require a special prescription from the doctor for iron. Full-term babies have a greater reserve of iron and normally require only the ingredients already mentioned.

One third milk with almond purée and lactose (milk sugar).

	Daily amount: metric (imperial) (depending on body weight)		
Volume:	600 ml (20 fl oz)	750 ml (25 fl oz)	900 ml (30 fl oz)
Number of bottles:	4–6	4–5	4–5
1 part cow's milk	200 ml (7 fl oz)	250 ml (8-9 fl oz)	300 ml (10 fl oz)
2 parts water	400 ml (13 fl oz)	500 ml (17 fl oz)	600 ml (20 fl oz)
4% almond purée	24 g (⅔ oz)**	30 g (1 oz)	36 g (1¼ oz)
6% lactose*	36 g (1¼ oz)**	45 g (1⅝ oz)	54 g (2 oz)

* Corresponds to the content in mother's milk and cannot be substituted by any other sugar.

** Weigh once and see how many teaspoonfuls make up this amount.

Preparation

Bring the milk, almond purée and water together nearly to the boil — up to at least 80°C (176°F). Stir in the lactose. Strain and pour into bottles. Seal those to be stored, and cool them in a bath of cold water before putting in the fridge. If you have not got a fridge, each feed must be prepared separately. Each bottle should contain no more than is required for each feed.

The following recipe is used after three months if the baby requires more feeding or is not flourishing. Introduce gradually, substituting for Recipe 1 at the rate of one feed per day over several days.

Recipe 2 (for over three months)

Half milk with almond purée, lactose and cereal-flour.

	Daily amount: metric (imperial) (depending on body weight)	
Volume:	600 ml (20 fl oz)	800 ml (26 fl oz)
Number of bottles:	3–4	4–5
1 part cow's milk	300 ml (10 fl oz)	400 ml (13 fl oz)
1 part water	300 ml (10 fl oz)*	400 ml (13 fl oz)
2% cereal	12 g (⅜ oz)**	16 g (½ oz)
3% almond purée	18 g (¾ oz)**	24 g (⅔ oz)
4% lactose	24 g (⅔ oz)**	32 g (1⅛ oz)

* To keep the correct consistency after heating, replace the water lost through evaporation (about 10%).

** See note for Recipe 1.

Preparation

Mix the cereal with water and boil for 5–8 minutes, or according to the directions on the packet. Add the milk and almond purée and heat up to 80°C (176°F) briefly. Then add lactose as directed for Recipe 1.

Recipe 3 (for up to ten months)

At 4–6 months, go over to a ⅔-milk feed. This ⅔-milk feed is to be used until replaced by a full-milk feed, between 8–10 months. With the latter, the cereal and sugar can be reduced or left out altogether.

The amount of protein in the left hand column of Recipe 3 with 500 ml (17 fl oz) of cow's milk is rather more than what is needed daily (the daily amount required being about 400 ml, 14 fl oz, of cow's milk in the baby's first year), while the amount in the centre column with 330 ml (11 fl oz) cow's milk is rather too low. By giving an extra 70 ml (2 fl oz) of cow's milk or some quark with the fruit purée, the gap is made up. The right hand column shows the amount for a bottle which may still be conveniently given in the morning.

Two thirds milk with cereal and sugar, with optional addition of almond purée.

	Daily amount: metric (imperial) (depending on body weight)		
Volume:	750 ml (25 fl oz)	500 ml (17 fl oz)	250 ml (8-9 fl oz)
Number of bottles:	3–4	2–3	1
2 parts cow's milk	500 ml (17 fl oz)	330 ml (11 fl oz)	165 ml (4-5 fl oz)
1 part water	250 ml (8-9 fl oz)*	170 ml (5 fl oz)	85 ml (2-3 fl oz)
2.5% cereal	19 g (¾ oz)	12 g (⅜ oz)	6 g (¼ oz)
3% sugar	22 g (⅔ oz)	15 g (½ oz)	7.5 g (¼ oz)
(1% almond purée)	(7.5 g, ¼ oz)	(5 g, ¼ oz)	(2.5 g, ⅛ oz)

* See note for Recipe 2.

Preparation

As for Recipe 2. The cereal can be increased to 2.5%. The almond purée can still be mixed in up to 1% or it can be left out altogether. The sugar can now be cane-sugar (muscovado or molasses, see 14.4 below on sugar and honey), or with older babies, malt extract or honey. In our experience most children only require 3% ordinary sugar to be added. This is important because by keeping the sugar content low, you can prevent the child from developing too sweet a taste. This problem does not arise with lactose (milk sugar) as it is far less sweet. In Recipe 1, the proportion corresponds to the content in human milk.

If any of the above feeds give rise to problems the following adjustments can be made:

In the case of constipation the sugar amount can be partly replaced by milk sugar or malt extract.

If the stools are too thin, replace the milk sugar by 3–5% ordinary sugar or full cane sugar and reduce the almond purée *temporarily*.

If the baby is not getting enough, you can change to recipe 2 earlier.

If the baby spits up or has too much wind, it is not always the ingredients in its food that are at fault but often other factors (see Chapter 2.7 and 4.1).

If the baby's wind is a result of too strong a fermentation of the milk sugar, the latter can be substituted by ordinary sugar or full cane sugar (3–5%).

If intolerance to the almond purée is suspected, it can be replaced by an equal number of teaspoonfuls of sunflower oil (stir in well or shake well immediately before feeding). For intolerance to cow's milk or cereal see above and Chapter 4.1.

Generally medical advice should be sought regarding any changes to the baby's diet.

Recipe 4
(temporary supplementary feed)

The following feed *without cow's milk* is for exceptional cases and for strictly temporary use (the baby will lose weight if it is used for any length of time). This feed can be used as a supplement when there is not enough mother's milk in the first three weeks of the baby's life, otherwise with other feeds only on a doctor's prescription to guard against lack of protein or minerals.

Temporary feed without cow's milk, with almond purée and lactose.

	Daily amount: metric (imperial) (depending on body weight)	
Volume:	300 ml (10 fl oz)	600 ml (20 fl oz)
Number of bottles:	2–6	3–6
Water	300 ml (10 fl oz)	600 ml (20 fl oz)
6-7% almond purée	18-21 g (¾-⅔ oz)	36-42 g (1¼-1½ oz)
6% lactose	18 g (¾ oz)	36 g (1¼ oz)

Preparation
Mix with boiled water.

Supplementary feeding with vegetables, fruit and pap

Bottle-fed babies should be given fruit and vegetable juice daily from the sixth week onwards. Give one to four teaspoonfuls (increasing later up to ten) of orange juice or better one to three teaspoonfuls of pure black-currant juice or other fresh currant or berry juice. Additionally one to four teaspoonfuls of carrot juice can be given (grated raw, with a pinch of sugar to draw the juice and pressed out through a sieve). Keep this up at least until the child is on to a vegetable and/or fruit meal.

Use oranges where possible that have not been sprayed and choose carrots that have been organically or bio-dynamically grown (see below). Sandthorn, sloe and other elixirs usually contain a lot of sugar and, in the quantities given to children, little Vitamin C. They can be used for sweetening if you know their sugar content. If the child gets a sore bottom from the fruit juice, stop giving it for a few days and start again with smaller amounts. With fully breast-fed children, the recommended times for introducing fruit can be put off by two to three months (see table on page 243). For use of carrot juice in cases of Vitamin K deficiency, see 14.1 above.

Preparation of vegetable feeds
Cook the vegetables until they are soft, and press through a sieve. Begin with carrots. Later introduce once or twice a week fennel, spinach, spring kohlrabi, cauliflower or lettuce mash. The carrots must be boiled for a long time, and this can be done without spoiling them. Either feed them with a spoon before the milk feed or mix them in with some of the bottle feed, or both. The baby has to be got used to the spoon as well as the new taste. Some added sugar or a little honey can help. Slowly increase the amount given to a half and then to a full vegetable feed without salt (but finally with two teaspoons of sunflower oil).

We do not recommend meat or other additions (see 14.4 below on eggs, meat and fish). Organic or bio-dynamic products are preferable. Vegetables preserved in jars are acceptable where nothing else is available, but in such a case carrots in jars grown organically or bio-dynamically are preferable.

Preparation of fruit feeds
Steep one or two rusks in boiled water or milk. Mix the softened rusk with grated apple (washed, peeled, pips removed) adding a little sugar or honey. In addition to apples the following fruits in season may be used: strawberries, raspberries, black and red currants (pressed through a sieve), peaches and bananas, and possibly even fruit juice. Older thin babies can be given a few spoonfuls of cream quark. Always begin with small amounts, increasing them to a full meal.

Feeding charts for the first year

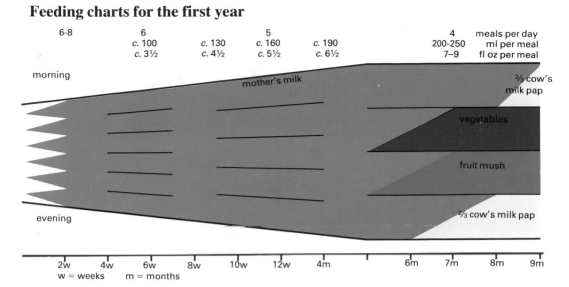

Age increase from left to right. Time of day from top to bottom. Horizontal lines indicate the number of feeds. The daily amounts add up to between 800 and 1000 ml, 1½ to 1¾ pints.

Table 1. Programme for a fully breast-fed baby. Between five and seven months vegetable and fruit feeds are introduced. Fruit and vegetable juice can be given earlier (from the sixth week) by the teaspoonful, but this is not essential. Give cow's milk preparations from the time the mother's milk is insufficient. The child should be fully weaned by nine months or twelve months at the latest. By then bottle-feeding is quite unnecessary. (For growth/weight table, see page 383).

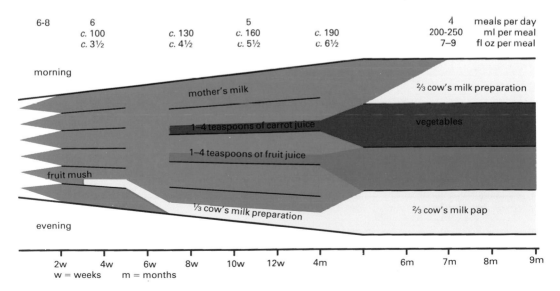

Table 2. If the child is not thriving, diluted cow's milk can be given as a supplement from the third or fourth week. If this is given in the evening, breast-feeding is then least disturbed.

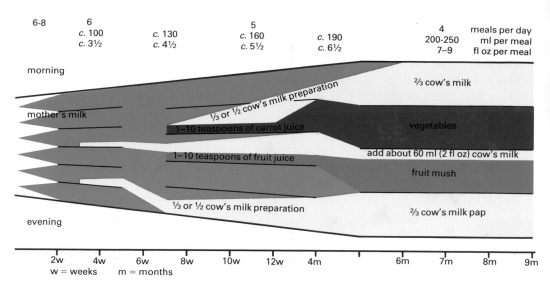

Table 3. Programme for supplementary (two-milk) feeding when the mother's milk is inadequate. Of course breast-feeding can still go on longer than five months.

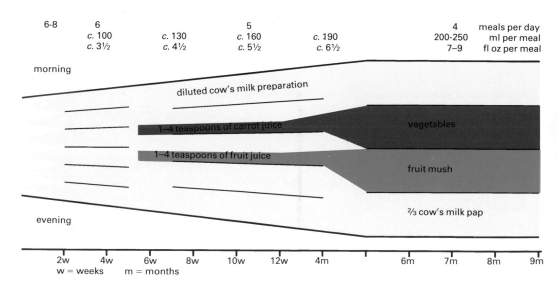

Table 4. Programme for bottle-feeding on cow's milk preparations.

Milk-pap

While breast-fed babies are being weaned, milk-pap can be used as an evening feed. Milk-pap can also be given to bottle-fed babies after they are a few months old, replacing their bottle at the evening meal. Use the same dilution of milk as for the normal bottle feed, and cook with semolina, fine oat-flakes or barley-flour according to choice; later millet-flakes or other cereals (do not give bran), adding about 3% sugar. In calculating the total daily amount of milk to be given, remember to include the milk in the pap.

Apple and semolina pap

Some parents supplement the pap feed with apple purée or compote or grated apple by the fourth month. For babies with a big appetite who are growing too fast, this is a good way of reducing their milk intake.

Should extra drinks be given?

Babies get a lot of liquid from their normal feed. If adults were to take in as much liquid in relation to solids per day as a six-month-old baby does, we would consume two gallons (ten litres) daily. Thus babies have relatively much more liquid in their normal diet than older people. The commonly heard advice that children and especially babies must be given lots to drink because they need it, is quite erroneous. Of course, extra liquids are in order in hot climates or during very hot weather, or with fever and, of course, with diarrhoea and vomiting (see Chapter 4).

Change of food in the second year

At the beginning of the baby's second year, the change-over from baby food to infant food should be made gradually. At first the actual food remains the same, only it is now taken in the high chair at table together with the rest of the family. The bottle is replaced with feeding from a cup, giving milk with bits of bread in it. Very soon it can be observed how very young children eat not only because they are hungry but also by imitation. Now you can give the child a piece of bread or crust to chew. Before long, the child will want its own spoon and so, with much mess and dabbling, the change-over is made to independent eating. The build-up of diet from milk alone, via the various cereals and paps, to the wide variety of adult food should be achieved gradually.

14.4 General aspects of nutrition

In the consulting-room, we are often asked when a child should start eating meat and eggs, and what kind of vegetables, cereals and so on, we recommend. We are also asked what anthroposophy has to say about various foods. It will be useful, then, to look at some general ideas about food before going on to discuss individual items.

Quality in nutrition

In the previous section, we discussed in detail the correct amounts of food to be given. Here we turn our attention to a wider aspect of nutrition: quality. Where quality of food is concerned, we are interested in *how* the food product is, how it stands in relation to nature as a whole. We are not so concerned with *how much* protein, fats or carbohydrate the product contains but rather with the different qualities of all these when found in various foods such as potatoes, rice and pulses. The question of *how* the produce is cultivated, stored and prepared is all important. Take, for example, the difference in quality of the starch in cereal and potatoes. This difference stems from the different life and growth conditions of the two kinds of produce as well as from all the processing and handling before they reach the consumer.

Quality in diet comes from a balance of different foods. Hence we make up our diet from different parts of the plant: root, stalk, leaf, blossom and fruit. Each of these has a different interplay with the surrounding forces in earth, water, air, warmth and light. Each part of the plant stimulates the human organism differently and so the more varied our food, the broader will be its stimuli — not only on our muscles but also on our thinking, imagination, instincts and feelings.

How these various stimuli have their effects is described by Rudolf Steiner in his lectures on nutrition. The functions of the human nerves and senses correspond to the activity of a plant root; the metabolic functions correspond to blossoming and fruition; while the rhythmic functions (circulation of the blood and breathing) correspond to the action of the leaves of the plant. This is why root-vegetables, root-juice or root infusions promote the activity of the nerve system, while the metabolic functions are stimulated by blossom-teas, apples and other fruits. Imbalance in nutrition should be avoided as it will eventually lead to a debility in the organ system which has been insufficiently nourished.

Another aspect of quality relates to the conditions in which a plant or animal will flourish. For instance, a pig that is allowed to live naturally, not deliberately restricted in its movement, and has not been subjected to hormone treatment, will provide pork meat or meat-products with quite different nutritional value from a pig which has been reared only for fattening without consideration for its natural needs.

The same applies to plants. Radishes and spinach forced on by nitrogen fertilizers have a high water content, taste more insipid than those not so fertilized, do not keep so well, have a higher nitrate content (spinach) and show atypical growth tendencies (this can be seen especially with radishes where the artificially fertilized radishes show quite a different type of root from that of the naturally grown ones). Furthermore it has been found that the plants grown with chemical fertilizers are late in blossoming and fruition or do not blossom and form fruit at all and so require, in addition to nitrogen, feeding with potassium and phosphor salts in order to guarantee proper fruiting.

For these reasons we recommend organically grown plant and animal produce. Cultivation which continually impoverishes the mineral content of the soil, thus requiring more and more inorganic fertilizer every year, and which further robs the soil by monoculture, is not a good omen for the future. Equally impoverishing of the natural environment is cultivation or breeding where quantity dominates and everything is geared to maximum profit. Such an attitude to nature will in the long run prove disastrous for all.

By contrast, bio-dynamic cultivation consistently aims to preserve and maintain soil, plant, animal and human being in a healthy condition with quality always in view. The significance for the future in these agricultural methods lies in the fact that they can be applied to poor soils and to those that have been impoverished and robbed. They bring about a gradual regeneration of the soil over the years, and reintroduce soil bacteria and micro-organisms; a fact that will in future be more and more appreciated as the damaging effects worldwide of chemical fertilizers, pesticides and weed-killers become more and more obvious.

Books describing bio-dynamic methods of crop fertilization, crop rotation, pest control, plant selection and stock-rearing are listed in the bibliography at the end of this book.

Digestion and diet

The fact that the child's intestines are very susceptible to upsets shows that the organs of digestion have not yet learned to function properly. We ask what do they have to "learn," what is it that the digestion actually does? It has to be able to destroy the particular character of a food; only when it has been completely destroyed can it be used to build up human substance. Food as part of our surroundings must "die" in order to generate human strength. For example, even if only a very little foreign protein gets into our blood, the body will react violently with fever or allergic symptoms. If malabsorption (as for instance sensitivity to gluten, milk-protein or certain sugars) occurs, then the organism is no longer sufficiently able to "humanize" the corresponding bit of "world."

With certain illnesses a diet excluding certain foods may be necessary. The aim, however, should be eventually to learn to cope with the foods that have been excluded. We are at our strongest when our digestion is able to transform all foods into human substance. If for example the body suffers from an enzyme deficiency so that particular foods are not easily or properly digested, it will help to reduce intake of the food in question. But by gradually and carefully increasing the digestive load the synthesis of the enzyme can be stimulated whereas if no demand were made on it, it would simply die away.

Generally speaking, then, a person who can eat almost anything is extremely healthy. Those who suffer from occasional digestive disorders, or who have supposedly fussy tastes, should aim to accustom the body to a variety of foods and so make it all the more efficient.

There is also a good social reason for ensuring that your diet is broad and unfussy. If you have invited guests and set before them a meal prepared with love and care, you will be glad not to find that half of them have brought their own wholemeal bread and raw salads and then dominate the evening's conversation with talk about nutritional values. In broad terms, we should be able to sit down and enjoy things which we would not normally buy or prepare for ourselves at home, just because we are with others. Any sort of individualized diet leads in some degree to social isolation and should be avoided. On the other hand, as hosts, we will of course be considerate for someone with a sensitive stomach — without making a great fuss about it.

In this connection, a misunderstanding frequently crops up: namely that, from an anthroposophical point of view, certain foods are recommended or forbidden. Rudolf Steiner always emphasized that he would not take sides for or against any particular food, and that he would only offer points of view which would enable others to make a more consciously selected diet. Our discussion here is aimed simply at helping readers to know better what they are doing when they choose meals to put on the family table.

Different types of food

Herb-teas
For babies and infants and later for children with tummy and bowel upsets, fennel and camomile tea are generally used. Fennel tea is made more effective by crushing the seeds. Pour on boiling water and leave to stand only for a moment or two, and strain when the colour has become a

faint yellow. Camomile tea should not be made from tea-bags but from dried plants which you have collected yourself or obtained from the herbalist.

Less well-known but very good are apple-peel tea and rose-hip tea, the latter being made from rose-hips which have been cleaned of their hair. Boil the hips for ten minutes, or leave them to soak overnight and then boil for three to five minutes. Rose-hip tea-bags always contain hibiscus (rose-mallow) and make a somewhat bitter tea with a fine red colour. Pure rose-hip tea, however, is a pleasant mild refreshing drink.

Children usually like mint tea with perhaps a drop or two of lemon in it, but it will not help in cases of an upset tummy. Lime-blossom tea has a somewhat distinctive flavour which is not to everybody's taste but with a drop or two of lemon and honey added, almost every child will drink it. It is especially good for bringing on a sweat and so is useful for colds and during a rising temperature. A good substitute for cough mixture is a tisane from coltsfoot blossom, ribwort and sage laced with honey and lemon.

We shall not discuss here the whole range of herb-teas which may be prescribed by the doctor for specific illnesses, as these must be selected for every individual case. Much of general interest, however, can be found in books on herbal remedies.

For children of nursery age and upwards, you can make a big jug of unsweetened tea on summer mornings and this can be improved by adding some fruit juice. The children can then drink this tea whenever they are thirsty and there will be no danger of them losing their appetite at mealtimes. Between meals, all drinks from the fridge and lemonade should be forbidden.

Except in the summer, it is better to limit drinking to meal-times. It is a bad habit to have a bottle of herb-tea (whether sweetened or unsweetened) standing by the baby's bed within reach. Apart from harming the teeth (see Chapter 15.1) children get used to drinking because they are bored or simply as an amusement, and then at meal-times there is a fuss because they do not want to eat. We refer to the "bottle-addict" when children appear in the consulting-room clutching a bottle to suck. The arguments are always the same: "Oh, but he's so fond of it," or "I thought children needed lots of liquids."

The stomach, bowel and kidney system are not a waterworks. They are a regulating system for the processes taking place in the body's liquidity. If we understand this, we shall see that we need to accompany the rhythm of this internal function with a corresponding external rhythm (see also Chapter 7.1, 17.4 and 17.9).

Milk
Easily obtainable, cow's milk has become one of the most important foods of our civilization. Mare's and ass's milk are much closer in kind to human milk, but are hard to obtain and very expensive. It is said that up

to the last century a she-ass was taken through the streets of Amsterdam to be milked on the spot for babies in need of milk.

Goat's milk and sheep's milk are still used in families who are too poor to keep a cow. How far goat's milk is suitable depends chiefly on how the goat is fed and whether it has freedom to graze. Milk from a goat in a pen should not be given to young babies.

In general terms, the smaller the animal the higher the protein content of the milk, and therefore for a low protein content you cannot find better than cow's milk. As far as the amount is concerned, a baby should be given 400 ml (13 fl oz) full milk per day and occasionally up to 500 ml (17 fl oz). As the child's range of food is extended to other dairy produce such as quark, yoghurt, kefir and, later cheese, it becomes impossible to say what the minimum amount of milk should be. But you should not be surprised if children don't eat much when they drink a lot of milk.

Chalky-soapy stools (grey pasty stools) can be the result of too much milk protein from milk itself or dairy produce.

The fresher the milk the better, so that it remains a living whole which cannot be substituted with any artificial product, though it does need certain additional substances to make it better fitted for human consumption. Properly prepared, it is a much better substitute for mother's milk than soya and cereal or meat and eggs.

There is no doubt that mother's milk is the best nourishment of all for babies. Rudolf Steiner refers to suckling at the mother's breast as "a bodily education" because the mother's milk being full of vitality enables the child's organism to learn to direct the forces of growth, providing a foundation for the rest of life. If at all possible, this "education" should not be denied to any child.

Fats

Butter is the principal fat to be used for children. Only in rare cases should it be necessary for health reasons to change to a margarine diet. Hard fats (lard, and so on) are not recommended as they do not contain any unsaturated fatty acids which act on the metabolism. Hard fats are found in many sweets (candy) which should therefore be almost totally banned. Oils to be preferred are those which are extracted cold, such as sunflower oil, olive oil and good quality thistle oil.

Cereals

The first cereals were developed from carefully selected grasses about 5000 BC. The cultivation of cereals formed the basis for agriculture and enabled mankind to develop forms of civilization requiring completely different conditions from a life of hunting and gathering. Mankind moved over to tilling the soil, rearing flocks and cooking and baking its food.

When grain is transformed into bread, the process not only involves water and air, but also fire. Baking is a kind of digestion in that it helps to open up the cereal, and this produces a food of a particular quality, as the process is a kind of extension of natural growth. It is interesting to note that bread is held in particular esteem in all the cultures which use it.

Until recent years, the consumption of cereals had declined considerably in the West. This was due to a higher consumption of fats and proteins as well as potatoes. But recently, there has been a marked return to home-baked bread and cereal foods have come back into favour. More and more families have discovered the good taste of home-baked bread in comparison with bought bread; and not only mothers but daughters and sons have become enthusiastic bakers. All sorts of different cereal mixtures, doughs and leavens are tried out.

In our consulting-room, the effects of some of these experiments are more and more obvious. In the enthusiasm for pure and natural high-fibre food, coarse meal and unground whole seeds are used for baking, thus causing distended stomach in children. We can often tell right away from the child's complaint that the parents are either baking coarse bread themselves, or giving their child morning and evening muesli made from thick oat-flakes, or making a pap with lots of meal in it. This sort of diet simply leads to giving the digestion too much cellulose to cope with. It is wrong to think that wholemeal bread has to be coarse. With finer wholemeal flour, the grain opens up in the baking and turns into an easily digested bread. Coarse bread can be eaten as an occasional treat or as an item of diet for an adult suffering from chronic constipation.

Grains of all kinds have great value for a family meal. If the grain is properly prepared, the children will eat it with enjoyment. A lack of protein and fat can be recognized if the children are soon hungry again. Then some adjustment to the diet should be introduced. Care should be taken especially during the period of weaning because the organism cannot be expected to cope suddenly with foods demanding more digestion.

In general, we recommend a greater use of grain in the diet provided that it is not overdone.

Potatoes

The potato was widely cultivated in South America over two thousand years ago. In the sixteenth century, it was brought to Europe where it spread rapidly and, in the course of the eighteenth and nineteenth centuries, the advantages of potato cultivation became universally recognized.

The potato belongs to the family of the nightshades: black nightshade, deadly nightshade, henbane, thorn-apple, bitter-sweet (woody nightshade), tomato and paprika are all related to it. Most of these plants are poisonous. The potato also contains a small quantity of the poison solanine which can be increased by an attack of bacteria, exposure to light, or becoming green, and this can lead to poisoning.

Potatoes and cereals show quite opposite tendencies. If a potato-plant grows from the seed of a potato-fruit the main shoot will grow up but the first and second sprouts will incline downwards and grow into the earth. The tubers then grow as offshoots under the surface of the earth like roots. In contrast to the cereals, there is a tendency to turn away from the light.

Like other roots and tubers, the nourishment provided by potatoes works on the nervous system. Rudolf Steiner, on more than one occasion, described the effects of too high a consumption of potatoes on thinking. Meditative, inward thinking is subdued while a more intellectual rational kind comes to the fore, so thinking becomes more sense-orientated and materialistic, with the attendant urge to maintain this condition by eating more and more potatoes. In children the result is a weakening of the mid-brain area and, in addition, weakening of the eyes in old age. Looked at in this way, it is not surprising that the advance of materialistic thinking so closely bound to sense-perception coincides with the spread of potatoes as a main food.

What conclusions can we draw from this? There is nothing to stop you from trying an experiment in your own family. You can try to limit the amount of potatoes eaten by gradually replacing them with cereals, roots and vegetables. A month or two after this change of diet, you will be able to observe an appreciable increase in freshness and mobility of thought together with a greater alertness.

During pregnancy and during the first year of the baby's life, while the cerebrum is still developing, we advise that no potatoes should be eaten by the mother. Also avoid potatoes in the case of nervous diseases and cancer.*

Vegetables and lettuce
Everyone knows that vegetables and lettuce are healthy. As we saw earlier, the health value of such foods does not lie in their constituents alone but in their relation to living nature. Only in certain limited diets or at times of want are the constituents and with them the trace elements and vitamins of special significance.

A number of items are worth special mention for a baby's food:

Carrots. Carrot purée when cooked long enough can be digested easily from the third to the fourth month. Before that it can cause flatulence. The raw juice is digestible earlier and is usually recommended from the sixth week. The yellow colouring-matter becomes partially deposited in the body or transformed into Vitamin A. Cooked carrot is good for forming the stools, and provides a good protection against diarrhoea. Raw grated carrots are suitable only for the baby's second and third year and not

* In the UK a connection is suspected between potato-eating in pregnancy and the incidence of spina bifida (neural tube defects) and anencephaly (being born without a brain) and this supposition is confirmed by laboratory experiments.

as a diet for diarrhoea. For breast-fed children carrot is a valuable source of Vitamin K (see 14.1 above).

Spinach. Spinach is usually given to babies later. It does not contain as much iron as was formerly believed. But where it has been carefully cultivated and freshly prepared, it may be regarded as a healthy vegetable. If it is taken too often it has the disadvantage that the oxalic acid in it binds calcium in the intestine and makes it insoluble. A shortage of milk in the diet could then result in a greater lack of calcium in the blood (see Chapter 15.2).

Even as we write we can see in our mind's eye the long faces of children and parents round the plate of leftover vegetables and salads, the child protesting, the parents pleading, demanding or resigned. How often "I don't like it," "I can't eat it" is heard. It is not always the child's fault. The problem can sometimes be the way the food is prepared: it may be tasteless if the vegetables are cooked too much, or just too salty or bitter for children's taste. Disguising the unwanted ingredients in a blend of other foods usually helps. The old saying that "the secret of a healthy appetite is enjoyment" is based on scientific reality: the secretions of the digestive glands are actually influenced by enjoyment or lack of enjoyment in eating.

Fruit

Most children seem to like fruit. If a child does not like fruit you can hide it grated or as freshly squeezed juice

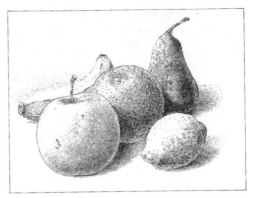

Figure 48. Untreated fresh fruit is best.

in quark or muesli. The child does not have to have very much. Half an apple and a little lemon juice per day is enough if your child doesn't like fruit. If possible children should be given untreated fruit so that they can eat the peel with it. It is sad these days to hear children ask: "Can I eat the peel or has it been sprayed?" What have we come to when food can be regarded as something dangerous and poisoned and we must look at the label to see whether we can trust the food or not.

Nearly all children like bananas, but they should not eat too many. Bananas contain good nourishment but not much vitalizing force. They are very filling but they do make the system rather sluggish. Furthermore the process used in harvesting and storing the unripe fruit leaves a lot to be desired. The bananas have to be shipped and stored in refrigerators with carbon dioxide to prevent decay. By raising the temperature and exposing the produce to ethylene gas, the fruit is made ready for sale. Citrus fruits are quite different as they keep well and have a freshening and vitalizing effect. Here, too, great amounts should not be eaten. For children we recommend the more expensive untreated oranges, or grapefruit or kiwis, only a few segments or teaspoonfuls per day.

Sugar and honey

Natural sugars are formed in the green parts of all plants and stored as a source of energy in root, leaf, stalk, blossom or fruit. In its refined and crystallized form, commercial sugar keeps for an unlimited period and also offers an energy reserve, one which can be absorbed without the digestion having to work.

Sugar does not stimulate the vital activity of the organs but provides the

Figure 49. Honey and unrefined sugar.

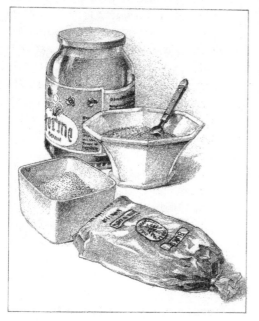

body with a substance which the body, when in full health, can itself create in abundance. When the organism is ill or overtired then the intake of sugar acts as an energy-producer and relieves the organism of the work of digestion. This can be seen vividly when a weak premature baby in the incubator, with only slight chances of survival, is given a drop of sugar water. As soon as the baby tastes sweetness, it is filled with life and movement and seems affected right down to the tip of its toes, pushing out its lips to receive more. The drops become the longed-for water of life.

Even if tasting sugar does not affect most of us healthy humans in quite this way, we do feel an immediate effect from the sweet taste. Sourness, saltiness and bitterness all have a more aggressive nature that prods us awake. Sweetness on the other hand comforts, consoles, calms and supports. It immediately strengthens our feeling of self, making us feel stronger and better in our bodies. This effect awakens the desire for more sugar. We enjoy the momentary increase in strength and do not notice the ensuing decline in strength which we seek to compensate for by an even greater sugar consumption. Sugar-eating children are marked by fidgetiness, lack of stamina and lack of concentration. Since the introduction of sugar in post-Napoleonic times, we all suffer from an increasing excess of sugar in our diet, with the consequent spread of diseases of civilization, such as dental caries (see Chapter 15.1) and the sugar-illness, diabetes mellitus.

As is well known, diabetes declined considerably during the Second World War (both in the UK and in Germany) and increased again as living standards rose. This was a direct result of a fall and subsequent rise in sugar consumption. All diabetics are aware that their condition becomes worse when they are ill, angry, upset, mentally overworked or under stress, or after indulging in alcohol or uncontrolled eating. They feel better and can achieve more when they can do their physical and mental work in an ordered careful rhythm. It has been observed that older diabetics have often had a history of mental and emotional stress during their childhood and adolescence. Heredity also plays a part. Everything that tends to weaken the "I" and hinders it from becoming master of its own domain upsets the metabolism of sugar. Sugar-metabolism is the vehicle of the "I" in the blood. When the individual becomes exhausted the intake of sugar can stimulate to further achievement. But this can become an addiction and the body no longer produces its own sugar from starch. If the "I" is then further weakened by environmental and hereditary factors, a disposition to diabetes can ensue.

But the conclusion to be drawn from all this is certainly not to ban all sugar from the diet. Many babies fed without sugar who are not thriving and have a pale complexion can be transformed into fresh rosy children in a few weeks by adding 3% sugar to their diet. Sugar is a very effective substance which promotes self-awareness, and should be given in reasonable amounts according to circumstances and taking into account the temperament and constitution of the child. Try to avoid always finishing off a meal with a sugary pudding. On the other hand, when a child comes in tired out from playing outside, there is no point in denying the child a sweet herb-tea or milk and honey with supper.

What kind of sugar is best for children? Be sparing with *white* sugar. Although bleaching is no longer used in its production, all the accompanying substances are eliminated by processing. Thus chemically it is pure, but it lacks all the minerals and vitamins of the cane or beet juice which are required by the organism in order to break down the sugar. Where these are lacking the organism itself must supply them but in natural foods, of course, these elements are generally present. The sugar in apples, for instance, brings with it enough trace elements to assist the breaking down of the sugar. Cane and beet sugars (molasses) are also healthier.

Ordinary *brown sugar* is not recommended by us. Only the final stages of refining are omitted, and so not only does the sugar still retain the last residue of its accompanying substances but it also contains deposits from the production process which cannot be eliminated.

If muscovado, molasses or other

pure cane sugar products are not available, you can mix white sugar with other foodstuffs. If it is mixed with milk, quark, grains, or muesli, or used in wholemeal buns in a concentration of 2–5%, it will do no harm as long as the teeth are cleaned regularly.

Honey should not be taken simply as a substitute for sugar. To give honey its proper value, we must consider how it is produced: foraging bees collect nectar from blossoms while other bees work in the hive to transform and store the valuable food on which the whole colony depends for its survival. A natural substance produced through such a variety of work stages has more the character of a medicine, such is its stimulating effect on the body (amongst other uses, Rudolf Steiner suggested that honey should be taken by ageing people who are inclined to sclerosis). In our practice we do not usually recommend honey for the first six months of the baby's life because its effect can easily lead to diarrhoea. Later on, one teaspoonful per day is sufficient.

Sweeteners are never recommended by us as they add a false sweetness to the taste which does not correspond to nature.

Eggs, meat and fish

Proteins are built up from amino-acids and so a lack of amino-acids in the body causes protein deficiency which gives rise to certain diseases. As the body cannot itself build up all the protein constituents, but has to obtain some of them through food intake, it is important to pay attention to the provision of protein in diet.

The essential amino-acids required to maintain life are abundantly present in meat, almost complete in milk, less in pulses (legumes), soya beans, almonds and nuts. Enough protein can be obtained without eating meat, fish, or eggs so long as enough milk products are consumed.

A number of things can be taken into account when deciding at what stage to introduce eggs and meat into the child's diet. The main development of muscles and physical strength takes place during and after puberty. During the first years of life, brain-formation is paramount and, at the beginning of this period, mother's milk is without doubt the natural nourishment. It seems obvious that the transition from milk food to meat should not be too hasty, especially as mother's milk (as a nutritional model for the early days) has a surprisingly low protein content. Therefore, for the first stage of the transition, we recommend cow's milk and the produce derived from it together with cereals and vegetables. This "lacto-vegetable" diet is suitable up to the end of the third year.

At this point, children will start to announce their likes and dislikes more clearly because they are able to talk and remember. The child's own instinct, and not just family habits or imitation, will also influence individual tastes. It is interesting to note that already at this age it can be seen whether a child will become a vegetarian or not; some children will simply refuse meat or even egg. For others, on the other hand, meat will be their favourite dish.

There may be genuine reasons for an individual child avoiding certain high-protein foods, such as intolerance to milk or problems of not thriving. A change of diet may be needed in such cases, which are exceptions requiring a thorough medical investigation.

A more general reason for avoiding eggs and meat in the early years is that a high consumption of protein accelerates the maturing of the body with which the developing soul cannot keep pace. Those animals whose milk has the higher protein content develop more quickly.

We shall avoid saying too precisely the exact quantity of protein which is necessary for a child each day. The requisite amounts of milk for babies have been indicated (see 14.3 above) and more precise calculations depend on local diets and conditions.

Salt and mineral water
In principle, babies should be given unsalted nourishment and young children should not get much in the way of salty foods. Bread and milk contain enough salt. Occasionally a child has a distinct liking for salt. That is not necessarily harmful, but for the doctor it can be an important indication of the child's constitution.

We are sometimes asked about using mineral water to prepare the child's feed, especially when travelling or in a case of diarrhoea. Mineral waters with a low sodium content are suitable. In France, Evian is widely used for babies. Italian waters are generally suitable and are also widely used for babies. In Germany only a few mineral waters are suitable; most German mineral waters cannot be digested properly by small babies.

To sum up our advice on diet:

In infancy provide a lacto-vegetable diet, in later childhood a diet suited to the individual's need, varied, of the best available quality, with not too much protein. In the case of children with unbalanced appetites, keep trying to rectify the balance and resort to subterfuge, if necessary, by mixing the unwanted items in.

15 Teeth and bone formation

15.1 Does fluoride prevent tooth decay?

In the consulting-room we are often asked: "Do we really have to give our children fluoride tablets or fluoride protection for their teeth?"

It is now known that fluoride checks dental caries. In regions where there is a higher than average level of natural fluoride in the water, there is less incidence of caries (tooth decay) in the local population. That is why it is now recommended in several industrialized countries that fluoride in one form or another should be given to the population. This can be done in a number of ways: by adding fluoride to the supply of drinking water in a concentration of one part per million: by adding fluoride to cooking salt; or by administering tablets of ¼ to 1 mg fluoride according to age.

In addition, fluoride can be applied as an enamel coating, or added to mouth-wash or toothpaste. It can be proved that the surface of the teeth is made more resistant to acids by fluoride coating. Particularly harmful are the acids that are formed in dental plaque when sugar is broken down by bacteria. Apart from protecting the surface of the teeth, a greater intake of fluoride during the time when the teeth are forming will, it is hoped, make the whole structure of the enamel more resistant. If fluoride is not given at all, the surface of the teeth begins to lose its natural resistance and caries can soon appear.

Looked at in this way, it is understandable why more and more dentists and health organizations want fluoridation of drinking water or the regular taking of tablets.

We however are not in favour of this policy because, in our view, giving fluoride only masks the real problem without solving it. Dental caries is caused *not* by lack of fluoride, but by unhealthy eating habits and by insufficient care of the teeth and poor dental hygiene. It is not right that the bad habits which give rise to caries should be retained with all the consequences for the whole organism; nor is it right that, in order to counteract bad effects on the teeth, fluoride should be added artificially to our food, for although fluoride works upon the enamel of the teeth it is an imposition on the entire bone system.

If we look at the amount of natural fluoride first in children's bones, then in the bones of adults in mid-life and finally in old people, we observe a steady increase. This means that the more fluoride there is in the bones the more advanced is the ageing process. If we give children extra fluoride on a regular basis, we force the organism to deposit fluoride in the bones prematurely.

Those who would like to see all children given fluoride maintain that long-term fluoridation is quite harmless and support this assertion by quoting from articles in medical and other professional publications. But it is still not clear at this stage of research whether existing findings have really taken into account the following questions. What are the effects of premature ageing of the bones in later life? What are the effects of fluoride on our consciousness? Can we assume that the addition or removal of a substance like fluoride has no effect upon the activity of the soul or the spirit? We should not ignore such questions simply because the answers cannot be measured statistically.

We do know about the unsightly patches appearing in the enamel which are called dental fluorosis. This condition can be caused by a fluoride concentration as low as one to one million, which is considered the best concentration for combating caries. As the bones consist of a substance similar to enamel and as most of the fluoride administered will end up in the bones anyway, some restructuring, however delicate, must take place there.

In this connection it is interesting to note that Nature herself is very sparing with fluoride towards human beings. Human milk contains remarkably little fluoride even when there is an increased amount in the drinking water. For example, with 0.2 mg fluoride per litre of drinking water, only 0.01 mg per litre emerges in mother's milk, in fact only a very little more than if the water had not been fluoridated. This shows us that the mother's organism actually screens the child against a higher intake of fluoride. As mother's milk has proved itself to be the best baby food, we must give some weight to this evidence which indicates clearly how we should regard fluoride during the baby's first months. If a baby is given a single ¼ mg fluoride tablet, it will get twenty times as much fluoride as from breast-milk. If a baby is fed on powdered milk and the drinking water used to mix the feed contains 1 mg fluoride per litre, the child will get eighty times as much as a purely breast-fed baby.

Taking all this into account together with the fact that tooth decay has causes unrelated to a lack of fluoride, we regard the statutory policy of adding fluoride as unjustified. The taking of supplementary fluoride should be the individual's responsibility, just like any other medicine. Caries should be combatted at source, especially by a balanced diet and by abstention from refined foodstuffs such as commercial sugar and white flour. It is common sense to see that, through keeping teeth clean and free of plaque by regular cleaning after meals and by avoiding sweets and sweet drinks, the problem of caries is tackled preventively.

Particularly impressive are the results of field research done by the Swiss doctor Roos on the harmful effect of sugar and white flour products. In 1930 nearly all the villagers in the high valley of Goms in Valais had good teeth. Twenty-five years after the opening up of the valley by a new road, the change in diet of the children had led to a catastrophic level of dental caries (see also Chapter 14.4 for increase in diabetes).

Teeth give earlier and clearer warning than anything else that something is wrong with the body's nutrition and needs correcting. As well as a balanced diet, good dental hygiene is of great importance. In addition to developing good habits at home, children should be encouraged to clean teeth at school as well.

After every meal and after eating sweet things, children should clean their teeth with a short-headed toothbrush. They should be taught how to use a toothbrush correctly, brushing briskly but gently with a rotary movement from the gums down (or up) on to the teeth and along the chewing surface. The gums should be brushed gently, too. After a snack that is not sweet, it is enough to rinse out the mouth with water.

15.2 Rickets

Rickets is an illness affecting babies which is caused by lack of exposure of the body to light. As it occurs chiefly in industrialized areas of the temperate zones, it is at the same time a disease of civilization. During the last century, living conditions among the industrial poor were so appallingly deprived that older children, too, were likely to get rickets.

Lack of light upsets the body's metabolism of calcium and phosphates and, if not treated, can result in severe bending of the bones, deformities and lowered resistance to disease. Acute forms are nowadays only to be seen in cases of grave neglect or congenital malfunction of the metabolism. Nevertheless rickets can attack all children if they are not exposed regularly to the light. Babies in their first winter are those most endangered and affected. Along with rickets, calcium deficiencies of the blood appear and these can be so severe that convulsions occur (hypocalcaemic tetany).

The beginning of rickets may be suspected when a baby starts to perspire increasingly over a matter of weeks without any other recognizable cause such as fever, drinking too much or wearing too warm clothing. A typical symptom is when the back of the head, hands and the soles of the feet become clammy. Further symptoms usually associated with an incipient lack of calcium are increased restlessness by day and night with no obvious cause, and signs of taking fright at little noises or even for no reason at all. These indications require urgent medical diagnosis. A thorough examination will make the situation clear at once.

Very occasionally there are babies with no early signs of rickets or tetany who are suddenly seized by convulsions. Pursing of the lips and the fingers becoming rigid can indicate a lack of calcium. Such cases require immediate clinical examination and treatment.

How Vitamin D works in the body
There is a progressive transformation of substance through the skin, liver and kidneys. Sunlight on the skin starts off the process. The liver produces a first stage of the activator (which only acts in abnormal conditions). The kidney reacts to the calcium content of the blood, assesses the amount of calcium required and allows the requisite amount of activator to be produced. In this way, a balance is established in the blood as a precondition for healthy bone-formation.

These processes should all be considered within the picture of the complete bodily environment. Each reaction depends on many others and they would all come to nothing without warmth and breathing. The "I" and the soul work upon all these events, and consequently we cannot regard the process as being purely mechanical (see Chapter 3.6 and 6.14).

Preventing rickets

There are several ways of preventing rickets:

1. The simplest method is prescribed by orthodox medicine and consists of giving 500 units of Vitamin D daily for all babies from birth until after the second winter. The vitamins are usually taken directly by mouth in tablet form. If the tablets are added to the baby's bottle, it is not certain whether all of the vitamin content will be taken as some of it can stick to the sides of the bottle. In commercially prepared baby-food, a small amount of Vitamin D3 is added in the proportion of 250-300 units per litre of the mixed feed.

2. A similar dose to the above is found in cod-liver oil which can be taken either in its natural form or in capsules. Cod-liver oil has the advantage that the Vitamin D3 was made in the fish's liver and not from ergosterol in the chemical laboratory. That is an important difference when taking quality into account. With cod-liver oil other substances such as Vitamin A are given at the same time, but this cannot be avoided. Cod-liver oil is not much harder to take than the tablets except that it has an unpleasant smell; this, of course, is avoided with the sealed capsules. Fear of contamination with heavy metals from polluted sea-water and other residues is unfounded with medicinal cod-liver oil as this is protected by controls. Remember that cod-liver oil is not vegetarian!

There are several brands on the market with names suggesting cod-liver oil, but they should be checked to see whether they are not an artificial substitute with vitamins added.

3. Those who prefer not to give Vitamin D pills — for reasons which we shall presently discuss — can take the following measures, bearing in mind that they should in any case consult their doctor for the baby's regular check-up at least every four weeks:

a) In temperate zones, expose the baby's head as often as possible to the blue light of the sky, beginning at the third week, for ten to fifteen minutes daily increasing to two hours and longer (see Chapter 11.3). If the city haze is not too thick, this will be sufficiently long in good weather to prevent rickets. See that the forehead is clear and that neither the eiderdown, blanket, veil, window-pane, or canopy intervene between the baby's face and the sky. Where possible, the forehead and face should be open to the sky immediately above. No ultraviolet light comes from a hazy sky near the horizon. Direct exposure to the hot sun is recommended only as long as the baby is carried in your arms, because it is only then that you can feel when it becomes too much for the child.

b) Breast-feed for at least six months. Breast-fed babies rarely get rickets while still at the breast, and never acutely. We have never observed a tetany (convulsions due to lack of calcium in the blood) during the time of breast-feeding. Both rickets and tetany can affect children after they have been weaned.

c) With bottle-fed babies be careful not to overfeed or underfeed. Over-fed children are more inclined to rickets because their plumper bodies require more Vitamin D. Underfed children on the other hand are more prone to tetany. Therefore do not try any experiments with milk-free nutrition or nutrition low in calcium. If the baby's consumption over a period is more than half a litre (17 fl oz) per day or less than 350 ml (12 fl oz), we recommend adjusting to between 400 and 500 ml (13-17 fl oz) per day as described in the chapter on nutrition (see tables on pages 243f, also Chapter 14.3 for feed recipes).

In countries where Vitamin D is already added to household milk, it would not be wise in our view to try to avoid taking milk. But take care not to give too many other nutritional sources of the vitamin.

Where bottle-feeding is concerned, it should be noted that phytin, a substance present in all cereals but especially in oats, makes calcium insoluble for nourishment and the calcium passes out again in the faeces. If a bottle-fed child receives enough light or Vitamin D, phytin from cereals will do it no harm as cow's milk contains enough calcium.

But if the child has insufficient light, there is a risk of calcium deficiency. This is one reason why we prefer the addition of almond purée, which is free of phytin, to the baby's feed for the first three months and only after that go over to cereals (see Chapter 14.3).

d) Motherly attention: take time to "shine upon" the baby and to play together, for loving human care provides its own hidden and health-bestowing light. We have seen rickets much more often where mothers have a job or when neither parent is at home. Few substitute-mothers can bring the warmth and interest to bear on a child which is really needed.

In addition to this loving care, the mother should have a regular routine of fresh air and sunlight for herself and her baby, always avoiding, of course, the worst extremes of weather and city surroundings which are simply not suitable for a child.

e) Medical treatment can be offered with a constitutional remedy to stimulate the "light-metabolism." The treatment includes external applications such as baths. When supervised by an experienced practitioner, these remedies rarely fail.

Particular care is needed where it is not possible to follow any of the above-mentioned recommendations, for then the risk of rickets is greater and one must be all the more alert. It may then be necessary to use Vitamin D tablets or cod-liver oil. Any decision should be made jointly by parents and doctor after looking at the particular situation.

Finally, it must be remembered that rickets is not just the result of a lack of Vitamin D; many factors are involved in its development and vitamin or hormone deficiency is only the final straw in a bad set of circumstances. The real solution to the problem lies in creating proper living and working conditions which enable mothers to obtain the right amount of light, air and warmth, and allow them to breast-feed and care for their children in peace and tranquillity. Merely prescribing tablets is no substitute — only a makeshift.

Part III

Education and Upbringing as Therapy

*Love does not rule
but shapes, and that is more.*

Goethe, *The Fairy Tale*

16 Fundamentals of education

16.1 Parental influences

The child's development depends enormously on the attitudes which mother and father adopt towards bringing up their children, and therefore parental influence is one of the first fundamentals of education. Looking at family structures today, we notice more and more how few children grow up with both father and mother: many live with only one parent or are exposed to emotional difficulties within the family. The reason for this is often that we adults put our personal problems before the welfare of our children. The types of personal problem which lead to separation and divorce frequently find an outlet in a struggle for the possession of the child. In this kind of struggle, it is quite common for both parties to maintain that their only concern is for what is right and just for the child. Rarely, in this situation, do parents recognize that it would be better for the child to be lodged with a neutral family than to be exposed to such wearing tension between two beloved and sought-after people.

Our starting point, therefore, must be to try to clarify the obligations and tasks of mother and father from the standpoint of the child. We begin with a scene from the consulting-room which may serve as an introduction to the whole question.

During a baby's general check-up, the mother suddenly asked the doctor which was better for the child in its early years: to be constantly with its mother, or for the mother to be happy and contented. The doctor did not understand at first what she meant. She explained that she had broken off her studies when the child was on the way. Now, although she wanted to do what was right for her child, she found her situation intolerable and was getting more and more depressed. She simply could not see why her husband could continue his life as before while, in her own case, she came under pressure as soon as she talked about continuing her studies, with people around her saying that she wanted to escape from her duty as a mother.

This mother's situation is merely one out of thousands like it, personal destinies which must each be assessed and resolved individually. All of them pose the same fundamental questions: how do you fulfil the role of being a mother? What part does the father play? What does the child expect of its parents? Finally each parent must ask, where do I stand in relation to this drama?

A number of studies of children in care have revealed what happens to children without firm human ties. The lack of these ties in the first three years of life, that is before children become conscious of their own self, leads to the most severe disturbances in body and soul. During a baby's first year in care, for instance, its development can come to a complete standstill for two or three months. Then the baby will cling anxiously to the various nurses looking after it. Finally its constant crying gives way to increasing apathy. Lethargy, whimpering, head-shaking, sleeplessness and proneness to infection appear and can often lead to death.

These signs show most clearly that the physical development of the human being does not depend entirely on heredity and good nourishment but also very much on the warm spiritual and soul attention paid to the personality of the growing child. If the baby's personality is not wel-comed, accepted and engaged, it cannot "come through," it cannot incarnate properly, and so the above-mentioned disturbances appear with serious consequences for both body and soul. This loving attention is no automatic activity which can be applied in the same way to every child; it develops out of the individual connection formed before birth between the child and the selected parents. The strength of connection here lies largely in the maternal and paternal instincts enabling the parents to welcome the as yet unknown being. This applies particularly to the mother who carries the child within her body, gives birth to it, and whose whole organism is linked for a time with that of her child. No one else can possibly be devoted to the child in quite the same way during these first decisive months of life. But does this relationship mean that the mother must be fettered to the child at all costs? Is there no way that the mother can get any sort of temporary respite? What is the task of the father, and how do grandparents, friends, aunts and acquaintances fit into the picture?

If you have ever taken over the care of an eight-month old baby because the mother urgently needed to be relieved for a time, you will notice that the child distinctly feels the change of people and things. It takes about a week for the baby to get used to the new mummy and her surroundings and to be as settled as he was before. When the real mother comes back, she will not be accepted by the child right away. It takes some time to reestablish the former relationship. Because the baby has no independent memory as yet, it still has no knowledge of its own identity. This awareness only develops when the child starts to refer to itself as "I" and so begins to form its own life of thought and memory. Up to this point, the child needs to keep seeing at least one intimate person and the same household objects around during the day in order to maintain a sense of continuity. At that early age, the child can experience self only through contact with the world. The more stable and lasting is this experience of self through the surroundings, the more strongly the feeling of self will be developed.

Interruptions and changes of surrounding such as a prolonged stay in hospital will disturb the growth of personality, especially if they happen frequently. For children this means the same as a grave identity crisis for an adult, the difference being that children lack the ability to work at it consciously. As a result, the child will feel insecure and will lack confidence in both self and the world at large in later life.

What should one do, then, in cases where it is unavoidable for parents to leave the child? It is a help to the stability of the child if a sudden change does not involve both the person or people mainly involved with it and the surroundings as well. At least one of these should, if at all possible, remain unchanged so that the child's situation retains some continuity. In some cases, we recommend that the new "nanny" should be brought into the familiar surroundings of the child at least one week before the departure of the parents, so that the disruption for the child is minimized.

What makes up the individual roles of father and mother? Does each have its own specific and different elements? How much can these elements be learnt and transferred to other people? After all the child reacts trustingly to every bit of loving attention, irrespective of who is giving it. Are "father" and "mother" not just conventional names for aspects of child-rearing which can be taken on by anyone?

This last question concerns us particularly in these times when we do so much consciously to free ourselves from received notions and situations. Belonging to a particular race, nation, family, class or sex is no longer the criterion for accepted behaviour. In this century, women especially have been fighting against the role in society assigned to their sex. Rudolf Steiner discusses this issue in the following way:

"It is impossible to understand a human being completely if one takes the concept of genus as the basis of one's judgment. The tendency to judge according to the genus is at its most stubborn where we are concerned with differences of sex. Almost invariably man sees in woman, and woman in man, too much of the general character of the other sex and too little of what is individual. In practical life this does less harm to men than to women. The social position of women is for the most part such an unworthy one because in so many respects it is determined not as it should be by the particular characteristics of the individual woman, but by the general picture one has of woman's natural tasks and needs. A man's activity in life is governed by his individual capacities and inclinations, whereas a woman's is supposed to be determined solely by the mere fact that she is a woman. She is supposed to be a slave to what is generic, to womanhood in general. As long as men continue to debate whether a woman is suited to this or that profession "according to her natural disposition," the so-called woman's question cannot advance beyond its most elementary stage. What a woman, within her natural limitations, wants to become had better be left to the woman herself to decide ... To all who fear an upheaval of our social structure through accepting women as individuals and not as females, we must reply that a social structure in which the status of one half of humanity is unworthy of a human being is itself in great need of improvement." *(The Philosophy of Freedom,* Chapter 14, pp. 204-5).

From the point of view of the child, what matters is not whether "being a father" is a male characteristic, or "being a mother" a female characteristic, but whether both parents offer the child the full range of human qualities needed for its development.

The more father and mother consciously adopt these qualities and make them their own, the more effectively they will promote the child's growth and development.

The terms "mother" and "father" have a twofold sense: a natural sense and an ideal sense. We shall try to show in detail how these two aspects relate to each other.

We become fathers by begetting and mothers through conceiving, carrying and bearing our children. The function of the father is to initiate the process of the child's becoming, and thereafter to watch over it. The father stands by the mother when she and the child are in need of external support. Male instincts incline him to fulfil this role: he is ready to act to protect, safeguard and provide for mother and child, and is affronted or ashamed if he is prevented or fails in this duty. The specific function of the father is to be *there,* both inwardly and outwardly, for mother and child. Outwardly it is possible for another person (say an older child or relation) to take over this function. But without the presence of the father, it is difficult to create that "protected field" in which the unifying bond of mother and child is fostered. It is the father who creates the secure haven in which all that is motherly can enfold. Freed from material wants and cares, released from occupational demands outside the home, the mother can devote herself all the more freely to her child and be available until it is able to stand on its own feet. Until that time comes, the mother should be able to stay with her child. Labour laws which provide a six-month leave for pregnancy and childbirth can be regarded as an important step in this direction. Through her maternal presence, she gives her child a feeling of trust and confidence in life. The specific function of the mother is thus to devote herself to her child and his needs and to be able to withdraw from all disturbing outward activities.

Looking now at the "ideal" aspects of fatherhood and motherhood, the devotion of both parents to a responsibility and a task held in common is by its very nature something beyond their own private and personal interests. In parenthood, we give without knowing whether we shall ever receive anything in return. Personal desires, needs and comforts are pushed into the background in order to meet the child's needs. As parents, we do all we can to respond to the demands placed on us by the child's helplessness.

Something of this impersonal selflessness is recognized by the child when it addresses its parents as "Mother" and "Father" (or "Mummy" and "Daddy"). These forms of address refer beyond what is merely personal to images and symbols of a profoundly religious quality. For children to call their parents by their Christian names thus deprives them of experiencing a fundamental pattern of relationship echoed even in our knowledge of the divine. For in the marriage between father and mother and in the child of their union, the interdependence and love between these three reflect the primordial principle giving rise to the very continuity of the world, a principle which finds its highest expression in the concept of the Trinity. It is of inestimable value for a child's later life if parents can give their children even a glimpse of this concept in the workings of their family life, an experience which will be remembered through life with gratitude no matter what the family's material conditions. Seeing, as a child, parents serve goals which are higher than mere personal interest can provide the individual with a standard of inner life and a model for a lifetime.

How does this picture of parenthood relate to everyday problems, as for example when roles are switched with the mother going out to work and the father looking after the house? How can it help the single parent? At what age does the child require more of the mother and at what age more of the father? How does our picture help parents to accomplish their task?

It is axiomatic that the "ideal" aspects of the maternal and paternal are interchangeable. The man can acquire the maternal qualities of intimacy and homeliness, and practise cherishing and caring; similarly, the woman can take her place fully in her profession or trade. What is important is that the two should complement each other, freely and without being forced. The tragedy of many young mothers is that they are quite ready to take on the task of motherhood to begin with, but soon find that they cannot adjust to the confines and limits of the household. This results partly from the limited structure of the small family in which the father is usually very much taken up with his work; but it is also due to the limitations of present-day education with its lack of training in deeper cultural values.

Finding oneself in this situation can raise fundamental questions: Why am I really discontented with my lot? Perhaps it is only because I cannot accept it freely. Perhaps I can apply myself freely in another direction? Can I find something to learn in this situation? What effect will it have on my child if I just put up with my situation? On the other hand what if I tackle my problems actively? Perhaps I could now take up things that I always wanted to do, like learning a foreign language or learning to play a musical instrument. I could make a start on something new seeing that I am so much at home. Am I using all the resources of help available to me, such as friends and neighbours, or grandparents who can mean such a lot to children? Or is there a elderly person who might be able to take the role of a grandparent?

Asking questions such as these can be a start to discovering a way out of the crisis through positive action or change. Of course some may reach the point of regretting that they ever started a family at all, in which case it is now time to take stock and work out these feelings in a way that takes everyone concerned into account.

What about the single mother? In the consulting-room, single mothers are always asking whether the child is missing out on something important because it is growing up without a father. Here it could be important to look around and see if there is anyone who could take on the role of father to some extent. It is even more important that the mother should see her situation positively.

Here is an example. A two-year-old child lived with his mother who had a job. She did not put the child out to a crèche but searched far and wide until she found a family who were willing to look after the child regularly. In this way a continuity of person and place around the child was maintained, and the child had both a Mummy and a Mum and called his foster-father "Daddy." In this way the maternal and paternal functions were shared amongst other people.

What about the child who was brought up by her grandmother because there was no father-figure, and the working mother performed the father role and was away from home a lot? Here it was the grandmother who took on the maternal role.

Even in the absence of a father, the child's relationship with him can be an important factor. The mother can create a picture of the natural father, taking every opportunity to talk about him and describing him as someone loved. The separation of the parents can be put down to circumstances beyond both of them. If she succeeds in creating a positive picture of the father, the child can actually experience something of the father's presence. Given this background, it will not be too hard to answer the sort of questions which the child may start to ask around the age of three or four. She can say that he is far away, is very busy, and cannot come because he is looking after another family that need him even more: "You have got Granny and me, and we don't need Daddy so much." The pre-school child accepts as a matter of course everything which the mother considers to be right. Problems arise for the child only when the mother says something which she does not really mean, or when she cannot accept her situation and is still harbouring resentment.

It is a good thing for the child without a father to have a male teacher at school for the child approaching puberty will increasingly seek some sort of relationship with a father-figure. The male represents more physical strength than the female, and boys and girls in puberty unconsciously look to the role-model of the man who stands firm, grapples with life's problems and masters them.

16.2 The child's temperament

The study of the four temperaments (sanguine, choleric, phlegmatic and melancholic) and their relationship to human health and character was handed down from the ancients in the writings of Hippocrates. But in modern times we have lost sight of many of these insights and become less and less able to use this approach in diagnosis and therapy.

"Temperare" means "to mix" and the word "temperament" therefore has to do with the mixing and balance of the bodily fluids and the corresponding attributes of the soul. The insights gained can be applied fruit-fully to medicine and education and, indeed, Waldorf education (see 16.6 below) uses a knowledge of the temperaments. In our discussion here, we have no intention of describing a rigid system of types in which people are instantly classified. The temperaments are rather to be regarded as aspects of the individual which offer both opportunity and danger: opportunity when they can be used to achieve a purpose; danger when the individual becomes trapped by their proclivities or weaknesses. In the case of education, which can to a certain degree affect a child's constitution, these insights can be used to help the individual to deal successfully with the peculiarities of his or her own temperament.

What do we mean in practice by the four temperaments? The three physical states of solid, liquid and gas, operate together with warmth in the human organism (see Chapter 1.4 and 3.6). Our bodily frame exists in the solid state. The complex biochemistry of our metabolism makes life possible in the liquid state. Our air-organism (see Chapter 3.6) expresses the soul in breathing, but also in the bodily fluids and even in the calcification of the bones. Finally our warmth-organism enables the "I" in us to act and realize our will.

The soul is involved with these four organizations, the balance and interplay between them giving rise to feelings of well-being or discomfort. If the solid element is predominant in the constitution the soul will tend to be heavy-hearted and gloomy. If however the airy element of the body is easily stirred the soul will be cheerful and light. These moods colour the soul's sense-activities, its perceptions of colour, form, scent and sound, and the feelings of pleasure or displeasure which arise.

We shall now take a closer look at each of the four temperaments in turn.

The choleric temperament

The choleric person appears somewhat pent-up and under pressure. Here the warmth activity is predominant. Napoleon was a prototype of this temperament: a somewhat squat figure with an imposing head, short neck, and short limbs in relation to a longer trunk. The choleric's gait is resolute and dynamic, generally stepping hard with the heels. The main characteristics are initiative, a readiness to act out ideals, persistence and stamina even to the extent of exhaustion, enthusiasm, intensity in everything undertaken, love of truth, punctuality. The choleric is easily roused if things do not quite go according to plan. Of course all these attributes can become negative if they are used for personal ends rather than idealistically. In that case ruthlessness, obstinacy and self-assertion take the upper hand. It is understandable that such purposeful people are to be found in positions of authority.

Choleric children are very strenuous to manage. They are characterized by flare-ups of temper, sudden changes of mood or emotional outbursts. They can rage, hit out, and even literally try to bang their heads through a wall. They can however shoulder responsibilities, stand up for other children, or try to rectify mistakes in a most exemplary fashion. In school they are always stimulating. They are usually the leaders in a class-discussion, they are pleased when their teacher singles them out to show the class something and they do not like coming late. On the other hand they are demanding and do not easily accept everything or always do what they are told.

The sanguine temperament

The sanguine type really feels best when surrounded by a circle of people. These children are open and interested in all that is going on around them and they have understanding for it. Their judgment is seldom formed on fixed principles, they do not normally harbour resentment and they like making new contacts. You can recognize sanguine children by the fact that they are always on the move and easily overspend themselves. This leads to them requiring more sleep at nights and an afternoon rest until well on into their school days.

In school sanguine children are generally popular as they are full of clever ideas. As adults, their stimulating conversation makes them valued and you like them because they always know you by name. The danger of this temperament is when gaiety leads to irresponsibility and a superficial "hail fellow well met" takes over.

Physically the sanguine child is of slender build with light fine bones, with strong curly hair and mobile expressions and gestures. The gait is inclined to be light and on the toes.

The phlegmatic temperament

People with a predominantly phlegmatic temperament have the ability to remain calm in difficult situations and to act even-handedly where a choleric has long since departed, slamming the door. Without their patience, faithfulness, equanimity and love of habit, as well as their exactitude in their work, no human society could exist. Among phlegmatic types are to be found ideal mothers and teachers: they are the pole at rest, they are not aggressive, always endeavouring to balance out, and they are exceptionally reliable. You can recognize the phlegmatic child often by their eyes full of wonder as they look out on the world. In the midst of hubbub they can sit there contentedly especially if they have found something to eat and are consuming it with relish. Phlegmatic children will not be drawn out of their reserve, least of all with a commanding tone designed to get them on the move, for then they settle down even more comfortably. They can easily drive their teacher to distraction when for instance they are still unscrewing the cap off their pen when the others have already written five sentences. This temperament becomes a danger when their calmness becomes a bore to others, their love of habit becomes pedantry and convention.

Physically the Phlegmatic is well-proportioned as long as a fondness for good food does not make them podgy. The gait is comfortable with the soles of the feet rolling along.

The melancholic temperament

Even in childhood the expressive eyes in the often narrow face of the Melancholic are striking. Experiences and encounters work on in these children for a long time, and they can still be weeping in the evening over something which happened in the morning. As a schoolchild and adolescent, they often feel misunderstood and not recognized for what they are. They readily identify themselves with tragic happenings and suffer particularly in surroundings marked by superficiality and indifference. When they grow up their positive attributes are: depth of thinking, earnestness and compassion. Melancholy becomes a danger when it becomes egocentric, self-centred, carpingly critical, or when the sense of justice becomes an envious comparison of self with others.

The build of the melancholic child is tall and slender, with often a slight looseness of the joints giving an "hung" appearance, accentuating the rather poor posture and carriage. The head is often specially well-shaped with deep-set eyes. the gait can be firm and measured, but also rather heavy.

From this brief description of the temperaments, it will already be clear that the individual's own inner activity determines whether temperament will come out as a positive gift or as a danger. Therefore the aim of education should be to strengthen character in such a way that the individual can learn to control temperament.

Education and temperament

Experience shows that it is no use trying to spur on a phlegmatic, or to restrain a choleric nor is it any use trying to tell a sanguine to pay attention, or trying to cheer up a melancholic with jokes. Usually the very opposite occurs of what one is trying to achieve: when goaded the phlegmatic will sink into even deeper calm, restraint will make the choleric even more angry, humour incite the melancholic to withdraw even more, while the sanguine will soon be as restless as ever. In dealing with the child's temperament it is better to work on the principle of like heals like. In school the order in which the children sit can be arranged so that children of the same pronounced temperament should sit next to each other. The cholerics can then thump each other, measure their strength against each other and so have the opportunity to grind down their temperaments slowly but surely. Unconsciously they experience the one-sidedness of their own nature and feel the need to counterbalance it in coming up against their fellows. Similarly when the phlegmatics sit together they bore each other and so feeling slightly uncomfortable they begin to wake up and become more active in stimulating each other and looking around at the other children. The melancholics need to find a friend in whom they can confide, are glad to have someone next to them who understands them and they then become more contented inwardly and more open to outward things. The sanguines soon get on each other's nerves and the ensuing discomfort makes them more reflective within themselves and so they become more biddable.

If the teacher succeeds in actively engaging the children's temperaments in the lesson, then the positive side of their temperaments will be cultivated and reinforced. Rudolf Steiner emphasized that teachers should train themselves to deal with all the temperaments, thus when dealing with a Choleric the teacher must be able to act with power and vigour, while at the next moment adjust to the rhythm and feeling of the phlegmatic.

There are a number of specific ways in which children of different temperaments can be helped in an educational context:

Choleric children are helped by learning to respect and value the achievements of great men and women. They should be set difficult tasks which tax their strength. It is good for them to learn to play a solo instrument so that their feeling of self-importance and pride can be applied to providing something beautiful for other people. The basic principle is to engage them positively without suppressing their surplus energy. If this energy is left unharnessed it will lead the children into mischief.

Phlegmatic children can be helped by having a stimulating friend whom the teacher can involve in set activities. The Phlegmatic will be induced to participate in a certain project much more readily out of love and interest for the friend than if there is a direct approach. The piano is an ideal instrument for this temperament. The tones are already latently there and need only to be struck. Furthermore the piano with its fullness and melodiousness meets the child's need for harmony and completeness. And it will be a useful achievement if the teacher can persuade the child to manage without snacks in between meals!

The sanguine child's flightiness is not to be overcome by reproach, threat or scolding. Much can be achieved if these children can be induced to persist with one thing out of love for an adult. They require a lot of personal attention and understanding for their difficulties which usually arise from a lack of perseverance. Their abilities are appropriately developed through learning to play a wind-instrument in the school orchestra. As they enjoy a wide variety of activities and quickly come to grips with them, they can be entrusted with a broad range of tasks. They should not be given too many sweet things which will only make them more restless.

It does the melancholic child good to learn how hard the lives and destinies of others can be. For these children the ideal teacher is one who has seen much in life. It helps the Melancholic's lonely soul-life to be allowed to sing — especially solos. The child can then express feelings outwardly. Learning a string instrument can also help. Unlike sanguine types, melancholic children should be allowed sweet things to eat regularly, and this will compensate for their somewhat "bitter" approach to life. They should not be burdened with food that is hard to digest.

Temperament and self-development in the adult

When discussing temperament in children, we are often asked whether adults can still work at their own temperament. This question can be answered with a definite "yes" even though it will no longer be possible to make such extensive changes as in the growing child.

A Choleric might ask forgiveness after an outburst of rage by saying: "You know I didn't mean what I said just now, it just came out." Or a Phlegmatic may remark: "Now do it nice and slowly, you know I cannot take things so fast." Both examples show how individuals are aware of how they react and how they begin to work at themselves. The aim of self-training is not to eradicate or suppress the choleric or phlegmatic in us, but rather to manage our characteristics in such a way that they are applied in a positive direction.

In his numerous lectures Rudolf Steiner gave a number of ideas for self-training, a few of which we shall mention here:

Cholerics who frequently allow an explosive nature to erupt seem to make no progress by merely getting annoyed with themselves for their lack of self-control and resolving not to get angry again. People with this problem should take on some small demanding daily task into which they can pour their concentration and energy. For example, they could saw up a piece of wood every day, or carry a loaded tray with one hand. By the daily practice of this kind of small peaceful task, carried out exactly as planned, they will find that they become more conscious of the use of their energy and acquire much better self-control.

Those who have too little of the choleric in them, who fit in too easily and who find it difficult to give an opinion or criticize until a matter is past altering, can do the following exercise for developing initiative: every day they should do something which they are not compelled to do by any exterior circumstance. It can be quite a simple thing like opening all the windows in the house at a given time, and then closing them again; or deciding to get up a quarter of an hour or half an hour earlier each morning and do something which they would really like to do. What is important here is that the will is not activated by any outward compulsion or necessity, but only by the person's own decision. If such exercises are practised regularly every day over a period, it will be noticed how much assurance and persistence have developed.

Sanguine people can train themselves in concentration by tackling quite uninteresting things and executing them punctiliously before going on to the next thing. In this way they will become aware of their tendency to be superficial and indifferent and will develop perseverance. If on the other hand, there is a noticeable lack of sanguine qualities (which is usually the case with Melancholics), the aim should be to train oneself in openness and cheerfulness by trying consciously to show an interest in everything that presents itself. For many people that is not so easy and requires a real effort of will. In carrying out this exercise the person concerned will have to look for an interesting slant to the matter in question. If this cannot be found at first it is a help to ask other people: "Why do you like this? How long have you been doing it?" Even people whom we have considered boring or insignificant can show an interesting side to their character when asked in this way. Questions always open up, stimulate and promote understanding. The ability of the sanguine type to find the right word for everyone can be acquired step by step and we become astonished at how much we have hitherto passed over unheedingly and how rich and colourful life can become through such an exercise.

The phlegmatic type can work on his temperament by taking on a particularly boring and uninteresting activity such as simply sitting in a room where nothing is happening. Soon boredom will make itself felt and then it becomes clear how much has been missed in life by passive behaviour. Another good exercise is to practise "love of truth" for, because of innate complacency, this type of character is liable to give utterance to a comfortable lie. Furthermore it is good to practise reviewing the day's events in reverse order. This exercise requires only five minutes at the end of the day, passing an inner eye over everything quickly and evenly. In this exercise, good and bad receive equal attention and the danger of savouring only pleasant experiences is avoided.

A person lacking in phlegmatic qualities of persistence and patience can acquire them by practising love and care of detail and making these an ideal. The task here is to become faithful to detail and to make perseverance into a positive force underlying all other abilities.

Melancholic people can exercise their temperament by watching tragic things, or things that fail to develop, in other people and in nature. By identifying themselves with the pain and suffering of others, they overcome the tendency to become self-centred. Through this exercise they will begin to feel an inclination to self-pity, introspection and brooding being transformed into helpful sympathy with other people.

The same exercise is good for the person with too little inclination to deep thinking and melancholy. It is good for such types to identify themselves with the problems and needs of others, taking them to heart and working at them as if they were their own.

16.3 Religion in childhood

In the consulting-room we have been struck time and time again by the depth of openness and trust in the eyes of very young babies. Anyone who has experienced this will never forget it. Picture, if you can, the general examination of a three-month-old baby. The baby lies undressed on the table with the mother waiting alongside while the doctor does various tests to see that all is in order. The doctor is about to begin when she notices that the baby is looking at her out of wide-awake eyes. The doctor feels that this gaze goes right into her innermost being. For babies fix their gaze upon the pupils of the observer, upon the "dark hole" where there is really nothing to see. This is where we encounter the "I" of another person most directly. So who is the child trying to encounter? What is it really looking at? How can a baby look so long, so steadfastly, so openly into the eyes of a strange adult? We only see such a gaze in later life at those moments when another person is confiding in us. The baby has this same openness and trust towards all people, a characteristic that will soon become visible in the rest of the child's behaviour as it grows: an uninhibited receptiveness to the world and an undiscriminating imitation of everything that happens in the surroundings. In the baby's eyes is expressed the touching and boundless expectation that it can depend on the adult for everything.

This acceptance of everything as a matter of course — this unspoilt sunniness that radiates out from young babies — begins to fade only when the consciousness of their own "I" appears. From then on repulsion and resistance begin to work into the child's further development. The unbounded ability to imitate begins to disappear (see also Chapter 13.4 and 13.9). In our early childhood we have all experienced this time of unbounded devotion, we have all had this primordial trust. In later life such an attitude to the world can be regained only by conscious effort, as when for instance we are totally absorbed in something; or when through religious devotion we acquire new trust in our existence and future life.

Often when we have remarked to parents how little children behave as if the world were thoroughly good and trustworthy, some respond by saying: "Should we not show the child as soon as possible that this is not the case, that the world is not perfect, but that we have to protect ourselves against the world and come to terms with it?" This question answers itself when we look into the expectant eyes of children. It is pointless to open a child's eyes to the want and misery of the world until its powers of mastering these problems have grown sufficiently. Premature awareness will lead to uncertainty and weakness, and later to doubting the meaning of one's own existence, a doubt which is hard to overcome. The parents' question ought really to be phrased thus: "What can we do to prevent this childish trust in the world from being shaken? What can we do to make the child feel there are adults who are trying to make things better. What can we do to strengthen the soul of the child to cope eventually with all that is not good in the world?"

Only during our babyhood is the mother there "as in paradise" doing everything for us, providing everything that we need, simply loving us because we exist. In later life such a relationship with another person is rare, and yet it resides in us all as a deep longing. This longing can become the criterion for developing a kind of loving that is not coloured by "I need you," "I want you for myself," "I want to enjoy having you and you me." Thus in childhood the noblest qualities for life can be engendered: trust in the evolution of the world, selfless love towards others, a true feeling of freedom (see 16.6 below). These qualities can be nurtured if our attitude and behaviour towards the child already embodies them, and if we foster the child's innate trust in us and in the world. In later life then the child will seek to develop these qualities further.

This view often provokes the comment that all this optimism seems very fine but it is extremely difficult to have any confidence or joy in the face of so many dangers in our modern world: the risk of nuclear warfare, the destruction of the environment, social disintegration and personal breakdown. All these are undoubtedly a part of our present reality but so is the experience that in a child's eyes there shines something which proclaims other realities. Through newspapers, radio and television, we are overwhelmed daily with problems of the moment, and thus easily lose sight of deeper issues such as the fundamental question of where mankind can draw strength in order to build up, to help and to further. Our concern should lead us towards an interest in those worlds from which the child's spirit and soul originate, out of which the child brings its ineffable trust and out of which flow those forces which inwardly accompany and strengthen man's true self.

So understood, religion is something that we can learn from little children. From them we experience the religious undertone that is common to all humanity. The unquestioning dedication of the child to its surroundings can become in the adult a religious devotion to the divine. But why is a consciously religious attitude so difficult for us today?

To begin with, our ability to relate the truths of the Bible to everyday life has declined in modern times. This decline must be seen against the fact that our consciousness is directed more and more to the things of the senses. Religious devotion is regarded as purely emotional and faith as hardly justified by a thinking person. Therefore it is objected that such unclear thoughts and feelings keep mankind in submission and allow us to be governed and directed.

Clearly a similar evolution has taken place in mankind at large as we find in the little child: imitative ability and ingenuousness decline as the consciousness of the "I" rises. Many people cease to pray at the stage when they begin to think for themselves and no longer merely accept what they are told. They begin to doubt and they no longer know to whom they should address their prayer. The fading of religious awareness in our times, then, results from the preponderance of thought and cognition in our modern life. It follows that a new religious consciousness can only come about through deepening and developing this very life of thought and cognition.

This links up with something which we have already touched upon in the introduction as well as our discussion of learning to think (see Chapter 13.4). Through thought we can apprehend the laws which operate in the natural world. In nature "thoughts" work directly as laws whereas our own thoughts and their execution as actions are separated. But it is this very shadowiness of our thoughts which gives us the possibility of freedom. After all it depends entirely upon ourselves, upon our own free decision, which thoughts we

put into effect and which not. We feel all the more free the more we understand and the stronger our will is to put into action what we have recognized as right. This freedom comes into play especially when we focus our thought beyond what is already created and on to projected notions and ideals. Ideals can only be effected through the human being when *he so wills*. As long as he does not do so they remain shadowy reflections. When however they become dedicated life ideals, ideals which can enthuse and motivate actions, then we experience the effectiveness of these thoughts in us as strengthening power. By devoting ourselves to an ideal, we experience directly that it is our will which lives in it and which helps the thought towards realization.

Just as there is a correspondence between our thoughts and the way that natural laws operate so too there is a correspondence between our ideals and the reality of the supersensory world. Natural science can make no pronouncement about the value of selflessness, peace or friendship; these cannot be measured quantitatively. But we can evaluate such things in philosophical, ethical or religious terms and, of course, the great world religions and philosophical systems are all based on a small number of important ideals. Through these, we become acquainted with a reality higher and more enduring than the transient world of the senses. Higher reality reveals to us not only the truth of natural laws but also truths connected with the soul and spirit worlds. The insights of Rudolf Steiner's spiritual science show that the forces which we invoke when we adhere to ideals emanate from beings who have no earthly incarnation.* In the Bible these are called angels, archangels or "the multitude of the heavenly host." Thoughts are thus not mere interpreters of an abstract world but bridges to a higher world and its beings to whom we humans may become devoted and allied.

In the spiritual world one being can live in another and reveal itself through another. This fact is borne in upon us usually when we begin to love another person. The community of friendship with a person, like the unity with a particular ideal, can be experienced as an increase in power. When Paul says: "Not I, but Christ in me" (Gal.2:20) he is referring to this potential union. Jesus, too, taught his disciples: "By this all men will know that you are my disciples, if you have love for one another" (John 13:35). And "For where two or three are gathered in my name, there am I in the midst of them" (Matt.18:20). Of himself he said: "I and the Father are one" (John 10:30). And again: "I have come down from heaven, not to do my own will, but the will of him who sent me" (John 6:38). All these sayings are evidence that things and beings in the spiritual world are not so separated from each other as in the temporal-spatial world in which we live.

If an individual learns to unite self with the supersensory world through thinking, then an attitude to life will establish itself, an attitude which may be called a religious one. The person will feel rooted in that supersensory world and no longer isolated or lonely. Feelings of trust and gratitude towards existence will be renewed, along a path of development which is in harmony with the laws of that higher world. As adults, we will then look with new confidence upon the development of our children, expressing a trust which has had to be achieved with difficulty. From this viewpoint, it then becomes possible for us to pray with our children with deep conviction and honesty, and to express in this prayer a real feeling of union with the sensory and supersensory worlds.

At present there are many people who are of the opinion that one should withhold religious upbringing from children in case they become brain-washed and lose their freedom of choice. But those who in childhood have not been able to experience qualities such as reverence, respect and devotion, have already lost a degree of freedom in not having been educated with regard to what is religious. They do not know that they lack essential human powers and it may be that later they will feel bitterly their lack of idealism. By contrast, those who succeed in arriving at an independent relationship with religious tradition will be able to find there an endless source of stimuli for inner development. They will also understand why in the field of reli-

* In *Knowledge of the Higher Worlds.*

gion, tolerance and absolute freedom of thought must reign.

Festivals and prayer

It is a common feature of our lives today that more and more people find it difficult to find meaning in the traditional religious festivals. For many, the festivals have lost their spiritual reality. The childlike acceptance of these festivals and the consciousness which accompanies that acceptance is being lost in modern society. Because of this, we wish to put forward some ideas which may help towards a new approach and a revitalization of these major events of the year's cycle.

In general terms, anniversaries celebrate a particular event in the past which we wish to commemorate. Birthdays, wedding anniversaries and remembrance days all reflect this. This is our way of remembering past achievements or victories, or of holding in memory the life and passing away of a beloved person. Then there are the great seasonal festivals, marking the cycle of the year. In ancient times, the solstices and equinoxes were all celebrated, and there were community festivals marking the arrival of spring, summer, autumn and winter. Associated with these were folk customs reflecting the principal events of the agricultural year: sowing and harvesting. Over the centuries, different regions and countries developed a worldwide variety of customs and practices to mark the course of the year. Some of these were re-interpreted to represent aspects of Christian faith.

Some of the great Christian festivals, like the ancient festivals before them, celebrate the passing of the year: Christmas and St John's Day mark the solstices of the sun, while Michaelmas and Easter mark the equinoxes. But more especially for the Christian, most of these festivals are also celebrations of particular events in the life and work of Christ. At Christmas we recall the birth of Christ, and in the Easter period, his death and resurrection. Whitsun commemorates the outpouring of the Holy Spirit. By their very involvement with the work of Christ, celebrations like these not only evoke the past, but also prepare for the future. In addition, they work as a living force for the whole world, not just for professing Christians, and allow every individual to be united with the guiding spirit of creation and evolution, that is, with Christ himself. To discover the way towards this union is the task of every adult and, as part of this process, through understanding the inner spiritual content of the great Christian festivals, we make these into moments of great spiritual reality. This is of vital importance in the education of the child. Through all the images and symbolism of each festival and in carrying out all the familiar customs and practices, the soul of the child will be nourished, so long as that spiritual reality is made present by the surrounding adults.

Of course the exact relationship of

annual festivals to the solar events will vary between the southern hemisphere and the northern hemisphere. This has led a number of people to propose that Christian festivals should always be tied to the natural cycle and so, in the southern hemisphere, be celebrated in direct opposition to the northern calendar. But, in practice, the seasonal events generally experienced in the southern hemisphere do not correspond exactly to those in the north, partly because the centres of population do not lie in the same latitudes and partly because of general geographic conditions. It should really be understood that, at their deepest level, the Christian festivals are more than just commemorations of Christ's life or celebrations of seasonal events reflecting what is happening in nature. Beyond this, they are festivals relating to the universal consciousness of man and as such should be celebrated universally even though this may mean that people in the southern hemisphere have to look harder to see the connection between the inner and the outer aspects. The essence of Christmas, after all, whatever the surrounding climatic conditions, is to think of all people on earth and, with our children, to celebrate our common humanity regardless of race, country or continent.

We should like to describe one example to show the kind of form a family festival can take. We shall choose the feast of Michaelmas on September 29 as it is one of those holy days which are not so often celebrated. In the Revelation of John there is an account of St Michael the Archangel's war with the dragon (Rev.12:7), a motif that plays a part in many legends and sagas reflecting the struggle of the soul as it contends with the evil in the world. How can the courageous spirit called forth by this struggle be presented to the child's experience? At this period of the year, too, we find ourselves at the beginning of autumn. The leaves are changing colour and starting to fall. In the stems of the leaves however we can already see the buds of the leaves of the following year. Again, how can we present to the child's imagination the promise expressed in the hidden buds when the leaves are dying and falling?

One possible approach to these ideas is to invite friends and relations to an "ordeal of courage." In the garden equipment is set up which will enable the children to display their courage: a high ladder, a see-saw, a sack or trough in which they have to probe blindfolded guessing what it contains (plants, sea-shells, mud and suchlike). For older children these ordeals may require a real self-conquest; for the little ones who are imitating everything the event may be more of a test for the mothers! A simple puppet show depicting the legend of St George and a few well-chosen songs on appropriate themes will contribute to the festival mood. Every year the ordeals of courage should be different and, as the children grow older, the tests should become harder: a tree to be climbed, a difficult expedition on foot in quest of something hidden. Perhaps the children will have to search for a hidden chest in which there are costumes for a St Michael and the dragon. All dressed up they come back home and can stage a little impromptu play showing the struggle with the dragon. In this example what matters is that the content of the religious revelation is presented in such a way that the children can combine the relevant experience with some sort of activity.

In the same way the mood of expectation before Christmas can be

Figure 50. A prayer, song or blessing at bedtime.

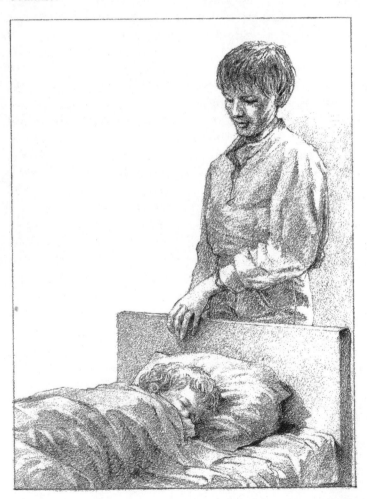

celebrated; by rehearsing a Nativity play through Advent which will finally be staged on Christmas Eve, the arrival of the feast-day is given quite a new emphasis. Epiphany, Lent, Easter, Ascension, Whitsun and St John's Day can all similarly be brought with meaning into the child's experience.

It is important that the adults themselves endeavour to enter deeply into the spirit of the festival and do not simply "get something up" for the children. It is also important that the framework or pattern of the event should be the same every year, consisting of special activities, songs, Gospel-stories and related customs. Children love and need these repeated customs for the cultivation of memory and will. But if the festival degenerates into a formal routine without inner involvement and effort on the part of the adults, then it will lose its soul-substance and become empty.

In the religious upbringing of the young child, another meaningful element is the cultivation of the time between waking and sleeping, that is to say between the world in which the soul of the child dwells during the day and that other world where the soul abides during the night. Here by means of a song or a prayer a mood of reverence can be created which enables the soul of the child to come to rest, raising it for a brief moment above everyday things. Children love such moments even though they may not understand the content of the words. Parents that we know used to say the following prayer every evening with their children:

From my head to my feet
I am the image of God.
From my heart to my hands
I feel the breath of God.
When I speak with my mouth
I will follow God's will.
When I see God
In Father and Mother,
In all dear people,
In animal and flower,
In tree and stone,
No fear shall I feel
But love will fill me
For everything around me.

James was two and a half years old and he had just learned to say "I." He now joined in the prayer and his enthusiasm grew from line to line. After the point at which father and mother were mentioned he would say after each word: "me too" and was only happy when the parents at the end of the prayer added "yes, and in James too."

Christian, two years old, loved to repeat the lines after his parents but he always left out the line where fear was mentioned. To compensate he repeated the previous two lines twice: "animal and flower, animal and flower, tree and stone, tree and stone." At the end he was so happy that he would jump up in bed and with the words "good, good!" throw himself down on to his pillow.

These instances do not mean that we can only start praying with children when they have learned to speak. Moments of reverence in the morning and at night can be observed by parents in the presence of their babies and very young children. Verses and prayers for these moments can be found in *Prayers and Graces* (see the Bibliography) together with a number of graces for meal-times.

To come to an understanding of the world of angels is important for children. Guidelines can be found in *Our Spiritual Companions* by Adam Bittleston (see the Bibliography). To know that every individual is accompanied by a guardian angel and every child in particular is protected by him can be a great support and comfort. The objection is often made that accidents and cruelties do happen, and the question then arises: why does the angel not protect in these cases? We can only reply that every day innumerable miracles do happen when accidents and cruelties are warded off. To be aware of this and to be alert and thankful brings us nearer to the world of angels. The guardian angel only allows those events to come to the individual which provide a way to learn and grow, and which are related to personal destiny.

Coping with death

Well before puberty, around the age of nine or ten, the child can experience a deep and real questioning of his own existence and begin to search for a feeling of what death signifies. For instance, in a family of five children the grandmother had died.

The father solemnly told the children about the last events in the hospital. All were listening attentively. The difference in each child's attitude could be seen clearly, showing what stage of maturity the soul life of each had reached. While the four-year-old was soon back in the sandpit and lost in play, the nine-year-old took everything in very attentively and clearly realized that she could not be sad in the same way as the adults. Deep inside, she knew that Grandmother would not come back and had died but she could give very little expression to this feeling. The reaction of the twelve-year-old was quite different. As the father was speaking she remembered her last meeting with her grandmother. It had been during an illness when the grandmother had looked after her lovingly. Now, as she remembered, her eyes filled with tears. Grandmother would never come again to comfort her during an illness. Where had Grandmother gone? The inexorability and yet also exaltedness of death remained in her soul for days. She felt in the face of this mighty reality both disquiet and trust at the same time.

Children are realists and take the world and the event of death as they come. It largely depends on the attitude and emotions of the adults whether meeting with death has something dramatic about it or not. If the anniversary of the death of a loved person is celebrated with the children as that person's "heavenly birthday" they will learn something important. They will come to see that a person's being has a visible and an invisible existence. They learn that we can meditate on the person who has died, their habits and characteristics, and can rejoice in them. Through regularly celebrating such heavenly birthdays, children will see that the spiritual world with all its beings projects into the visible world. To give another instance, in a family of six children one child had died early. His heavenly birthday was always a special festival when the family did something special. Even the visit to the grave had nothing oppressive about it. The grave was cared for and a prayer was said. At mealtimes stories of the child's short life were told, and it was not distressing when the mother was often moved to tears. If the event of death can be experienced as something belonging to life, something solemn and yet serene and trust-inspiring, then it will bring into everyday life an element of true piety which can contribute something important to religious upbringing.

16.4 Punishment and reward

Many of the questions facing parents are concerned with punishment and reward which are opposite extremes of a whole range of educational measures including: yielding and resisting, promising, asking, distracting and threatening. We regularly get stories like the following, listed at random:

"My child (four years old) stole something from me."
"My two and a half year old is so aggressive that I slapped him once or twice. Will it do him any real harm?"
A five-year-old says as confidently as his elder brother: "It wasn't me!" But the mother knows that he is lying. What should she do?
"I think that children ought to be praised or rewarded every day — that strengthens their feeling of their own value."
A three-year-old yells: "I won't" and brings his mother to the end of her patience.
Another child in a temper kicks in a window pane.
A child barely three years old picks up a special flower-vase that he has been forbidden to touch, and now it lies broken into bits.
Although they have been called twice to come to lunch, one of the children still has not appeared at table.
"We often have quarrels over the pudding although everyone gets enough."

Usually, stories like this are brought to us with the question: "What is the right thing to do in such situations?"

Hardly any subject touches so centrally upon the problem of human social life and development as that of punishment. In the Old and New Testaments we read of the God who judges and punishes and of the Last Judgment. Does man need the threat of punishment in order to strive for good and to turn away from wrong? Is not love of goodness sufficient?

To act in harmony with our environment is something which has to be learnt. We help the child to learn this harmony from babyhood onwards, by playing together so that it learns to grasp and release objects, by weaning from the bottle to the cup, by teaching how to eat with a spoon or to put on clothes and shoes. All these skills have to be acquired laboriously through repetitive practice. After a while the child begins to use a spoon properly, gets its arm into the right sleeve unaided and no longer curls up its toes when putting its shoes on.

Through learning all these little

routines of daily behaviour, the child gradually acquires greater and greater assurance in its environment. But at the same time these routines form habits and customs which set certain limits to the child's development. Of course all this happens at a time when the child cannot decide independently what or even whether it wants to learn. Therefore parents cannot ask *whether* they ought to influence their child's will but rather *how* and to what end they should help and influence.

Just as they must set clear guidelines to prevent toddlers from playing with a hot iron, from falling downstairs, from pulling the saucepan full of soup off the stove, or scattering oatmeal all over the carpet, in the same way parents must help their children through all the troubles of their school days and later with important decisions in which the child cannot yet foresee all the consequences.

In the end it boils down to this: we give direction to the child's as yet undirected will, for the child cannot truly direct its will until feelings and thinking have matured. The educator, then, must act as proxy for the personality of the child until it "comes of age." In the educator the desire to be the boss, the demand for absolute obedience, threats such as "just you wait till *I* come" are as out of place as an attitude that lets the educator be tyrannized by the child through the adult's unwillingness to "influence." Education, then, takes on a different aspect at different stages depending on the age and maturity of the child.

"Punishment" at pre-school age should simply mean that we let the child experience how *we* put the matter right. All learning at this stage is from the example set.

At school-age, as well as putting right what was done wrong, we can explain things to the child who can now help to think out how the damage can be repaired. There is however no point in appealing to the child's conscience until the inner life is developed deeply enough. That is hardly ever before the child is ten years old (see 16.6 below). If we start to preach before that stage we simply devalue the meaning of important words and contribute nothing to solving the immediate problem. Even later than this, appealing to conscience does not help very much unless some indication is given of how the damage or wrong can be rectified.

In puberty and adolescence, punishment should become a sense of failure in something which the youngster has laid upon self, while the adult should adopt a more advisory and helping function. The youngster will feel punished by failure and rewarded by success (as does the adult, too) and so tries to act in harmony with environment, at the same time setting personal aims in learning and in work against which to test and train self. If a person has to be punished as an adult for breaking the law, in most cases it is because the individual's development has suffered severe disturbances.

Against this background, let us return to some of the situations raised above to see how they may be dealt with.

Punishment

Let us look now at some possible attitudes to punishment in the incidents referred to above:

1. The larger broken bits of the vase which the child has smashed are carefully gathered up by the adult. The child helps to sweep up the smaller bits and tip it all into the dustbin. The mood all the while is serious but not unfriendly. Perhaps the parent will say: "A pity about that lovely vase — but now we shall take care that it won't happen again," and she removes similar objects from the child's reach.

2. In the case of the smashed window-pane, a piece of cardboard or a curtain is put over the hole and left for several days to remind the child of the damage. The mother may say: "We can't see through there any more but in a few days we'll have another pane put in." She will think through how the situation arose leading up to the event and she will reflect how she could have acted differently.

3. All hot and bothered, the child arrives fifteen minutes late and breathlessly explains that he had to finish his game of football. The child shows that he knows he ought to have come punctually but he really wanted to finish his game. That is understandable, and so the matter can be ended by the mother simply saying: "I'm glad you've come after all, I thought we'd have to eat without you."

This is not the same as a case where the children out of habit pay no attention to what they are told. Here they will simply have got used to being called several times to meals and only come when they feel like it. Things have gone so far because of the adult's own inconsistency that the line has to be drawn in the form of a threat: "Tomorrow if anyone comes late to the meal after I have called once, and once only, they will have to eat alone." Of course such a threat must really be carried out the next day.

4. The four-year-old who takes money out of the drawer usually does it because she has often seen her mother doing it. She is simply imitating, not stealing. It is the same with the boy who "steals" toys: he has not yet learnt that the world does not belong entirely to him. So when the child is going home after a visit an adult should help him put the friend's toys back in their place.

5. How do we deal with a situation where children quarrel or misbehave during meals, climbing up on to the chairs and table in spite of the mother telling them to behave? The problem here is that the mother's word has lost its authority. It may be that the parents have often been indulgent and have laughed at their children's other tricks, or that one of the parents has said to the other: "Never mind, let him do it!" Parents can

usually regain control in such a state of affairs only by recognizing that the cause of misbehaviour lies in their own lack of consistency and by rectifying their own attitude.

6. What if a five-year-old tells lies? And he knows that he lied. At first the parents show that they are shocked. But then they realize that the child really wishes that he had not done it and the child will sense the adult's insight by the change in response. With older children, parents can discuss how to make amends by some small pleasurable act towards the person who was hurt by the lie.

We shall now look at the effects of punishments which with hindsight may appear unjust. Here it is important to remember that a child who is left on its own and misunderstood after an incident will retain a deep sense of insecurity for a long time (see also Chapter 18.6).

And what about the possible effects on the child of an injudicious smack? Parents who frequently let fly with their hands should realize that, whenever they let themselves go, they are behaving just like their wild unruly child. They should decide to set the child certain agreed limits and in this way avoid exposing the child defenceless to their own spontaneous emotions and temper which can only have a harmful effect. The fright associated with this sort of incident affects a child badly at a deep organic level. Furthermore the child experiences a bad example which has no bearing on the matter in hand. When the child gets a chance, it will then imitate the parents and hit a smaller weaker child, thus passing on the injustice which was done. Perhaps as an adult, the same person will wonder why their hand is so ready to strike.

Reward

Now some illustrations of ways in which adults can offer reward:

1. "When we get to the top, there will be some juice for everyone." This will cheer up the tired members of the family on a hill-climb and it is the kind of reward that relates directly to the effort beforehand and to the goal achieved.

2. "If you're quick getting ready for bed, there'll be another story." That too is right, because otherwise there would not be time for the story.

3. "If you'll go and get the bread for me you can buy yourself an ice-cream as well." Here there is no connection between the action and the reward. But it would be different if the situation had developed as follows: "John, please go down to the shops on your bike and buy me some bread." John hates to stop work on the model aeroplane that he is making, but he goes without a fuss. When he gets back, he sees how glad his mother is because he helped out. And on going back to his bedroom, perhaps he finds a new brush for painting his aeroplane, as a surprise present.

4. And what about praise? Praise and affirmation strengthen a child's

sense of his own personality. While experiencing pleasure over something in which she has succeeded, the child learns something about the effects of her actions. Exaggerated praise, however, comes as a surprise to a child in a situation where the action came naturally and was completely in character. Overpraise here would make the child re-examine the action and realize that it could have been performed less well. This distancing of self from action is not good at pre-school age.

5. When a child has an earnest wish, this should be treated seriously. It may be that her toy shop needs a hinge for the door and this is required urgently. At other times the child should have to wait for a birthday or for Christmas, because "we might manage it by then." Or in some cases it may be advisable to transform the wish, as for instance when the eagerly desired gun becomes a bow and arrow. A child's special wish should never become a bargaining chip or used for punishment or reward.

6. Is "earning money" a suitable reward? If we pay our children for household tasks such as washing-up, clearing-up or shopping, we are cultivating a wrong social attitude. We are training them to think that we do work for our own material advantage and not to help others and to bring them pleasure. Furthermore, the children will use their money to buy things that they think they will not get from their parents anyway, and so come to the view that everyone has to look out for himself and that nothing can be expected from anyone else. On the other hand if children know that their own needs and wishes will be registered by their parents and that their own work is useful to others then the basis will be laid for a different social attitude: we serve others with our work and others interest themselves in our needs. Our present-day attitudes based entirely on self-serving egoism might then gradually be transformed into a more sharing social attitude. This would of course affect the whole structure of our working world.

To summarize our discussion of punishment and reward, we have to see that both can have bad effects when administered badly. Excessive rewarding leads to a selfish attitude to life. Things are no longer done for their own sake but because of the recognition, honour or financial profit which they bring. Ambition, envy and selfishness are engendered. Excessive punishment leads to the attitude that to make mistakes is wicked and so one must be "good" and not make mistakes. This attitude cannot recognize that it is man's prerogative to learn through experience, to work at mistakes and imperfections, indeed to be allowed to make mistakes. Instead the attempt is made to create an appearance of infallibility and moral perfection which is doomed to failure, for it is not possible to become fully human without mistakes, errors and ordeals.

On the other hand, avoidance of all reward and punishment and making a premature appeal to the child's judgment will lead to a loss of orientation, instability and indecisiveness in later life.

Finally, it should be remembered that every error or misbehaviour on the part of a child can be the starting point for a valuable lesson designed and taught by the adult. Wherever the child can be shown how to make amends in a suitable way, another step forward in the child's development will have been achieved.

16.5 Sex-education

Understanding sexuality

Nowadays many people refuse to accept "moral" laws and conventions imposed on them by religion and society especially in their attitude towards everything that has to do with procreation. This is a sign of modern man's increasing independence and responsibility for his own actions. It follows that not only does the child require "sex-education" but that the adult, too, must determine personal actions with regard to sexuality much more than before. No longer can we hold blindly to rules, commandments and prohibitions, without deciding about them for ourselves.

Here we shall begin with observations which can help us to understand sexuality itself and then go on to discuss possible ways of approaching the subject in conversations with children.

The sex of the human being is determined genetically at conception. But every new organism has the initial potential of both male and female development. The gonads develop in a hermaphrodite form in the embryo until the sixth or eighth week when they become differentiated into either male or female. Further development of the abandoned sex stops at this point.

What happens to the growth forces that are no longer required to build up the organs of the abandoned sex? In Chapter 13.9, we discussed how growth forces are transformed into thought energy. Rudolf Steiner's research indicated also that the growth forces released by unisexual development become engaged in the development of the cerebrum. Once this has matured, only a small proportion of the building forces are required for regenerating the nerve-system and the greater part is available for thought activity. This insight into human growth throws light on the fact that development of the reproductive organs takes place simultaneously with that of the cerebrum. We may also find the same events patterned in the story told at the beginning of the Old Testament where the separation of the sexes coincides with the knowledge of good and evil. The "Fall of Man" may, then, be an image of that early stage in our development at which the division into the two sexes also marks the emergence of our ability to distance ourselves intellectually from the world, to stand back, observe and reflect.

Significantly, the English word "sunder" meaning "to separate" is related etymologically to the word "sin." The reality is better described in terms of "separation" or "splitting" and the word "sin" has unfortunately come to be associated with fear, compulsion and manipulation. These are not necessary to a knowledge of good and evil. It may be asked why animals do not develop a similar consciousness of thought as they, too, are divided into two sexes. But in their case, the released intelligence is closely bound to the organism. The instinctive behaviour of animals is much wiser and more perfect than that of humans who have first to find the right way of doing things. In animals, there is no conscious separation of self and world. Their integration with their surroundings is directed by wisdom and their lives and behaviour are at one with nature. But humankind is destined to a dual separation: from the opposite sex on the one hand and on the other from the world and its needs and demands. The human being is an individual striving for truth. Only humans suffer this dual separation which must be overcome in either of two ways, both of which are described in the Bible.

Full humanity is recovered in the sensory world by the physical union of the two sexes. The sanctification and guarding of this sexual love is described in the Old Testament. Strict rules of behaviour and marriage laws served to elevate sexual urges to a level worthy of the human being at a time when the individual's capacity for thought was not yet sufficiently developed. The abandonment of polygamy meant that sexuality was no longer lived out in a group but became individualized and took place on a personal level between *one* man and *one* woman.

Love between man and woman, although based on the individual, was still subject to the laws of the group. From ancient times, those who broke the sexual conventions were cut off from the social structure and marked with guilt and shame. Our present-day ideas of morality still tend to reflect this ancient tradition and not be dictated purely by individual circumstances, which gives rise to a great number of tensions. Conflicts are created when people have very strong but not necessarily well-founded views about what is sexually permissible or not. Rising above social, racial and ideological barriers, what unites two people can only really be judged by themselves and criteria for "sin" based on received social attitudes no longer apply. A morality based on the individual will find "sin" only where the sensual and the soul-spirit do not work together, that is to say that when the physical and emotional love-life is lived primarily only to gratify personal lusts and there is no search for the other's being in the physical union. The "I" strives towards what is enduring and indestructible for that is its nature. Responsibility and faithfulness are its qualities. Sexual intercourse without involvement of the "I" becomes merely selfish pleasure-seeking and thus an activity sundered from the true being of the individual. But where there is a true meeting, a true finding of each other, that experience lives on in an enduring and indestructible way.

We find the connection between creative thought and the physical act of procreation expressed in language. In Hebrew, for example, the same word "yalad" is used for *to know* and *to procreate,* a homonym which is carried over in older translations of biblical texts into Greek, Latin and English. Freudian theory of the sublimation of the sexual urges only obscures this vital connection. The forces related to the reproductive organs are not "sublimated" but, freed from the work of growth, become available for the cultivation of our life of thought. If, in adolescence, these forces are thoroughly engaged in an absorbing interest in the world and humanity, this will help the young person not to be led compulsively by sexual urges.

The second way for mankind to overcome dual separation is through cognition. Through cognition we achieve spiritual union with the world and our fellow-men and so conquer the separation inherited from our birth. The path of cognition is the path to inner freedom. In the biblical terms we have already discussed, we overcome sin by freely knowing good and evil. It is this freedom which is described in the New Testament: "and you will know the truth, and the truth will make you free" (John 8:32).

Neither of the two ways which we have described excludes the other. A sensual or passionate relationship between a man and a woman may well develop in depth when both individuals really learn to know and appreciate each other at a spiritual level. Indeed unless this takes place the union is doomed to failure. This is why the modern liberal outlook on sexual matters has not much helped our social relationships; instead, the problems of living together have become more difficult and insoluble.

Our social attitudes depend a lot on how we regard ourselves, our fellow human beings and the unconceived human being. The much discussed question of birth-control and family planning is involved here (see Chapter 10.2). Through sexual union we give a third being the opportunity to enter existence and so we connect with human souls who are about to incarnate and who need us. We decide to accept them or exclude them according to our circumstances and outlook. A sexual relationship which takes no account of the unconceived child acquires a selfish character, and where this selfishness becomes predominant then irritability, discontent, insensitivity and moodiness assert themselves. Of course the purpose of a partnership between a man and a woman will not always be to bring up children! It can be the sharing of a common activity or the realization of a common goal. The more a relationship is founded on motives which are above purely personal wishes and interests, the more beneficial it will be. Today we are almost entirely free in the way we form our relationships with the opposite sex and conduct our married lives. Accordingly what we have said would be misunderstood if it were construed as pontificating on what is permissible and not permissible (see Chapter 10.2 on birth control).

We shall end this discussion by looking briefly at the differences between male and female on the soul level. The physical differences between man and woman are obvious but the specific differences between male and female soul attributes remain subject to debate. First, though,

we realize that there must be a fundamental difference between the soul-life of a man and that of a woman. The forces which in the man are tied to sperm production and to the function of the male reproductive organs are available to the woman for thought activity. Conversely the man's soul-life is largely determined by the released forces which in the woman are engaged in the monthly ripening of the ovum and the building up and breaking down of the mucous membrane (endometrium) of the uterus. The dynamics of the functions of both organ systems are entirely different. Thus we can see that the soul-life of the man and that of the woman must be differently affected by the reproductive forces freed from their bodily functions. The woman's varied, enthusiastic and creatively stimulating life, her way of reacting impulsively and emotionally, her ability to digest impressions flexibly: all these are related to the transformed male reproductive forces. These soul characteristics correspond to the rapid and mobile qualities of the spermatozoa. By contrast, the man's characteristic ability to think abstractedly and to concentrate on one thing more easily, as well as his greater equanimity of feeling, derive from the forces which in the woman are used in the more peaceful ripening of the ova. At the same time the man's soul-life is more shut off from his surroundings and is by nature less variegated than that of the woman. The man does not get emotionally upset as easily as the woman and reacts more slowly and thoughtfully. Physically and emotionally, the two sexes are polar opposites and so can stimulate and compensate each other in many respects. Spiritually, however, each individual is a full human being with complementary sex-characteristics of soul and body, and the more freely we can stand above these the more our actions will bear the stamp of true individuality.

Practical aspects of sex-education

Here is a common family situation: the children are five, eight, ten and eleven years old, and the next child is expected. Many family conversations centre on the coming baby. Will it be a little brother or sister? What will be its name? When will we be allowed to take it for a walk? And so on. All the children know that the new baby is cosily tucked up inside their mother's body and is growing there safely, and will be born when it is ready. The children ask lots of questions but their questions are all very different. The oldest wants to know exactly how the baby manages to come out of the mother's body when it is ready and whether it starts to grow right away. The youngest on the other hand is only interested in how things are in heaven and in what the soul does until the body is ready for it to live in. The eight-year-old is fascinated with the idea that there might be twins; otherwise she does not ask about anything in particular. Much that is discussed together as a family emerges when the two youngest are playing with their dolls. Almost every day the mother hears that there is a wedding and a child is born, and of course there are often twins.

The important point in all these conversations was that the parents answered only questions which the children were asking themselves and in which they were really interested. Generally speaking, everything you explain which is not asked for will turn out to be a dead weight on the soul of the child and may disturb the thoughts and feelings about the question of the child's own origin.

One day the ten-year-old secretly showed his mother a piece of paper which he had brought home from school. On it was an obscene drawing and an equally unpleasant rhyme. The mother said calmly: "I don't think that's nice at all. It's good that you showed it to me, but now I should like to throw the bit of paper away." The matter ended there. When the boy saw that his mother did not make a fuss like his teacher (who had turned scarlet and made the class stay in after school), he was greatly relieved. Now he knew this was something to be avoided like other things that are unpleasant and that the fuss at school was unnecessary. At supper time the father told the children how he and their mother had got to know each other and how much they had looked forward to having lots of children.

The following examples of behaviour in young children are typical of many told by parents. Playing at doctors in the kindergarten, the five-year-old discovered that it created a great stir when he showed other children his penis. In another inst-ance, a shocked mother reported that when she went into her little boy's room, he was lying on his little playmate and told her with pride: "We're playing at man and woman in bed!" Games of this kind are mostly played by children between the ages of three and eight, that is to say, at the age of imitation. When we hear such stories we begin by asking the parents about possible examples of this behaviour in video, television or in their ordinary surroundings. Usually it turns out that the children are neither sexually precocious nor depraved, but that they quite simply absorb, play and imitate what they have seen in their surroundings. Therefore the most important part of what we call sex-education is the example set by the parents — that is to say the way in which they them-selves speak about the subject and how they behave. If situations such as we have described arise they can be met either in the way in which the mother did with her ten-year-old or they can be played down or treated with humour. Complexes or feelings of guilt only come about in children if the grown-ups react unnaturally and get worked up and do not know how to deal with the situation. One thing is certain, the more fuss the adults make about this type of incident, the more often it will be repeated, for children love it when they attract the attention of the adults. If the adult does not react in a positive way or denies the child sufficient attention, the child will try to force the adult's attention by this kind of provocation.

The story of the stork bringing babies is an image of the as yet unembodied soul seeking to come to earth. In former times these images were more easily understood but if today adults use them when talking to children, they should first try to acquire some insight into the truths they are describing. Otherwise it is better not to talk in such terms at all. If asked, parents may simply say that they know nothing about life before birth. Or else they should find some-one who can speak to the child about these things.

It poses difficulties for children if the conversation is kept purely on a biological level. Children feel this cannot be the whole truth and they may take in the details without being able to digest them inwardly. Curios-ity is initially assuaged but the ques-tion of origin is not really answered. There are also many children who keep their thoughts to themselves during talks on this subject by their fellow-pupils or parents and refuse to join in.

Adolescents often ask about the pill and other contraceptive methods. Many young people's magazines propagate the view that the pleasures of sex should be kept quite separate from a possible pregnancy and that this is quite normal. If this subject is discussed, young people should be made to feel that this conflict and its resolution are matters ultimately for their own decision. Boys must become aware of their responsibility towards their girlfriends, towards the unconceived child, and towards themselves. And of course the same responsibilities are borne by girls.

It is important for young people, too, to be aware of the more fundamental differences between the biology of man and woman. A woman cannot influence her monthly cycle and the development of the ovum which follow their own strict rhythm dictated by nature. With a man, however, the production of semen depends on the frequency of ejaculation and this can to some extent be consciously controlled. Through concentrating his interests in other directions, the man reduces his production of semen and the forces thereby released can be employed on a cognitive level. Young girls should be aware of their responsibility in this respect as the young men are much influenced by the way in which girls show their love and interest.

As adults, we can help young people to see how wonderful it is that these questions of sexual responsibility are now largely within our freedom of choice owing to progress in scientific knowledge. But freedom means neither that we simply follow our natural urges nor that we submit to strict conventions and moralities. Freedom is deciding responsibly what is right for our own situation.

In such talks with young people, they will not on the whole betray their own idealistically coloured and delicate love-experiences. Often they only ask questions to see how the adults react. They may have had experiences which they find in stark contrast to what they have read in their magazines. Then it is all the more reassuring when the adult adopts an honest open stance, neither excessively permissive nor shocked and horrified.

A sixteen-year-old boy casually asked his biology teacher (a woman) as he was leaving her classroom, "Tell me, is it actually harmful for a woman's body to take the pill?" "Yes," was the short answer. "Mm, I see, thank you." End of conversation! Exact explanations were to be found in the appropriate books but what mattered here was an assessment of the facts by someone whose judgment was respected.

With so much public airing of sexual matters these days, many young people harbour secret doubts as to whether they are normal in regard to their own sexual feelings and behaviour. This is especially the case where they may know that among their friends there are close relationships involving sexual intercourse. They need to know whether it is abnormal at their age to have no desire for complete sexual union but to want love on a more spiritual-soul level. We have repeatedly found this in talks with sixteen-to eighteen-year-olds who tell us that they prefer waiting until they meet someone they wish to "know" fully and with whom they would like to bring up children. They are always greatly relieved to hear that this is quite normal.

If adults are fully aware of the connection between "knowing" and the reproductive forces, they will do all they can to further the soul-life of the growing child: music, handwork, painting, botany, zoology, other cultures and people, ecology. All these provide abundant food and areas of activity for the awakening consciousness of self and interest in the world. If young people are given the opportunity to travel and to get to know foreign people and customs, to go mountaineering and hill-walking or to do drama, the awakening physical interest in the other sex will not become obsessive or imprison them. An excessive focus on sexuality is always the result of an upbringing and education which does not sufficiently encourage spiritual interests or take them into account.

16.6 Educating to freedom

Waldorf school (Rudolf Steiner School) education

The first Waldorf school was set up in Stuttgart in 1919 under the guidance of Rudolf Steiner and was to lead to a rapidly developing educational movement. There are now Waldorf schools in many different parts of the world. Waldorf education, through its curriculum, methods and teaching content, aims to promote healthy development in the child and adolescent and is therefore therapeutic in nature. Of course pupils are eventually required to study for public examinations and to acquire the necessary leaving certificates but the school is not regarded primarily as a place where knowledge is imparted but rather as a place where the human being can develop fully.

The kindergarten age

Children come into the kindergarten at about the age of four. A typical day starts with the children taking off their coat and putting on their houseshoes. They greet their teacher who may be already busy at work. While the youngest ones prefer to stay near her watching, the older ones start playing together. Tables and chairs are arranged and hung with cloths to make a house, fire-engine, dust-cart, ambulance or ship. Some play at horses and carriages or trains. Others dress or feed their dolls or take them for walks in their prams. Some dress up as fathers and mothers, nurses and doctors, and so on. And so this first hour of the morning passes in varied and concentrated activity. The teacher is present as the tranquil centre. Although busy herself, she shows the greatest interest in all that is going on around her. She sees to it that the life of this "large family" runs in an ordered but lively fashion. From all the many possible activities, she chooses those which are simple, can be easily grasped and imitated by the children: washing, baking bread, making breakfast and so on. From time to time she leaves her work in order to take part in a dolls' birthday party, or to make a crossing in the ferry-boat, or simply because a child needs her attention. She will deal with quarrels or with difficult behaviour.

When playtime is coming to an end, the teacher will begin to put away her own work. This is noticed by the children who then prepare for a general clearing-up, which takes a

Figure 51. In the kindergarten.

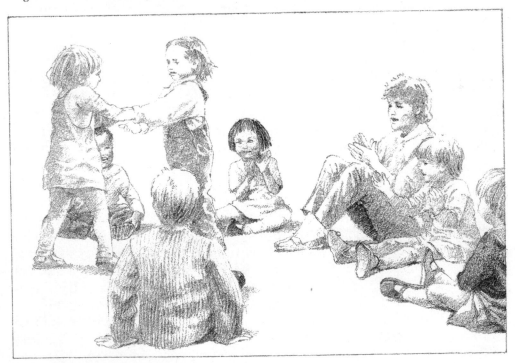

few minutes. Then the room is swept and the children wash their hands in preparation for the rhythmic activity which follows: verses with acting or movements, songs and singing games, all of this being generally orientated towards the seasons and what the farmers are doing at that time of year, or what is happening in nature. The festivals of the year are another important feature. As the same singing games and songs are repeated every day for a longish period, the children acquire a rich store of poems and songs. In some kindergartens, this activity starts off with what is called a "morning circle" when the children and teacher stand in a circle to recite a prayer-verse or to sing a morning-song. After this communal activity, there is a break for a bite to eat and something to drink.

There now follows a period in which the children can again play by themselves, usually outside in the garden. Then at the end of the morning, the children gather in a circle around their teacher to hear a story. The smallest ones love to sit near her, and such closeness is an inner need.

The teacher does not tell the story dramatically, but rather in an epic almost monotonous tone, yet with warmth and vitality. She tries to give expression to every familiar word and sentence. Every day over a long period she tells the same well-loved fairy-tale without the least variation, otherwise the children would notice it and correct her. Often the story is one of Grimms' fairy-tales which in

style, composition and content, are particularly well-suited for children at this age.

Thus the morning's timetable contains two main periods during which the children are occupied in different ways that are natural for their age. All sorts of things are offered to encourage play: not only in the form of toys and things to play with but also through the example of the teacher who, like the mother at home, is busy with some useful household activity: making "breakfast," baking bread, washing clothes, darning, ironing, mending toys. Or she may be busy with some cultural activity such as painting with water colours. Through this wide range of things offered, every child can then find in its own time and way what it needs to imitate and what is appropriate for its development. Thus the child is left free in how, when and whether to imitate.

Two shorter periods are devoted to a common activity (rhythmic activity, the morning break and story time). In this way, the programme alternates between active and passive activity in a natural rhythm which may be likened to breathing in and out.

A Waldorf kindergarten requires parents to understand and support its aims and objectives perhaps more than other forms of education. Some parents, for example, may not accept the important influence of fairy-tales in a child's development. If the parents take this attitude, their children will find it difficult to listen to a story at school without being disruptive and making remarks like: "There isn't any such thing as fairies!" In such a case, perhaps the parents would do better to choose another form of education.

Again there are children whose parents have given them extensive and rational explanations of things. Such children with their precocious remarks and readiness to argue and contradict can disrupt school activities. Children who, at home, are used to a regular diet of television or stories on tape tend to be disruptive at school during free playtime and even more so during group activity. It can take up to six months for these children to integrate with the group and no longer disrupt with their "machine-gun rattle" or other behaviour copied from the television.

After some weeks of Waldorf kindergarten, parents will start to notice how their children come home in a calm and positive mood. They will bring ideas home which can affect the family's everyday life. For example some children may start to ask for grace to be said before meals. Others will want to repeat singing games with their parents or brothers and sisters or hear their favourite fairy-tale again.

Education in the kindergarten is based on a deep understanding of the needs of the young child who wants to embark on the conquest of its surroundings. The child remembers yesterday's or even last week's events and it wants to repeat them in play and so enlarge and deepen experience. A child at this age is never content with a once-only experience. Experience is kept alive, repeated and united with it. In this way the will is strengthened, just as a muscle is strengthened by daily use; and it is precisely at this training of the will that the morning programme in the kindergarten is directed. At this stage of the child's development, feeling and thought are not as pronounced as the need to be active. The will requires constant stimuli, hence the child's need to imitate external models. It is therefore the teacher's concern to organize the programme in such a way that the children learn to use all their senses and abilities and acquire good habits at the same time. The more wholeheartedly the teacher fulfils her role, the more the children will respond to the stimuli.

There is a German proverb which says: "What little Hans does not learn, big Hans will never learn." This means that in later life the will moves in the tracks that have been mapped out in childhood. Good habits learnt when young are a great support in later life. But it is very important that this early learning takes place in an atmosphere of busy contentment and that the children are allowed to develop their play *freely*. The teacher's order and discipline should never be applied so as to hamshackle the children, nor should she bring any activity abruptly to an end. If the child is deeply engrossed in its play and it is time to come and eat, the teacher should try to effect a harmonious transition from the child's "work" to the meal. That can be quite difficult even with a very young child. All of us know the moans and groans when a child is hauled away from its game because we have something more important or necessary to do. The child finds this quite incomprehensible because it is happiest when active in its own way. Much harm is done here through lack of imaginative insight on the part of the adult, for our sense of freedom in later life is based on how we were able as children to live out our urge to play and do. If the child's activity is interrupted too often by the adult, this will adversely affect later development. Furthermore being happily engaged in doing something promotes the building up of a healthy body, while frequent interruption disturbs development. In a whining child the circulation of the blood is impeded, whereas before it was pulsing happily. This fact must be taken in all seriousness, for the individual has to live all his life with the organs that have been developed between birth and the change of teeth. This is the period when the organism and its functions receive their stamp, and when the will is adapting itself in many ways to its surroundings. It is the time when skill, persistency, endurance, bodily strength and the ability to concentrate are implanted for life.

At the beginning of the change of teeth, a great part of the growth forces are transmuted into forces of memory and thought (see Chapter 13.9). Once this transformation has been effected, the child's organism cannot be harmed so much by upsetting or neglecting the development of the will. Indeed the body has reached a certain maturity by the time the child is ready for school. If it were more widely appreciated how flexible and malleable the body of a little child is, much harmful upbringing would be avoided.

When we give a toy or plaything to our child we should ask ourselves whether it will stimulate the child's imagination and help the whole child to develop healthily. Everything ready-made, mechanically perfect, cripples the child's imagination and stamps its own form upon the imitative defenceless organism.

Our choice of toys and pictures has a physiological effect on a child right up to school-age. After that the imitative faculty declines. It will not harm a ten-year-old to build with Lego but if a five-year-old presses the standard pieces together in the prescribed manner, its imagination will be denied an important field of exploration. The material allows the child to build contrary to the usual laws of physics and so the child's developing awareness and insight into this area is thrown right off course. Where ordinary blocks would have long since fallen down and shown the child the weakness in the construction, the Lego pieces stick together and give a completely distorted impression.

If we look at the abundance of computer games, remote-controlled cars and railways, we can see right away that these things are really for the adults who thought them up.

When playing with these things the child can neither imitate anything nor develop its own creative activities. With such playthings, the child can only watch fascinated, work things out and manipulate them, and so it behaves in an unchildlike way.

From seven to fourteen

During the period between the change of teeth and puberty, the training of the will is not as paramount as it was at the kindergarten age. The child is now ready for the cultivation of feelings and the psyche which take foremost place. The growing person develops a sense of justice and injustice, of beauty and ugliness, and confronts the whole range of emotion between acceptance and rejection, between love and hatred. This development culminates in the passionate extremes witnessed during puberty.

Together with feelings, the faculty for judgment is developed. Mature judgment requires well-developed feelings as a precondition for evaluating the play of sympathy and antipathy and weighing several possibilities. Education should now take this stage of development into account using speech as its chief instrument. Great value is therefore set upon the use of speech in teacher-training. The teacher must be able to express nuances which will let the child experience through the teacher's words all the various shades of soul-feeling. Direction is thereby given to the awakening but not yet cultivated life of feeling, mostly through the way in which the teacher stands before the children with her views and judgments of the world. Her whole teaching needs to be built up artistically. She cannot use concepts and definitions which are so dry that the children feel nothing there. Science subjects, too, must be taught in such a way that the pupils can attend with all their hearts to the description of a plant, to the accounts of physical and chemical experiments, much in the same way as a work of art is experienced.

Here is an example from an arithmetic lesson of Class 3, dealing with prime numbers. The teacher might have said to the children: "A prime number is a number that can only be divided by itself or by one." Instead he provides a pictorial image of some sort, as for instance: "Prime numbers are the beggars among the numbers. They are the poorest of the poor. They have nobody in the world except themselves, and so they can only be divided by themselves, because they are not friends with any other number."

Here we can mark the difference in feelings engendered by these two ways of presenting the prime numbers. The German proverb: "You can only see properly with your heart" *(Man sieht nur mit dem Herzen gut)* has real significance for this age-group. This means too that the teacher cannot just teach from ordinary text-books but must be able to convey personal enthusiasm for the subject. Such a teacher will be loved by the pupils as an authority. What the teacher says is right: they can be sure of that. In their love for the teacher's authority, there is a focus for their own fluctuating life of feeling.

This close connection between teacher and pupils is further cemented by the class teacher retaining the class for the first eight years and teaching them all the main subjects during that time. The first two periods of the morning (main lesson) are taken by the class teacher. In this way the children feel that their teacher truly belongs to them.

It is not always easy for the teacher to manage the pupils' devotion in the right way. It would be wrong to seek their love for one's self. The teacher

Figure 52. Already leaving childhood behind.

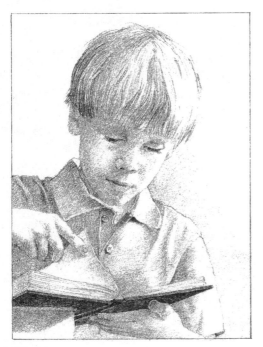

must realize that the respect and devotion which the pupils have will develop into interest for knowledge and truth. A child who was able to look up to someone with veneration will find it easier in later life to take something seriously, to love truth and ideals and to feel obligation where it is due. The child, through loving the teacher, will love the views which the teacher holds. Later the child will learn to regard things objectively.

Seen against such a background, what could be worse than boring instruction, especially if the teacher is indifferent to the subject and not particularly likeable by nature. The child's feelings are starved, there is a negative undertone. If this persists, especially right through the school years, it has a dispiriting effect which lasts into later life. The intellect is forced to absorb something which does not interest the heart and so the life of the soul is split, with feelings and thought going their separate ways.

To end this section we should like to draw the reader's attention to a particular turning point in the child's development which takes place around the age of nine. Rudolf Steiner called this point "the Rubicon of a child's development." Just as Caesar crossed the river Rubicon which made turning back impossible, so children between their ninth and tenth birthday leave childhood irrevocably behind them. The point at which this happens is often observed by parents. Anyone sitting in a lesson in Class 3 or 4 can see this change which is taking place. Whereas formerly the child used to look around unselfconsciously and naively, it now appears suddenly more earnest, more introspective and even quietly assessing the teacher. For the first time the child feels that it is not in the world just as a matter of course belonging to mother and father. There is a sudden insight into the loneliness of personal destiny. At this point, many children start to ask about their own origin, not so much looking for "sex-education" as inquiring about the exact circumstances of their birth: whether for instance they have been adopted or exchanged. Now to the *thought* of one's own self, which was expressed for the first time by the two-year-old child, comes the *feeling* of one's own self, the awareness of one's own individuality which cannot derive from father and mother. This feeling is accompanied by the sense of loneliness. The feeling of self becomes stronger. Children now test whom they will obey and who can be trusted. Unfairness is more strongly experienced than before. Conscience emerges and can be appealed to.

From fourteen onwards

During this phase of life, there comes a further critical change in the growing person. Will and feeling have been developed to a great extent and now need the direction of the intellect. Parents and teachers have in a certain sense finished the job of "looking after" the young person. Whether they are exemplary or be-

loved authorities does not matter so much any more; from now on the adolescent consciously turns away from many things and goes his own way. His thinking, now self-sufficient, helps him to distance himself from unpleasant happenings. He is no longer bound to participate and imitate. Now he can discuss and philosophize or follow his own happy and interesting thoughts during a boring lesson. Many good ideas, poems and drawings have come into being in such lessons! That is quite different from the idle scribbling on the desks of former years. Education now has to try to meet this new situation by stimulating thought-life in all directions. A staff of specialist teachers now replaces the more intimate class teacher.

In the art lessons certain techniques are now worked at: drawing in dark and light, veil-painting with water colours, modelling of heads and sculptures; and in woodwork, making small articles of furniture. In all this the teacher ensures that the pupils' thinking is engaged in a personal manner; that is, that the teacher treats the pupils as fully-fledged associates, stimulating them to work things out for themselves. Here personal freedom is anchored in independence of thought.

In this way Waldorf education takes into account the laws of human physiological-psychological development. Its whole manner of teaching is geared to the stage of development that each age-group has reached. Just as learning to walk, talk and think follow in sequence so likewise the training of will through imitation, the direction of feeling through love for authority, the stimulation of thought through independent search for truth and forming of judgment. Even in the most disturbed human development, this fundamental sequence is recognizable. The aim of this education can be seen as a way of awakening and challenging the child and, seen in this light, the true value of any educational method or means is to show the way and remove obstacles to the child's own progress towards the discovery and emergence of a more fundamental Way.

16.7 School problems

Hyperactivity

Since the end of the sixties hyperactivity in children of kindergarten and school-age has become the most commonly diagnosed disturbance. The diagnostic term "hyperactive" has been applied to an increasing number of children whose behaviour shows an exaggerated urge to move, poor control of impulses and of emotional reactions, as well as poor concentration and attention. These children are inclined to be aggressive and uncontrolled. They do not control their feelings towards people — they will hug and kiss complete strangers without any inhibition. Teachers and parents, who are unaccustomed to this behaviour can be driven to distraction. We should like to make some suggestions concerning the course and treatment of this increasingly problematic condition.

Causes
Up to the present, no one definite cause has been found for hyperactivity. Neither early damage, nor disorders of the blood-circulation, nor digestive defects, nor food allergies have been isolated as the main cause.

As it is most doctors agree that there must be several causes working together and linked to our modern way of life which is becoming more and more hectic and inimical to the child.

If we look at this complex condition from the knowledge of man gained from anthroposophy, we can see that the child's "I" has lost control over its soul-life. Attentiveness, concentration and readiness to act are uncontrolled, and balance of feeling is lost. There are physiological processes corresponding to these soul abilities (central nervous processes, sense impressions and thinking), rhythmic functions (expansion and contraction, sympathy and antipathy) and metabolic processes (readiness to act).

In all cases there is malfunctioning of control, namely a disorder of the will: effort of will in thinking indicates attentiveness; effort of will in feeling indicates directed reactions to sympathy and antipathy; effort of will in the sphere of will indicates self-control and control of actions. All therapeutic efforts must therefore have as object the strengthening of the "I" in the child's physiological and emotional functions.

Remedial treatment
During infancy (age two to seven) the most important remedial measures are the examples of the adults who can control their thinking, feeling and will. Very often however the child is up against rush, worry and tension in the family: mother always harassed, father irritable. Instead of giving the child loving care the parents do not know what to do with it. At the same time the parents treat each other with indifference and take no thought about the ill effects of our times. To top it all the child is swamped with masses of toys, sweets and all sorts of presents, is subjected to endless television, cassettes and videos, all of which destroy powers of concentration and make the child continually seek diversion.

Against all this to cultivate attentiveness and strength of will, we must create the right environment for the child to be occupied in a peaceful and sensible fashion. It is important for the child to have regular mealtimes, regular times for going to bed and getting up, and generally speaking life should have a regular rhythm. We do not recommend a special diet. In our opinion the only effective thing about the so-called low-phosphate diet is the tremendous effort of will required by the parents to control and select the items of the diet, for then the child has the example of the adult acting with purpose and decision. But if this clear lead can be given freely regardless of diet it is better for the child altogether.

In the chapter on Nutrition (see Chapter 14) we have already shown how artificial colouring and additives are an unnecessary burden on the metabolism. Our observations on food there also apply to the hyperactive child.

For the hyperactive child religious education is very important (see 16.3

above). Such a child enjoys nothing better than to experience with the adults true moments of religious devotion. Although the child does not understand much of the content of the spoken prayer, the mood of the adult is felt intensely and this has a soothing effect.

We see hyperactivity as a typical disorder of our times and civilization, being also closely connected with adult problems. In modern life sensation follows sensation, memory is impaired, the life of feeling is torn amid stress, rush and panic, and becomes superficial, lively interest diminishes and people become indifferent to their work, unable to identify themselves with what they are doing. The "I" is less and less active in thought, feeling and will. No wonder that the children reflect these disorders which we adults have ourselves, and hold up to us a mirror in which we can see what is wrong with ourselves. If we can take ourselves in hand, and work to remedy these adult defects, then we are on the way to helping the children effectively.

It is often asked where the line can be drawn between restlessness and hyperactivity. This can be done easily. A child who is simply restless *can* concentrate and be attentive the moment it becomes really engrossed in something, but a hyperactive child *cannot* even if it really wants to. Only patient attention on the part of the adult, attention that never flags and fails, and love and readiness to act can help the child. We have also had

good results from curative eurythmy (see 16.8 below on curative eurythmy) as well as constitutional treatment with homoeopathic and anthroposophical remedies.

One comfort for parents of hyperactive children is that the children lose most of these symptoms by the time they reach puberty.

Left-handedness

In Waldorf schools, left-handed children are encouraged to write with their right hands. This often leads to heated discussions which on occasion even reach the consulting-room when the doctor is called upon to help. The problem is made more acute because in state schools children are mostly given a free hand on the grounds that branding the children as left-handed and making them change over leads to traumatic problems. This view seems to be supported by abundant evidence of psychological disorders: neurosis, fear of school, fear of failure, refuge in fantasy and stammering. However, we see these symptoms as the result of changeover methods based on compulsion and pressure, aggravated by the timescale in which writing has to be learnt in most state schools.

Another objection to teaching left-handed children to write with the right hand is that it may cause a restructuring of the brain. But this could only take place if an attempt were made to alter the dominance of the left hand by training it in all kinds of other activities as well.

A further objection is that the speech organs will be impaired. It is however an incorrect notion that the speech centre is developed in the half of the brain opposite to the dominant hand. We now know, through different areas of research (including operations on the brain) that in about 98% of *all* people including those who are left-handed the speech centre is on the left. The location of the speech-centre clearly does not depend on which hand learns to write and on which side of the body is dominant.

There are three reasons for learning to write with the right hand, and we shall try to explain why it is encouraged in Waldorf schools. These reasons apply to all left-handed children regardless of whether they are totally left-sided (using not only the left hand, but also the left eye, ear and foot) or cross-lateral (using for instance the right eye and foot but the left hand).

Strengthening the will

Every conscious repetition of an action, however small it may be, strengthens the will. Learning to write with the right hand is therefore an exercise of will for every child; but for the left-handed one it is especially so, for by constantly overcoming a slightly uncomfortable feeling the child practises control for the entire period of learning to write. The child makes an effort for the sake of the teacher and parents (who should of course be in agreement) and is encouraged by them. The interest which they show enables the child to feel increasing satisfaction in overcoming the difficulty. In the end the child emerges strengthened and enriched by the experience of having successfully overcome something.

Qualities of right and left

It is not a matter of indifference whether it is the right or the left hand which is used in writing. In many cultures, we find clear expression in language and customs that right and left are considered to have different qualities and values. Generally speaking, the right-hand side is associated with external life, practical

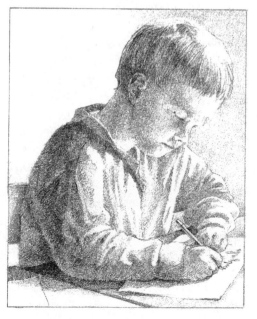

Figure 53. Learning to write.

and warlike qualities, while the left is associated with the inner being of man, happy, artistic, magic and religious qualities.

In English, for instance, we have expressions like "to have two left feet," "to be someone's right hand man." Values of right and left are expressed in the words "dexterity" from the Latin *dexter,* a right hand, and "sinister" from the Latin for left hand. Many more examples of this kind can be found in other languages and cultures.

We find a similar disparity when we study the human organism and the distribution of those organs which are not in pairs, like liver, gall, heart and spleen. The liver and gall which deal with breaking down and converting foodstuffs are on the right side of the body, while the heart lies to the left, regulating the amount and speed of the circulation depending on the demands made by the organism. It reacts sensitively to emotional conditions such as joy, fear and grief. The spleen, too, is on the left and likewise has no direct task with the outer world but is concerned with controlling the make-up of the blood.

Summing up we may say that not only are there cultural and linguistic values given to left and right but related qualities are to be found in the bodily functions. The organs lying to the right deal with what comes from without and work beneath consciousness, while those lying to the left are more concerned with the inner life of the organism and we are more conscious of their activity.

It follows that there is a correspondence with our organism when an activity such as writing is performed with the right hand, as this activity is concerned with the outer world, and in later life is performed to a high degree automatically and unconsciously.

To take another revealing example, the fingering on the violin together with listening for purity and quality corresponds more to the qualities of the left side, being nearer to consciousness and more receptive to the artistic and emotional. It is interesting to note that there has never been a serious attempt to teach right-handed children to master the complicated finger-play on violin or cello with their right hands. Here it is taken for granted that the right-handed child has certain disadvantages over against the left-handed.

Aspects of destiny

A left-handed person enters life with tasks and qualities different from those of a right-handed person. In a lecture to teachers, Rudolf Steiner describes how left-handedness of varying degrees is the result of a former earth-life in which the individual has overtaxed himself either physically or emotionally. The right side is then weakened and allows the left to seem stronger. Thus it would appear that the dominance of the left side allows the individual to develop more inwardness and clarity of mind. Education has the task of developing these latent qualities and of preventing the powers of the left side from being weakened. However, the left side *is* weakened if the left hand is trained in writing because once this complicated technique has been mastered, the action of writing is then almost completely unconscious. Furthermore the prime aim of writing is to communicate with the world. If the left-handed child learns to write with his right hand his left side will be relieved of the burden of this activity which is not of its nature.

Waldorf education takes into account the insights of Rudolf Steiner's research and advises parents to let their children learn to write with their right hands. Other activities such as painting, sewing and cutting may be carried out with the left hand if the child prefers, but the teacher will encourage these activities to be carried out wholeheartedly and with full attention.

Practical guidelines

How can learning to write with the right hand be made less arduous once the decision has been made?

1. Parents and teachers must be in full agreement over the decision.
2. We should not pity the child when it changes pen or pencil from the left hand back into the right with a sigh of distress and says: "But I can write ever so much better with the left hand." We should rather say: "We're looking forward to when you can do it just as well with your right hand. Your right hand wants to learn to write too."
3. Give the child plenty of time. In Waldorf schools this should be no problem as the learning of writing and reading is introduced much more slowly. If a completely left-handed child has particular difficulties with learning to write, it will be given one, two or even three years in which to learn without pressure.
4. Do not offer any reward of a material nature. The true reward is the adults' pleasure at each little step forward and the child's own pride when it sees that it is really learning to write with the right hand. This can be helped by giving the child a precious stone or shell to hold in the left hand while writing. Material rewards counteract the training of the will because the child will then perform not for its own inner satisfaction but for the rewards.
5. If a child (or an older person) decides to change over to writing with the right hand, it is best to do this in the summer holidays. We would recommend writing something in a good note-book every day: diary-entries, poems or passages that have appealed.
6. If during the period of learning to write, nervous symptoms or tension arises, the teacher and parents should investigate whether the problems are really connected with learning to write or whether there is some other emotional cause.

In this section, we have dealt mainly with the problematical aspects of left-handedness. But it should be remembered that there is a positive side which shows itself in a greater sensitivity for all that is beautiful and harmonious in life. Many poets and painters (including Michelangelo and Leonardo da Vinci) and other artistic and imaginative people have been left-handed. They may not have been quite so practical in regulating their everyday affairs but this weighs little against what they achieved for mankind in general. While there are more realists among right-handed people, the left-handed are more idealistic, artistic and spiritual by nature and in our materialistic and unimaginative world they have a distinct contribution to make.

Dyslexia

By the term "dyslexia" is generally understood any difficulty in reading or writing which is incompatible with the child's intelligence. We shall not go into precise definitions of these difficulties but simply give some basic principles for understanding and helping with such problems. To be able to recognize the form of different letters and write them entails a complicated interaction of motor, linguistic and thought activities:

1. The use of both eyes. Separate pictures from each eye have to be fused into one. One eye is generally the stronger and the other is subordinated. This coordination of both eyes does not function properly with a number of dyslexic children. For them eye-training in a good eye-training school is recommended.

2. Distinction of difference in form.
3. Correct visualization of the form in the mind.
4. Reproduction of the form by the movement of the hand.
5. Retention of the form in memory.
6. Recognition of the form from memory.
7. Correct pronunciation of the sound belonging to the letter-shape.
8. Aural distinction of the different vowels and consonants.

Any one of these activities can be faulty and cause dyslexia. Once the cause of the problem has been recognized effective help can be given. It is interesting to note that many Waldorf schools claim that none of their pupils suffer from dyslexia, for writing and reading are introduced slowly and practised for three years. In this way, children who are inclined to dyslexia do not suffer when learning to read and write. Some Waldorf schools do have dyslexic children, especially children who have been sent there because they were already found to be dyslexic.

In handling the problem, we must first find out the cause of the trouble and then, through our loving assistance, give the child fresh courage to keep on trying and practising. The following approaches have proved successful in a number of cases, depending on where exactly the problem lies:

1. Exercises in perception. Giving exact descriptions of things, also looking at the form of objects together (pictures, plants, stones).

2. Walking along forms and their mirror-forms on the floor:

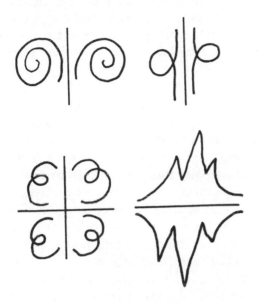

3. Drawing forms with the foot (pencil between the big toe and the next toe; writing on wrapping paper or with a felt-pen on newspaper).

4. Drawing forms with the hand in the air with the eyes closed.

5. Writing forms from memory the next day on paper, after repeating the whole process mentally.

6. Repeating all the steps until one letter-form is retained.

7. Reciting evocative poems, or even amusing rhymes, in which the problem-sounds recur frequently.

How can dyslexia be prevented?

Reading and writing are activities which can be practised at the end of a development which took place before the child went to school. Earlier in this book the stages of this development were enumerated as learning to see, to walk, to speak and to think (see Chapter 13). If at any of these stages, there is not sufficient activity and because of inadequate practice the ability is not fully acquired, a disability in reading and writing can ensue. This is because the metamorphosis of growth forces into thought forces (see Chapter 13.9, 16.5 above and 16.9 below) should take place without disturbance.

A prerequisite for a healthy intellectual ability is a good training of the perceptions:

Vision: gives the picture content to conceptual thinking.

Sense of balance: gives thought the correct relationship to space, for instance, three-dimensional thinking with the coordinates of up, down, back, front, left and right.

Sense of movement: enables thought to grasp the mobility of forms.

Hearing: enables thought to grasp the sound represented by a series of letters.

Many children are not encouraged sufficiently to develop these sense activities. Consequently we frequently find disturbances and inability to use these activities properly. It is important therefore to have the children tested and to use the kindergarten time to remove these difficulties. Orientation in space, and sureness of movement can be practised in play (see 16.8 below) and these form the basis for later mental orientation and mobility of thought.

Acquiring speech

Many children having difficulty at school with reading and writing also have problems with speech. Certain sounds are not properly articulated, vocabulary is poor, and we notice that the children have not been spoken to much or well. These children still retain expressions from baby language and do not formulate their sentences grammatically. The only remedy is to practise speech with them thoroughly, joyfully and lovingly. This can be done in the kindergarten too with singing, telling fairy-stories, reciting verses and sayings, as well as careful conversation with the children at breakfast, on walks, and so on.

Memory development

Sometimes dyslexia is due to a faulty memory. The children cannot write the letters properly because they do not recognize them again. This problem, again, can be tackled in the kindergarten. In Waldorf kindergar-

tens not only the short-term but also the medium-term and long-term memories are thoroughly cultivated. This is not done by thought training but by forming good habits: for example certain things are done at exactly the same time every day (see 16.6 above). Certain activities are performed only once a week as for instance, cleaning, washing, eurythmy and painting, then every month a new fairy-story may be told and a new song belonging to the season learnt, and finally there are the great festivals coming around only once a year. In this way the children enjoy seeing again all that they have forgotten in the meantime, and this provides a sound basis for the process of remembering and forgetting over longer or shorter periods later when the thinking has matured. Before the metamorphosis of the growth forces (see Chapter 13.9, 16.5 above and 16.9 below) has taken place children do not have an abstract memory, that is to say they are only conscious of the sense perception and they experience remembering only by actually seeing the thing again. If an infant can repeatedly see something with joy, in later life he will be able to remember a thought which once interested him.

It is important that in dealing with dyslexic children we give them the feeling of hope and confidence that they really can be helped. Very often the existing problems are accentuated because the children suffer from their failure to cope, and do not get enough encouragement, experiencing only indifferent or discouraging adults. In all slight cases of dyslexia a complete cure can be achieved. In severe cases this is not always possible, but with dedicated practice a marked improvement can be achieved.

16.8 Eurythmy

Eurythmy is the art of movement developed by Rudolf Steiner in the years 1911 to 1924. There are forms of movement corresponding to the sounds of speech and music and these forms are expressed in eurythmy. Both speech-eurythmy and tone-eurythmy are practised in three different areas.

Artistic eurythmy performs poems, stories, drama and music on stage.

In *educational eurythmy*, pupils practise agility and grace of movement in artistic sequences, learning to make their body movements express inner feelings and experiences. Through performing with others and discovering that the performance will only succeed if they all contribute selflessly to the whole, pupils also refine their social attitudes.

In *curative eurythmy* exercises of speech and tone eurythmy are repeated to help strengthen the body and counteract pathological tendencies.

The speed and intensity of each exercise is so devised that a particular exercise strengthens an area of weakness. Some exercises are designed to curb overdevelopment, others are for harmonizing, stimulating, developing concentration or calming. For left-handed people there are exercises to develop dexterity, orientation and symmetry. Curative eurythmy can also help in the treatment of physical disability, deafness and blindness. Treatment is prescribed by the doctor in consultation with the curative eurythmist.

Training in eurythmy usually lasts four years with a further year in the case of curative eurythmy. At present there are over twenty eurythmy and curative eurythmy centres in various countries.

Fundamental to all types of eurythmy is the precise evaluation of qualities in speech and musical tones. The vowels and consonants as well as the tone intervals from prime to the octave are studied in their connection with the human form. The basic movements of eurythmy underlie a whole range of movements of the human body and relate closely to movement elsewhere in organic and inorganic nature. We find correspondences with the growth-forms of plants and animals, and in the play of movement between the solid, liquid and gaseous states. Thus we may describe eurythmy as "a visible primal language." The eurythmist finds a way into the workings of visible nature, seeing in every form a movement come to rest and, in eurythmy, converts that form once more into movement.

Tone eurythmy is more concerned with showing the proportional relationship of the tones to each other. The human form is built up on these same proportions, as can be seen in the skeleton.

Both educational and curative eurythmy directly influence the growth and proportional development of the body, especially in the pre-school period. The practice of sound and tone movements has a harmonizing and humanizing effect upon the child and contributes to a strong and healthy foundation in life. Eurythmy will also help in later life where individuals suffer from a lack of harmony between body, soul and spirit. Practised regularly, it also has a beneficial effect on those whose lives are subject to pressure or stress and who need a calming and civilizing discipline.

16.9 Growing older

Until we reach the twenties, we all like growing older. Then sooner or later anxiety and uncertainty start to emerge. This is not the place to deal with the crises of adult life but we should at least like to show the connection between childhood and later life. In the section on Waldorf education (see 16.6 above), we explained some of the important stages in educating for freedom. There the measures described took into account the child's physical development. But how does our human development continue after the physical body has attained maturity? We need education and upbringing when we are children but after that what we make of ourselves is our own personal responsibility. Physical development takes some eighteen to twenty years. There follows another period of about the same length in which inner development takes precedence. Those who have been educated in awareness and skills of self-development have an advantage in dealing with the questions that now arise:

"How do I find my place in life?"
"How do I learn to deal with other people without confrontation? Should I always be the one who backs down?"

"How can I be uncompromising in what I recognize as right, and yet be tolerant of people who think differently?"

"To what extent does having a social conscience mean sacrificing my own personality?"

These are problems arising from relationships with other people, with our work and with the world at large. If we have developed a love of learning in early life, we will not suffer later when we find ourselves in situations where for instance we may be either totally rejected or universally admired. We will ask ourselves: "How can I learn from this situation? How can I stay human without despairing, without withdrawing or becoming vain and superior?" With this sort of outlook, we will have achieved some stability in the knowledge of ourselves, usually by the age of forty. This will give an inner assurance which is founded on all the previous work of maturing at an inner level. But once this stage has been reached human development still does not stop. There is no resting on one's laurels, but rather a new dimension of spiritual development opens up. Now our interests are strongly directed to aims beyond the personal and quite new questions arise:

"How can I use my experience in a way that is useful to society?"

"What does the world require of me?"

"What do I owe to my upbringing, to my fellow-men, indeed how have I become the person I am?"

"What can I do to assist the development of my fellow-men?"

At this stage, too, we begin to look more closely at young people growing up. We take pleasure in them as individuals and we may become involved in helping them. A deeper interest develops in the achievements of those who have already died. Now our endeavours start to focus on the deeper meaning of events. Our attitude to time also changes; where formerly we were impatient and frustrated, now we allow things to take their own time and course.

Those who spend their lives seeking and working in this way will be a blessing to those around them. They will inspire confidence because they are not following personal ambitions or striving for power and because they are dedicated to whatever they undertake. They will be able to advise and weigh up a judgment in a way that no twenty or thirty-year-old can. They will sit calmly during discussions while others fly off the handle. They can forgive and allow others a second chance because they know how hard it is to persevere with self-development and not give up. The older they get, the more benevolent and mild will be their whole manner.

This view of a human life reveals the shallowness of a materialistic outlook. If the soul was a mere extension of the body, then the life of our soul and spirit would suffer as the body degenerated in the second half of life. But the very opposite is the case: even though degeneration sets in and our powers of physical regeneration decline, the soul and the spirit can become more and more rich. Women especially can experience this: once the change of life is over they are not poorer in soul than before but, on the contrary, feel freer and able to achieve more then ever before in spiritual terms. This phenomenon may be understood better in the light of the transformation of growth forces already described (see Chapter 13.9). Thus the increase in spiritual vitality is directly related to the body's declining powers, as forces no longer required for physical regeneration become available to the soul. All this is summarized in the diagram opposite.

It is one of the tragedies of modern life that many people spend their childhood and adolescence in such a way that their ability to learn throughout life is not sufficiently cultivated, with the result that their development may simply to come to a halt. If this happens, physical or psychological disorders will ensue

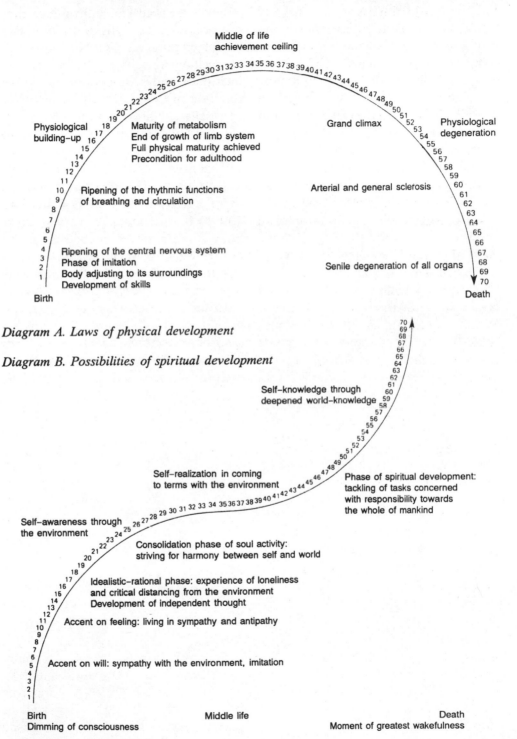

Middle of life
achievement ceiling

Physiological
building–up

Maturity of metabolism
End of growth of limb system
Full physical maturity achieved
Precondition for adulthood

Grand climax

Physiological
degeneration

Ripening of the rhythmic functions
of breathing and circulation

Arterial and general sclerosis

Ripening of the central nervous system
Phase of imitation
Body adjusting to its surroundings
Development of skills

Senile degeneration of all organs

Birth

Death

Diagram A. Laws of physical development

Diagram B. Possibilities of spiritual development

Self–knowledge through
deepened world–knowledge

Self–realization in coming
to terms with the environment

Phase of spiritual development:
tackling of tasks concerned
with responsibility towards
the whole of mankind

Self–awareness through
the environment

Consolidation phase of soul activity:
striving for harmony between self and world

Idealistic–rational phase: experience of loneliness
and critical distancing from the environment
Development of independent thought

Accent on feeling: living in sympathy and antipathy

Accent on will: sympathy with the environment, imitation

Birth
Dimming of consciousness

Middle life

Death
Moment of greatest wakefulness

leading to a illness. This usually begins after middle age when the biological decline of the body sets in. Instead of witnessing a spiritual upsurge, we observe in such people how their inner forces are consumed in brooding over their own rights and wrongs, in criticism of others, in mistrust, in domination or bitterness. Senile obstinacy, a sense of persecution, consuming fear and meanness, all these can appear. Here the forces released from the ageing organism cannot be absorbed through creative thinking. They lie fallow, as it were, and become complexes, emotions and illusions which keep the soul in bondage and the "I" imprisoned. Such a condition is often accompanied by the appearance of organic disease such as calcification of the arteries.

Even a successful upbringing cannot prevent all the ills of old age. But it is often possible for a good upbringing to have a positive influence on the incidence and progress of disease. In the case of those who cannot happily reconcile themselves to growing old, we usually find that their education and upbringing did not prepare them sufficiently for the necessary self-training later. On the other hand old people who are spiritually active are able to find benefits at every stage of life and have never been tempted to mourn the passing of time, least of all youth with all its imperfections, sorrows and joys. Each period of life has left them abilities which they can now use. Childhood, youth and young adulthood continue to live on in them and are in no way regarded as "paradise lost."

16.10 Can you learn to bring up children?

We shall begin by looking at three types of parental attitude towards children. Two of them represent opposite extremes while the third is a happy and healthy mean. We encounter all three almost daily in the consulting-room.

The first type of parent takes the attitude that good behaviour can only be achieved by chiding and admonition. "Sit there and be quiet!" the mother says to the child as soon as she starts to talk to the doctor. The four-year-old immediately begins to explore the room, touching everything it can find. The mother interrupts her conversation every two minutes with asides to the child, sometimes even before it has done anything: "Stay here! Don't touch! That's not yours, that's the doctor's. Stop fiddling with that! Have I got to put you on my lap?" And so on. The child's will cannot flourish here because it is not allowed to try anything out.

The second type of parent shows no will or decisiveness and simply gives way to the child in everything. This child constantly interrupts and seeks attention. Here is a flavour of the sort of conversation that ensues:

Child (looking at picture on the wall): Mummy, is that a bird?

Mother: No, that's supposed to be an angel. Now let me talk to the doctor.
Child: I want a drink.
Mother (giving the child a drink and trying to get back to her conversation with the doctor): And she never wants to eat anything at lunch. Of course I don't force her.
Child: But if there are chips, I like those. Mummy, I want a biscuit.
Mother (giving the child a whole packet of biscuits): But we only have chips once a week. Apart from that, though, she won't eat anything.
Doctor: But she must eat something. (To the child) What do you like to eat?
Child: Jam!
Mother: Yes, she'll eat half a pot of jam at one sitting.
Doctor: Do you let her do that?
Mother: Yes, should I stop her? I thought children always knew what was best for them.

In this case, the child's will cannot flourish either because there is no resistance from the parent, which the child needs and so does everything it can to provoke it.

So now we have two opposite attitudes: the authoritarian (often reproduced from the parents' own childhood) and the indulgent. In the authoritarian attitude the parent crushes all attempts of the child to develop an initiative. In extreme cases the child then becomes subservient or aggressive. With the second, permissive, attitude the child finds no support and becomes restless, insecure, disorientated, tiresome and demanding. Inwardly the child seeks the good example which it cannot find.

Now let us look at the third type, again in the familiar context of a visit to the doctor. As the mother and doctor begin to talk, the child settles down quietly and plays in the place which attracts him most. After a while he notices that the adults' attention is on quite other matters, so he comes to his mother with a question to see whether she has forgotten about him. The mother shows him that he hasn't forgotten him, either by quickly answering his question, or by taking him into her arms until she gets a chance to whisper the answer. He then leaves for a while, depending on how tired he is getting. Words like "you mustn't," "leave me in peace," "stop that" are not necessary, nor are long explanations because the child has trust, and clearly the mother's word carries weight. She did not have to prepare her child in any way specially for the visit to the doctor.

There is of course a background history to this case. The mother here had a feeling for the emotional needs of the child in his second and third year. She was open, responded to him, and offered resistance when it was needed. In many little trials of the second year she did not harass herself unduly by constant chiding, forbidding and running after the child. She gave him something interesting to play with and settled him in his play-pen while she got on with her work. She knew when he was hungry or tired, when he needed her attention and what he needed for his own activity. If anything had to be forbidden, she would only have to say it once, or twice at the most. If the child still had not got the message, he would find himself gently put somewhere else, where he could still see his mother, but could no longer get at some forbidden object such as the desired electric plug. The mother's acts all bore the stamp of matter-of-factness and decisiveness. The child therefore grew up in an atmosphere in which he felt himself belonging and in which word and action coincided. He was always included in his mother's soul-space. As he grew more independent he could create his own soul-space more or less under the aegis of his mother's. If the mother had to show opposition she did not do it out of emotion but from an overview of the situation. This the child felt as something mysterious and valuable, something that belongs to adults. At one time he would be enfolded wholly by his mother when he needed her protection and nearness, and at another time he would find himself confronted by her when she said "no." This alternation developed his character and fortified his self-awareness. Furthermore the child was never faced with decisions which the mother could make far better.

We may assume that even this

mother may have wondered at times whether she was making the right decision, but if so she never let the child share in her doubt. When she acted she did so as surely and as well as she could.

What can you do if you feel that you simply do not possess the capabilities of this mother? If you have done things wrong? If you do not know what you ought to say or do in a particular situation and are afraid that the child may turn out badly or later reproach you? What helps here is to follow good examples. Through practice, the right skills will gradually begin to show themselves. Here are three suggestions:

1. *Love your own work.* Try to see the sense and meaning in it even though it seems insignificant and worthless. Develop some activity which is not directed primarily at the child but has as its object something which gives you personal satisfaction.
2. *Keep your spoken word and let your actions speak.* This applies to the rest of the family, too.
3. *Review the day in the evening.* How was my child today? What has he experienced? Did I handle him in a way that corresponds with the stage which he is at? Where does he stand in his development? What has he gone through, and what has he still to face? What does he require of me? If it is possible for you to talk to your spouse about these things, you can both agree to tell each other if your words and acts do not agree, if for instance a

threat has been made but not carried out. If both parents are in agreement on upbringing, the child is fortunate. Hardly anything so disrupts a child's upbringing as when the child itself becomes the focus of disagreement between the parents.

Larger families

We should now like to give two more examples of characteristic attitudes, this time from life in a larger family where many of the problems discussed above do not arise. In families of more than three children, the younger generation are together much more and educate each other mutually, while demands are made on the parents in ways which a small family does not experience.

Quarrelling
An experienced mother knows that she must see what her children are up to when they are as quiet as mice for then she may be just in time to prevent a possible flooding or similar disaster. But if a row has broken out in the playroom with chairs crashing down and yells and screams, the parent will probably go to check out the situation here, too. The children are probably out of control and are trying to say: "Please come and help us, we can't solve the situation by ourselves!" Now the mother stands calmly in the doorway surveying the riot and asks herself: "Have the children got tired of playing for such a

long time? Do they fail to "mix" well in this particular game? How can I reorganize things to save the situation?"

One of the children rushes up to her crying. The other quickly says: "I didn't hit her." The oldest cries angrily: "I'm not allowed to say what's for dinner when it's *my* dolly's birthday, and now Annie won't come when I invite her," and off she goes with angry tears.

Scolding will not help in this situation. The children are ashamed anyway. Nor does it help to enquire how it all started, that only leads to louder vociferation, but questions like the following will calm them down: "How old is your dolly now? Is she three? Then you can have several courses for dinner! What are you going to cook?" Now the game takes on a new direction and the children learn to take into account the wishes of others. Then the mother says: "You two help me to get supper ready, and the rest of you tidy up the room again so that I can read you a nice story after supper. And mind that all the dollies play quietly so that they don't get too tired to listen to the story."

In this way the antagonists are separated, the game brought to an end, tasks allocated and attention directed to the mother's plans for what is to follow. If one of the children is still sulky, this question can help: "Are you still cross with her?" If she still is you can whisper to her so that the others will not hear.: "Listen, we don't go to bed angry. Can I tell Annie that inside you really love her?" And even if she cannot yet say "yes" the mother knows it and whispers into Annie's ear.

Envy

Ten-year-old Sarah had yet again cleverly helped herself to the biggest apple in the bowl for dessert. Thirteen-year-old Tommy watched disapprovingly but did not say anything. Katie, however, who was twelve, remarked in an accusing tone of voice: "She always takes the biggest and you just let her, I don't think that's fair!"
Father asks: "Who should have it then?"
Silence.
Katie: "Maybe you ... or Mummy, or we should have turns."
Father: "The smaller apples often taste better, but one thing I must say and that is, yesterday Sarah did the gigantic washing up after dinner all by herself without grumbling at all. Do you really grudge her the big apple today?"

This episode shows the many-layered problem of jealousy and envy. It often appears with particular vehemence among people who basically love each other. We do not like to admit that we are envious or jealous but we prefer to think that we are suffering injustice and have a better right to the thing in question. In this way envy and jealousy are masked. If however we realize their true nature we can avoid much conflict and accusation in the family circle.

Through sensitive handling of these incidents, children also come to realize that in life there are no generally applicable moral principles but rather individual situations in which the correct attitude has to be found afresh each time. The scene of the family at table might have the following sequel. Next day Sarah is allowed to choose the biggest and best apple and give it to the person who she thinks ought to have it, or she is allowed to share out the dessert. If misdemeanours are exposed without a chance to make amends, the child will in the long run feel insecure and character will be weakened. If, however, incidents are used to broaden the outlook or to awaken some ability or insight, then the child's character will be strengthened.

17 Problems in child development

17.1 Sleeping problems

Disturbed sleep

Sometimes babies and young children will open their eyes when mother or father tip-toe quietly up to the bed and yet go on sleeping peacefully while another child is screaming in the same room. A screaming infant will usually calm down when given attention by a calm adult. But equally the child's distress can be increased if the adult is tense or preoccupied.

Here are a few typical situations we have experienced in which children's sleep was disturbed:

A nine-month-old baby woke up every night between eleven and one o'clock and whimpered unhappily. Nothing would settle him in his bed. As a last resort he was often taken into the parents' bed where he went to sleep right away. One day the parents noticed that the bed stood right against the outside wall of the house and only the bars of the bed were between the child's head and the wall. They put a veil over the end of the bed and the very first night afterwards, the child slept right through the night. The cause of the child's waking was that, as the outside wall cooled at night, a cold draught passed over the child's head.

A few-months-old baby would wake up every night punctually at twelve minutes past eleven and fall asleep again after about thirty seconds. it was some time before the parents realized that the cause was the slight noise of a high-flying aircraft passing over regularly at that time.

A young child used to sleep happily with the door closed. One day however there was a dull booming noise caused by the wind in the chimney, sounding like a ship's foghorn. The child woke up screaming and after that would not sleep in the dark and certainly not with the door closed.

A baby was moved to the parents' room after disturbing its older brother every night. But the child cried in the parents' room every night and even in the parents' bed it was so restless that neither adult could get any sleep. For hours the parents went through the usual routine: feeding, singing, playing and so on. But each time success was only short-lived and soon the whole fuss started all over again. Then as a final desperate resort the baby was put back again into the other room with its older brother. Strangely enough, as soon as it had been put back there was peace in the household once more. Both children slept deeply and neither woke up any more.

These situations illustrate a number of ways in which a child's sleep can be disturbed. In these and similar situations, parents should ask themselves the following questions:

What is the general disposition of the child by day and by night? Are there any signs of flatulence, constipation, sweating, feeling the cold, envy, jealousy or irritability?

What is the mother's general condition? Are there signs of overtiredness or discontent? Does she feel unappreciated by others? Is she employed outside the home? Is she unhappy or overworked, or worried about anything: family problems, neighbours, security?

What is the child's environment like? Check for the position of the bed, sources of noise (radio, television, and so on) and toys (see Chapter 11.3 and 12.6).

Has the child had a particular desire or need for a time (such as being allowed into the parents' bed during an illness) and has this become a tyrannizing habit?

Is there a younger brother or sister who is just learning to walk? This can be a typical moment when jealousy occurs.

Is there an atmosphere of constant scolding and prohibiting during the day? This can lead to restlessness at night.

Once the parents have discovered why their child might not be sleeping right through the night, the next thing is to decide what should be done. The most important rule for parents whose sleep is constantly interrupted is to ensure that they both get enough sleep to do their work during the day. So do not worry so much about the child: it can easily make up for lack of sleep. Parents should arrange things so that they get out of bed as little as possible during the night. Do not let a young child sleep in an open bed which it can get in and out of. With this sort of freedom, the child will be an endless nuisance. One arrangement is to put the child's bed at the mother's side of the bed so that during the night she can simply put her hand through the bars if the child cries. Most children are quite satisfied with this and go to sleep again. The mother may whisper once only: "Go to sleep now, Mummy is sleeping too," and then not say any more. After a few minutes, the child usually begins to suck its thumb, lies down again and falls asleep.

Things will be quite different if every time there is the slightest noise from the child the mother leaps out of bed and dashes off to the child. Then the child sits or stands up in bed and starts to make all the usual demands. Only bring the child into your own bed as a last resort, and only then if you yourself can sleep. It is sensible to do this if the child is ill, but it is important that at least one parent gets enough sleep. It is useful to know that children quite normally wake up periodically during the night. Most settle themselves down but some demand attention and parents must then carefully weigh up their response.

Once children are about eighteen months old, they intuitively learn the behavioural limits set by their parents. We advise parents to meet the child's needs sensibly and with understanding but to set limits and keep to them. Meeting a child's night-time needs can take one or more of the following forms: leaving the bedroom door open, leaving a light on, letting the child go to sleep in the parents' bed, sleeping on a mattress beside the child's bed, or putting the child to sleep beside the parents' bed. If the child still disturbs the parents' sleep then give a gentle but firm warning, given only once: "Go to sleep now, Mummy has got to sleep too," and after a slight pause, "If you don't let Mummy sleep, you will have to go back in your own room."

It would be wrong to think that the child will understand the actual content of the words but it will im- mediately sense their intention. It is therefore of the greatest importance that the mother always means what she says. If the warning works right away this is fortunate for everyone. If it does not work, then the parents must follow through and take the consequences. To cause unhappiness to the child will, for many parents, create a sense of failure but where children never encounter firmness, they are eventually unhappier, more disoriented and more difficult. The important rule, then, is to let your actions speak and do not beg, explain or threaten.

Let us suppose that you have put the child back in its own room, or somewhere else so that the others will not be disturbed, and it is still screaming. The parents must put up with this for ten minutes, at most. Then go and open the door quietly and ask: "Are you going to be good now?" If the child is quiet, you can take it back with you. But if the child screams louder than ever then you say: "When you're good I'll come back," and you shut the door. After another five minutes you repeat the action, whether the child is yelling or not. This readiness to show the child that you are still there is important. If previously your actions have not matched your words, the process will last longer. But usually after a couple of times, the eighteen-month-old child will get the message that it is no use carrying on. Sometimes you can try standing near the bed and putting up with the screaming for a bit. If this is of no avail, then after five minutes.

you must leave the child and start all over again. It is important that your attitude towards the child is calm and deliberate and quite different from usual. Do not try sweet talk and mollifying. Obviously you want to reach the point of reconciliation and your attitude must reflect this, but never depart from the limits you have set.

Disturbed sleep is not helped by the habit of giving something to drink during the night. It helps to put the bottle for the child to reach, but not to come and give it. One day you can say cheerfully: "From now on you won't need your bottle any more and here is somebody (a soft toy or teddy) to sleep with you and tell you a story if you wake up in the night."

Difficulty in settling down to sleep

Children can get into bad habits of not settling down to sleep and going to sleep in the evening. As with other sleeping problems, the basic approach should be to change the routine and start to draw the line at the right place.

To begin with, make some attempt to give the bed and its area some new attraction for the child. For example, try hanging a blue cloth with some golden stars on the wall or over the bed, to represent the night sky. Offer a new soft-toy as a bed-companion. At bedtime, sing a song by candle-light or play a tune on a gentle instrument such as a guitar or a recorder.

If however, you have tried all these things without success, you should now stop and introduce some new routine. The new activity must give the child pleasure and may take a little longer, such as letting the child sit up for a while beside you on the sofa looking at a picture book. The child now feels that he is being treated as if he was older. But once this time is over, it must be straight to bed!

If the child gets out of bed, then take him back, lay him down and tell him that if he does not stay in bed, the door will be shut. If he gets up again, take him back once more and shut the door firmly. If he then gets out of bed and switches on his light this can be stopped either by removing the light altogether or, if it is a ceiling light completely beyond the reach of the child, taking the bulb out. But some light should be allowed into the room from the window. Leave the child shut in for five minutes and then proceed as already described in the section above. Only leave the door open finally when the child stays quietly in bed.

Children are not stupid. By the second evening the child will have accepted the new order of things. These measures only fail — and for the children it is then a great disillusionment — if the parents are not consistent and lack the will to see the thing through.

A different kind of chronic difficulty in going to sleep arises from a nervous disorder. Some children end up with the idea that they cannot go to sleep. This may have any one of several causes: overtiredness, hot weather, excitement, mother going away, start of holidays. Try sugar-water (not normally allowed because of its effect on the teeth), or a song, or bring one of the absent mother's things such as her woollen cardigan or a rug from her bed. Or tuck the child up a second time, stay with him a bit, stroking his hair so that he feels cosy, loved and protected. If the child is very wide-awake you can even let him get up for a bit, sit in the living room and look at a picture-book by himself. You can say to him: "When you're tired just go back to bed." But do not talk to him as you are clearly busy with other things. Boredom and the pride of knowing when he is tired usually send the child back to bed.

Night terrors

If restlessness, fright and crying occur frequently at night this is known as "night terrors" *(pavor nocturnus)*. The child cries out in sleep or tosses around in bed groaning and can neither wake up straight away nor go on sleeping properly.

Crying in the night may have various causes. The doctor will look for different causes in a baby under eighteen months from those in a three-year-old. When a child starts to cry in the night, the parents should first look to see whether the child is wide awake or dreaming. If the child is asleep, caress him or wake him gently. Then check whether he has any pain (tight tummy), fever or a blocked nose. Here too you can think through the events of the day by asking yourself: What did the child eat before going to bed? Did the child get a fright some time during the day, or did he appear frightened about something? Decide then whether to call the doctor or not. Ask yourself, too, whether the disturbance occurs in any sort of regular cycle (for instance, a four-weekly cycle could be connected with the phases of the moon). Usually this condition can be treated satisfactorily with anthroposophical or homoeopathic medicines.

Sleepwalking usually coincides with the full moon. It can be dangerous if the child wakes up while sleepwalking. Anthroposophical or homoeopathic medicines can be used in treatment. Neuroleptics (tranquilizers) are not needed either for sleepwalking or for night terrors.

17.2 Refusal to eat

Let us first look at some scenes from the consulting-room:

A happy-looking three-year-old is brought in. The mother says:
"He won't eat anything at all"
"What does he eat then?"
"Nothing. He won't touch anything I offer him. But he can drink milk all day and eat yoghurt."
Closer enquiry reveals that the little fellow does consume some sweet things at odd times as well as the milk. Even so the mother is right; he will not touch anything which she makes for him.

Solution: All milk products are completely banned for a week, then rationed to two mugs of milk or yoghurt per day. No sweets or confectionery are allowed between meals and no sweet drinks. Then appetite is left for other things.

Another mother says much the same for her boy, the only difference being that he does not drink milk.
Further questioning shows that he does eat cottage-cheese, eggs or meat as well as ice-cream and lemonade at regular intervals, but at table he will hardly touch anything of the main meal.

Solution: The child should be starved for three days. No sweets are allowed and at table the child is overlooked. After three days the child's love of sweet things can be met by allowing him a dessert.

Now a thin bony girl with fine features and delicate hands comes into the consulting-room. The doctor makes some enquiries: what was her weight at birth? What were her parents like at her age? The child takes only a very little of anything and is not even tempted by good home-made soup.

Solution: The parents should arrange for the girl to go on holiday into the country or into the mountains with other children. It is important for the mother to "let go" and allow her child to decide what and how much she eats. No one should expect anything from her. Her appetite however will come back by itself through the change of air. No special attention will be paid to the child. Afterwards when she is back home she will not eat much more than before but the atmosphere will be more relaxed.

Now along comes a mother with a rather mulish and sulky-looking boy. He will not do what is expected of him, and he will not eat either.

The solution in this case will only be found after a few confidential talks with the parents. They will have to be made to see that children are not just there to live up to their parents' fond expectations, but flourish best when they can shape their own behaviour on that of their parents and are not continually exposed to questions, exhortations, explanations and demands.

Now there comes a child who does not like anything at all — except red grape juice and a special kind of biscuit. The mother's example is the problem here because she is a weight-watcher. As long as the mother cannot sit down at table in peace and enjoy eating what she herself has cooked, this child cannot be cured. The mother will have to find a different way of keeping her figure.

Many of these problems arise because the mother is overstressed, the children make demands on her and she feels unappreciated. To keep your head above water, to love cooking, to stop children eating sweets between meals, and yet at the same time meet every demand and always be in a good mood — easier said than done!

To conclude, let us take a glimpse into that perfect home which children's doctors dream about. When the thirsty children come in from school, they drink a glass of the unsweetened herb-tea standing ready while they are waiting for the meal. All the sweets that they were given or swapped with their friends on their way home from school are put in a box. When the box is full, it will be exchanged for a new football or something useful. There is no radio switched on in the house so that everyone can talk in peace and exchange news. Like this, the mother can all the better tune into the mood of each child. Before the meal which is always eaten together, the family join hands and say a blessing on the meal. During the meal, they chat about the events of the day and tease each other a bit. They do not talk about the food. Everyone eats just as much as they want, usually a bit of everything. Each child may be allowed to leave one thing. Anything else that is not liked is cut up and mixed in with the rest of the food. Or there may be a rule that everyone must eat at least three spoonfuls of everything on the plate. Conversation is so interesting that everybody stays at table till the end of the meal. Then once again the family take hands and say a thanksgiving.

17.3 Bed-wetting (Enuresis)

If a child wets the bed after the age of four, medical examination and advice is necessary as the bed-wetting may be due to constitutional, organic and psychological causes. Provided that an organic cause has been excluded, there are some measures which can help. By wetting the bed the child is really saying to the parents: "I want to be a baby again, be cared for and wrapped in nappies."

First investigate to see if there are possible emotional causes: shock, fright or jealousy. Once the possible cause has been established, try to meet the child's need to be treated as a baby again, by comforting and protecting. Go back to habits of earlier childhood and at the same time try to bring a greater consistency and regularity into the daily routine. Also try to be much more conscious of the child during the day. If the child is of pre-school age, do not speak directly about the problem which started the bed-wetting, but try to find a solution to it. It may be that a baby sister or brother has just been born or has just learnt to walk. This might result in giving the older child less attention, so make a point of taking the child into your arms and sharing your pleasure over the new baby or its achievements. Show that you are equally proud of the older

one being so big now. It may be time to give a sign of this by letting the child graduate to a new mug or eating with a knife and fork. You can also tell stories which act as parables for bed-wetting, such as the tale of the little Dutch boy and the hole in the dyke. Stories like this can help the child unconsciously to control bed-wetting through an increased sense of responsibility.

Condemnation and disapproval of bed-wetting only increase the child's need for more positive attention, and will only lead to the complaint becoming worse. Parental disapproval is as bad as beating the child or subjecting it to cold baths as a punishment for wetting the bed! On the other hand by meeting the child's intrinsic need, by accepting the problem with a positive attitude, and by proper care, the complaint can be cured.

As for practical suggestions, if the child regularly wets the bed at half past ten at night and again at six o'clock in the morning, try the following approach. Accompany the child to the bathroom before bedtime to observe that the lavatory is used properly. One or two hours afterwards, lift the sleeping child and set it on the lavatory with a whispered encouragement. Do the same at six o'clock in the morning. In this way you take upon yourself the responsibility for the child's toilet habits and when you think the time is right, you can pass the responsibility back again.

This method is not suitable for children who wet their beds at frequent intervals during the night or who struggle and yell when they are woken up. The effect is doubtful also in the case of children who go on sleeping deeply while on the lavatory. In these cases, you must decide whether the child should go back to having a nappy or whether a rubber sheet is enough.

A regular routine in the child's daily life is beneficial and strengthening. First see that eating and drinking habits are regular. You cannot cure a "drink-when-you-want-child" of bedwetting, so begin by ensuring that the child drinks only at meal-times. Then you should experiment carefully with how much the child can be allowed to drink after five or six in the evening. It would be counterproductive to allow the child to drink freely at this time of day.

It is important that the child is kept warmly dressed in woollen pants or tights of a thickness suitable to the time of year. The trousers should reach well up the trunk. If the feet get cold and wet they should be treated with a hot foot-bath and rubbed with massage oil. Giving the legs a good rub with, say, St. John's wort oil, every morning has a good effect. Finally see that the child is being stimulated sufficiently by watching activities suitable for imitation. The feeling of "running in neutral" encourages a relapse into earlier stages of development. Other possible causes such as quarrels in the home, both parents out at work, conflicts arising through divorce and other things may require professional advice.

If a child wets by day as well as by night and organic causes are ruled out, the same methods should be used with the addition that during the day you must establish an "inner alarm" which is how we normally train a child to be dry. Without discussion, simply put the child on to the lavatory or potty at regular times.

Damp pants as opposed to wet ones require some investigation. Often it is just a sign of carelessness. In such cases you should accompany the child to the lavatory to ensure that the bladder is completely emptied. The child will not enjoy this kind of attention very much.

Once children are six to eight years old, the problem requires different handling. They are now old enough to listen to adults whom they respect, such as teachers, godparents or doctors. A direct injunction however would still be requiring too much of them. What, however, has proved effective in such cases is telling a little story as a way of increasing the child's awareness. The story might be about a little bird or fairy that keeps watch while the child is asleep and whispers in its ear to remind it to use the lavatory. The person telling the story should not be the mother or father, but the parents may play their part by saying quietly to the child at bedtime: "Remember the little bird and see if you can hear it tonight!"

The truth behind a story of this kind is that the child really does not want to wet itself. The fairy or bird is an image of the child's still weak intention to wake up. The image makes the child more aware of its own intention and through the trick of being reminded every night, the habit of waking up will come more readily. We consider it too soon at this age to admonish the child directly.

Appealing to the conscience is not appropriate before the child is ten. Then it is better to leave this to a third person, preferably the doctor. Sometimes a change of scene for a short while is recommended. This makes the child feel more independent and at the same time strengthens self-awareness.

The use of a "buzzer" (an electrical device which can be inserted under the sheets) can be successful but does not directly help the child in its self-development since there is no increased responsibility.

17.4 Fouling

By fouling we do not mean the dirty pants of irregular or careless children, but the deliberate depositing of excreta in the pants or in a corner of the house. Dirty pants require only the humorous attention of the parents and getting regular habits to fit into the rhythm of the day. Few readers will have encountered true fouling (encopresis) which may occur as a result of stress which the child cannot resolve or arise from a desire to put the parents to the test, or from fear of an unfamiliar lavatory or potty. These things are easily understood and rectifiable. But if fouling drags on for weeks and months, this indicates a more serious loss of will on the part of the child and the parents. Without professional help, this situation cannot usually be remedied. If the parents themselves are reluctant to seek help, a friend can act as go-between in obtaining guidance either from a psychiatrist or from a doctor.

17.5 Thumb-sucking

If you find a two-year-old sucking its thumb and you pull the thumb out and let go, the thumb will pop back into the mouth as if attached to an invisible piece of elastic. But if you keep hold of the thumb, the child will wake up reluctantly, noticing that the blissful peace has been disturbed. If however the child's interest is drawn to the sounds of lunch being served or the push-chair being got ready for a walk, the thumb will come out all by itself, pushed out as strongly as it had been pulled in before.

Thumb-sucking means screening oneself off from the world and being comfortably by oneself. As thumb-sucking can lead to deformity of the jaw, specially designed dummies are often recommended, but we advise

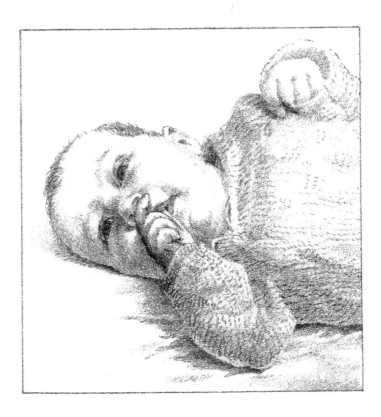

Figure 54. Thumb-sucking

against them because they encourage children to suck when they would not have done so of their own accord. The dummy hanging round the child's neck becomes a sedative, a presage of food to come and a means of self-indulgence. The thumb at least has the advantage of renewing its surface, is not so infectious and is always handy but never kept in the mouth when the child wants to play. However, if you do decide to go in for a dummy, secure it with a loose elastic or tape around the body, not around the neck.

As regards malformation of the jaw, this occurs not only with thumb or finger sucking; we have also seen it with the use of a dummy. The malformation fortunately straightens up by itself with the coming of the second teeth when thumb-sucking gradually ceases.

After all this, readers may be wondering whether anything at all should be done about thumb-sucking. We say that children should be allowed to suck something before going to sleep. For more persistent sucking, we recommend that you have patience. Some children when they reach the age of about five suddenly declare: "I'm not going to suck my thumb any more," and the habit stops overnight. One mother even noticed how her child's arm jerked away from the mouth when the child was asleep.

Action may need to be taken sooner, however, if a raw patch develops on the thumb or finger. It will be necessary to bandage the sore area and this can sometimes help to break the habit. Put plenty of ointment on the sore, cover with lint or gauze and then a bandage. First bandage the sore thumb (or finger), then all the fingers and then the whole hand. Now put the hand into a bag made from a handkerchief or cotton material and attach the bag by two tapes under the jacket and fastened around the body (not around the neck!). The child will observe its new limb with astonishment while the parents look pleased, thus reassuring the child that everything is in order. Change the bandage daily and remove finally after a week. By then the child may have given up the habit of sucking. Do not use a plaster as it can be sucked off and swallowed.

Sucking the thumb is the prolongation of an earlier phase of development, namely, sucking at the breast. Therefore it is not right either to forbid or to encourage sucking the thumb. The child can be encouraged to move on in development by the parent stimulating more interest in activities and the surroundings.

17.6 Nail-biting and scratching

Nail-biting has nothing to do with a calcium deficiency but is one of the many nervous habits resulting from emotional pressure, tension, embarrassment, boredom or tiredness. Children give up the habit when they themselves wish to, but never because their parents tell them to. Indeed, parental pressure can only make things worse. Parents should check to see whether they themselves are demanding and tense in their behaviour towards the child and whether the child is not getting enough stimulation. The child will respond to being given a shiny new nail-file and a pair of nail-scissors as a present and then shown how to file the nails so that all sharp corners, superfluous skin and roughness are removed. Afterwards the nails should be liberally treated with ointment. Dry, itchy skin is the most common reason for putting the nails into the mouth to moisten them. With older children, if the itch is removed with use of a moisturizing cream, then the habit will disappear.

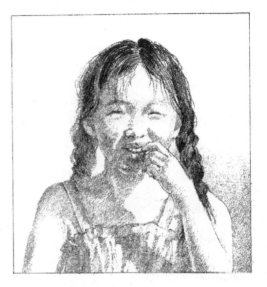

Figure 55. Nail-biting

17.7 Harmless urges

From time to time, nearly every child will walk *only* along the kerb, or step *only* in the middle of the flagstones of the pavement, or *only* on the cracks, whichever happens to be the rule at the time. But if a child really cannot move without keeping to certain rules and breaking them causes fear, this is a true compulsion. In a child of school age, compulsive washing of the hands, pirouetting, counting and so on, will require a visit to the psychiatrist or doctor. All habits and repeated movements have a tendency to become compulsive but compulsion manifests itself once the movement or action is taken out of context and is being executed for its own sake. The remedy lies helping the child to achieve greater control by using educational or medical treatment.

17.8 Pillow-thumping and rocking

Many children rock themselves to sleep. These movements may be compulsively repeated at the time of waking. The behaviour is more marked in handicapped, mentally ill or neglected children. In our experience, however, it is parents whose children are neither neglected nor mentally handicapped who come to the consulting-room with the problem.

As with thumb-sucking, these habits strengthen children's awareness of their bodies but here the chosen rhythm which relaxes can send the child into a trance-like condition. Whatever the cause of the inner tension may be, it can usually be dispelled by singing quietly to the child before it goes to sleep and by gently stroking the brow. Do not expect immediate success for this type of response to tension is also determined by constitution and will only change over time. A constitutional remedy is therefore often given over a longer period. When the child reaches school age, the behaviour usually disappears by itself.

17.9 Restlessness and tics

A little boy, hardly five years old, is very noticeable as soon as he enters the consulting-room. He runs to the window, looks quickly at the things on the desk, picks up the telephone receiver, loses interest in it and then sees the toys on the table. He picks them up but soon puts them down again. Now he inserts himself into the conversation between the adults and standing by his mother's knee he comments on what they have to say. In between whiles he makes grimaces and shrugs his shoulders. Finally his behaviour dominates the whole consultation and conversation is no longer possible.

Parents and doctor together must often analyse this kind of behaviour and arrive at a correct therapy. First we have to find out whether the parents regard the disorder as such; perhaps they have come to the doctor only because there is disturbed sleep or lack of social contact. The child's restlessness, running about from one thing to another, they took to be because he was so interested in everything, and on top of that, they may regard him as highly intelligent because he grasps things so quickly. They have not noticed that other children who approach things more slowly are able to form stronger attachments.

We try to look more deeply into the child's behaviour. Why are the movements so automatic and jerky? They interrupt or prevent contact with the surroundings and have no real meaning for the child itself. They are mechanical and stereotyped, mere vestiges of willed movements. The soul can no longer express itself freely through them. The sort of behaviour we are talking about here includes a variety of jerking motions and rudimentary movements like pulling grimaces, shaking the head, blinking or clearing the throat. Those who suffer from such involuntary movements usually feel something like a brief tension before the twitch starts. The tension disappears when the person starts concentrating on something else but, when he stops concentrating, the twitch comes on even more strongly. The twitch is also aggravated, rather like stammering, whenever the person feels watched. Susceptibility to this kind of automatism may be hereditary, organic or constitutional, and is aggravated by overstimulating the senses and by emotional stress which the child cannot deal with. When we examine children like this more closely, we often observe a slight restlessness in all their movements which leaves them generally rather clumsy. At home and at school, they will be characterized by this clumsiness and by their bad handwriting or disturbed behaviour. If in addition, they are growing up in surroundings exposed continually to the media and entertainments, their chances of developing inwardly dwindle rapidly.

From talks, observations and further examination of the child, the doctor can build up a picture of all the factors causing the restlessness. Once this is done, a therapy can be arrived at. Whether the disorder is neurolo-

gical (that is, physical and organic) or psychological, the following measures can help:

Establish a regular daily routine alternating between activity and quiet: keep to regular bedtime, getting-up and meal times. Concentration and attention improve through games with rhythmical movements, clapping and singing. In this respect eurythmy and curative eurythmy (see Chapter 16.8) are particularly good. The child should also be read to aloud from stories

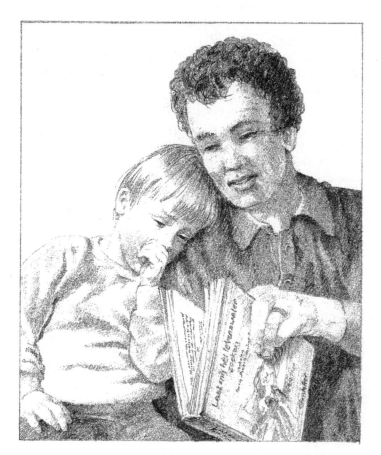

Figure 56. Establish quiet daily routines such as reading together.

illustrated with clear but not too formalized pictures.

If you are always telling your children to be good, learn to leave them more inner freedom. This usually happens only after several talks between parents and doctor. It helps parents to understand why the child is as it is. After calmly looking at the condition of the child, parents can often find the right approach to the problem.

Ban all exposure to television, radio and cassettes, including taped stories, as well as comics. Instead introduce a daily diet of structured games and playing, such as shadow-theatre or puppet shows. The stereotyped images filling the child's mind will gradually be supplanted by new images which do not deform the child's mind and stimulate, rather than compel, the imagination.

Such a programme of activities would probably be too much for the parents alone without the support of kindergartens, advisory centres and, in acute cases, children's clinics. Parents' groups may also be a valuable support.

It is a matter of debate whether such restless behaviour can be cured by simply avoiding food that contains certain phosphates or additives. It will always help to take the quality of food into account and to avoid foods with artificial colouring and other chemical ingredients but we advise against adopting extreme diets. With any behavioural problem of this kind, we would certainly not recommend the use of neuroleptics and tranquilizers.

17.10 Masturbation

In childhood masturbation is a symptom and not in itself a disturbance or a perversion. In babies the problem can often start with the healing of a sore. Sometimes the habit arises as a "discovery" and disappears again after a while. Lay the child down on its side rather than on its back and give it some favourite toy or object to hold.

With an older child, look for external causes if masturbation is practised excessively and habitually. Rejection, friendships breaking up, boredom or moral pressure, are all possible causes and require attention, the aim being to restore emotional balance. The child's attention should be diverted from its own body and directed to new interests, especially physical activities such as sport and hiking. Too much mental work should be avoided. Read the child a story at bedtime.

17.11 Mischievousness

True mischievousness has nothing to do with aggression or malice. When children get up to tricks — for example taking the neighbour's gate off its hinges and leaving it down the road, or ringing other people's front-door bells and watching their faces from a safe distance, or putting salt in the sugar-bowl, or thinking up really good April Fool's Day tricks — all these are a sign of intelligence and readiness to act: in other words, proof of a certain strength of character and of a budding sense of humour which will later be highly appreciated. Mischievousness shows that the child has an excess of energy, that intelligence is at work and that there is a need for activity which has not yet found a sensible outlet. In later life this energy will show in a readiness to take on work, to look at reality with a clear eye and with understanding for the many and varied pitfalls of everyday life. Of course this sort of mischievousness is not to be confused with sadistic, destructive and evil actions which result from a barren upbringing.

The child is fortunate indeed who grows up with adults who were once themselves inclined to mischief. Such adults will react to misdemeanours with understanding even while meting out punishment or giving clear warning that limits have been reached. In practice, we should worry more about the well-behaved children than about the mischievous ones as the latter always turn out well in later life.

17.12 Anorexia and obesity

Both anorexia (under-eating) and obesity (over-eating) are on the increase amongst children entering puberty. Growing too fat is generally more inclined to affect boys while growing too thin more often affects girls. In order to understand these problems, we should look at what is happening to the child as he or she enters puberty.

The adolescent girl (and what follows applies to boys also) feels not only that her body is becoming bigger and bigger but also that it is developing more and more out of her control. Movement becomes awkward and poorly coordinated. The girl is not as she wishes to be and, in emotional terms, is subject to violent extremes, veering from ecstasy to despair. Inside herself, she may feel older and more mature than she actually appears to others, or the reverse, and she may feel misunderstood, unaccepted and lonely. These feelings are aggravated if the parents allow her too little freedom and privacy, and are constantly pursuing her with their love and care right down to the smallest detail. In these conditions, the adolescent can no longer breathe emotionally and has no personal space in which to build up her own life. As a result, she takes refuge in an illness such as anorexia. This gives her parents. who already have too close a connection to her, an immediate object on which all their care and worry can fasten, namely the concern with food. The same basic pattern applies equally, but in the opposite way, to those children who are growing too fat.

These illnesses may also be a sign that the child, for one reason or another, is afraid of growing up. The child tries to revert to the chubby round form of the toddler, or else wishes to become less and less substantial until she disappears completely from the earth. It is distressing to see how often girls have allowed undernourishment to go so far that they can only be rescued from starvation by artificial feeding and intensive hospital care. By contrast, growing too fat can be a sign of too binding a connection with things of the senses and of the earth. Eating as a form of gratification, as sensual enjoyment, takes on a disproportionate focus and substitutes for spiritual interests which have not been developed.

On the one hand, then, we have a flight from the earth and a fear of life, and on the other too strong a bond with the earth and an excessive indulgence; the cure can only be to find again a healthy middle way. For this, it is nearly always necessary for the child to be completely removed from the home environment and admitted into a child-psychiatric clinic for a considerable period. This prolonged absence gives the parents the opportunity to review their child's whole development and upbringing in consultation with the doctor, child guidance specialist or counsellor.

In exceptional cases, the condition can be cured after a single stay in hospital and the child's development continues healthily thereafter. But experience shows that there is a great danger of a relapse with these two problems for the simple reason that it is not easy for the parents to change their behaviour towards the child in a few weeks. The prognosis is made more unfavourable if in the background there is a divorce conflict or an unresolved school problem.

In conclusion we should like to mention an aspect which is often overlooked these days. In adolescence, religious longings arise with special intensity at the critical stage where the soul desires to maintain its purity, not to sully itself, not to lose its innocence. These longings, sometimes openly expressed, sometimes concealed, are often to be found behind cases of anorexia in older girls, and they need to be handled delicately and confidentially. With the right sort of guidance, a true recovery can be achieved and the girl's life directed towards real depth of purpose and awareness.

18 Problems of modern living

18.1 The effects of television and video

In recent years, there has been widespread debate on the subject of children and television. In the first instance, we should like to describe our own experience in the consulting-room and the conclusions we have drawn. We have noted that young children who watch television regularly develop certain behavioural patterns:

They meet other people without shyness or reserve but do not attempt to have real personal contact with them.

They cannot meet someone's calm gaze without staring or making a face.

They ask superficial questions without being particularly interested in the answers.

They respond to questions with superficial or stereotyped answers.

They do not develop a very deep interest in anything.

Their emotions are primitive and inclined to be heartless.

Their thinking moves in rapid and predictable patterns.

Often parents of such children find their behaviour amusing and funny, so that it is difficult for the teacher or doctor to make the parents realize that there is anything wrong with their children.

There is much published research on the effects of television on children and the descriptions confirm to a great extent our own findings. The main known effects can be summarized as follows:

Speech remains primitive.

The ability to make sense of what is read is diminished. Even the spoken word hardly evokes the child's own mental pictures and the child's imagination is stamped with ready-made pictures and associations.

Such children read less and prefer to confine themselves to pictures mostly in comics and comic-strip books.

Active assimilation of what has been read and seen does not take place, with the result that the ability to concentrate is reduced.

A tendency to addiction to alcohol, drugs and medication is induced, as children become used to getting stimuli and mental content without effort, simply as it were by pressing a button.

The development of will is radically disrupted, because the children sit inactively in front of the screen and cannot occupy themselves actively and by imitation as they would otherwise do. After a period of watching television, the children are prone to release unused energy in a chaotic and aggressive outburst.

The problem has taken on a new dimension in the last few years with the increase in circulation of video-cassettes giving children access to a whole range of unsuitable entertainment, including horror films. Without close supervision, many parents have not the least idea of what their children are absorbing in the way of nonsense and perversion.

In the light of all the evidence about the bad effects of television and video, it is surprising to hear parents still express opinions like the following:

"It can't be as bad as all that!"
"Why then are there broadcasts for school and TV programmes specially for children?"
"I'd rather the children watched television at home than in a friend's house."
"After all we have to know what's going on and the children want to be in with the crowd."

But in response, we should like to ask:

Which helps development towards independence more — to follow the crowd in order to be "with it" or to have the courage to say: "We don't watch TV at home, we prefer other ways of entertaining ourselves"?

Is all television good simply because there are special broadcasts for schools and children's programmes?

How much do children gain by not seeing animals and insects as caricatures but watching them in nature and reading about them?

The best policy is to cut out all television until the development of the will and feeling has come to an end around the age of thirteen to fifteen. At all events watching TV should be absolutely taboo until the child is ten (see Chapter 16.6). Between ten and fifteen, there is room for compromise to individual circumstances. Generally speaking, the more sure the parents are of their beliefs, the more the children will accept what they say. But if one of the parents thinks that their children are missing something by not being "in with it" then there will be endless discussions and finally an unsatisfactory compromise.

If the child does watch a programme or the news, you should make the effort to help the child digest what has been seen by talking about it. This at least helps the child to absorb the material personally and not just passively lap it up. Up to the age of sixteen, it is best that parents choose, watch and discuss the programmes with their children. After that age, the children should be left free to choose. If they have sufficiently developed other interests, television will not have the same fascination for them.

Ideally, the television should be kept in a room which the children may not generally enter. Children will accept that there are things like smoking, drinking and television which are only for adults.

Many educationalists and child specialists take the view that we must accept the technological realities of the world and simply try to exercise an element of control. This view is of no use whatsoever where television is concerned in the development of the child. It only masks the problem and allows the acquisition of bad habits with all their consequences. Like other bad influences in civilization which experts tell us to tolerate, television will only be put in its place by ordinary individuals making their own decisions with the benefit of their own insight.

18.2 Comics

As the effect of comics is on the child's power of forming mental images, their influence is not as easily observed in the child's behaviour as that of television. If however, while we are having a talk with the mother in the consulting-room, we let the child draw a picture, the poverty and lack of originality in the child's effort can often be deplorable. After listening to a story, these children cannot create their own pictures of the story but instead reproduce comic-style drawings, consisting of distorted and unattractive caricatures. Why do children become so fascinated by the picture sequence of the comics long before they can understand what is written in the "bubbles"? It is because they can in fact only think in pictures. Every picture attracts them, and the comic pictures with their bright colours and sharp outlines have a particular attraction. But because the comic pictures are self-contained and finished products, they imprison and fetter the imagination. The child's mind cannot develop anything through such images and the psyche cannot flourish. Adults, with their mature abstract thinking, can distance themselves from the pictures of comics and television and shake them off, but a child cannot.

These comic caricatures often carry messages that are morally sound, with the result that ideals and pure ideas are stamped with these pictures on the mind. When for example a hero like Tarzan rescues a lovely girl from the claws of a beast, then such important human values as courage, beauty and love are tied to false and shallow images. In later life this can lead to distorted and superficial views about fundamental spiritual truths.

To sum up, comics and cartoon pictures prise the child out of a natural and direct relationship with the world and substitute an apparent reality where moral values are presented in a distorted form. What a contrast with the effects of true story images such as those inspired by Grimm's fairy-tales, which the child creates out of its own activity (see Chapter 16.6). The fairy-stories reveal a spiritual reality which is just as true as the reality of the sense world. If children take these pictures into their minds, they will feel themselves lifted up to and involved in the spiritual world around them.

The more our minds have been dominated in childhood by unreal or fantastic mental images, the less we will feel rooted in the world as adults and the more we will be liable to fall prey to inner doubt, insecurity and existential fears. In addition, we will become detached from the world more than is healthy and will tend to form cynical and mocking judgments about situations in life, with a tendency to find it hard to take anything seriously or to relate to things with any depth or commitment.

18.3 Overstimulation of the senses

The infant or young child focuses its attention more easily on a single prominent object than on an abundance of simultaneous impressions. When flooded with impressions, the child's mind quickly tires, cannot assimilate any more and sets up a protective wall; the child will start to suck its thumb or will fall asleep. Despite this protective response, the child still has to digest unconsciously the kaleidoscope of impressions experienced when awake.

It is clear, then, that a child does not gain by seeing and hearing as much as possible during the course of the day. For instance, a baby being taken around town in a transparent "panorama-pram" will have impression after impression thrust upon it and its attention cannot rest anywhere. But compare a child in a properly enclosed pram, looking up towards the mother's face as she pushes the pram along. The child has time to watch the mother's changing features: her smile, her pensiveness, her joy at seeing something beautiful, her conversation and animation when she meets a neighbour or friend. Now the child is experiencing the connection between what he sees from one moment to the next for it is one and the same mother that is seen and she represents continuity amidst the changing perceptions.

Similarly if a child hears its mother moving things about in the next room and singing a song as she works, there is an experience of connection between the work and the mother's mood. So it is not the amount of sense impressions that matters but that they should have a real connection with one another.

A mass of unrelated impressions has the opposite effect on a child, amounting almost to a training in superficiality and a devaluation of the senses. When sense impressions are devalued like this, the accompanying alienation from reality cripples genuine interest in the world. Things no longer receive a name which expresses something of their inner nature, but simply a label, while the child regards things only from the angle of the stimulus or pleasure that they offer. The activity of thinking comes to serve only the satisfying of personal desires, a marked tendency which we observe in the modern world with its emphasis on advertising and propaganda. As such influences are increasingly exerted on children, there is a real danger that the adverse effects of overstimulation will become even more pronounced in the future.

18.4 Early intellectual training

Early intellectual training has become extremely popular with both parents and educationalists, something which is reflected in the toymaking and educational materials industry. You can of course train single skills in the early stages of child development and, as the majority of people live in a state of scientific credulity, toys and materials for early learning are welcomed as the latest advances in education and psychology, and allowed to flood into the lives of children without `the least reservation. Froebel's methods are structured along these lines. He wanted to encourage creativity in the kindergarten with his play materials. Quite rightly he observed that children understand a totality first and from there go on to recognize parts. Consequently his programme provides the child first with a spherical object, then a cube, and then a cube of eight equal parts. We can see the direction of his thought: the child is to be trained in logical-mathematical concepts. The child has little alternative but to use the cube in the way that the adult intended and its imaginative powers are constrained by a mathematical principle which is inappropriately restrictive. The cube is followed by small blocks to be laid on a prepared surface representing the concepts to be recognized: number series, aesthetic forms (stars and medals), useful forms (furniture). It is clear that this material which is intended to develop the child's creativity defeats its own purpose: creativity never flows from a rigidly pre-designed scheme.

Similar ideas inspire the Montessori material, which consists of purpose-designed units each with a particular educational aim. Artistic and moral influences are to come from the teacher, independently of the learning material. Here we do not question the value of the teacher's contribution. Very often this is much more effective than the theory which is being put into practice.

An extreme form of this early learning is found in the "logic blocks" which have been introduced into kindergartens. The harm which these blocks can cause is twofold. Firstly mathematical concepts which in themselves are not sensory are made perceptible to the senses; and secondly the child's logical faculty which at that age should be passive and subject to sense-perceptions is now activated in isolation. The result is a further alienation of the child from the reality in which it lives.

Just as overstimulation of the senses leaves the child with only a superficial connection to the world, and comics and television lead thought into illusion, so premature training in logic sets up a false relationship between the world of pure concepts and the world of sense-perceptions. Thus a triple misguidance of the human mind takes place and millions of children bear the consequences in the form of feelings of meaninglessness and a sense of unreality in life. What we observe today is only the beginning. There is little doubt that, in future, psychological illnesses and crises resulting from these developments will become an increasing concern of medicine, psychology and education. Against this trend, those parents who make an effort to introduce their children only gradually to the complexities of modern culture, and above all to introduce them at the appropriate time, will spare them such a fate.

18.5 Computer games

The majority of computer games revolve around themes such as football, war, science fiction, chasing criminals or driving cars. In an atmosphere of sensationalism and excitement, all too often characterized by cynical indifference and cruelty, quick reactions are certainly stimulated, but at the expense of deeper reflection and true understanding. All young people need for their development moments of stillness, of listening and reflecting on what has been experienced, accompanied by a reverent and serene attitude. Computer games tend to train the attitudes and responses in completely the opposite direction. As a result, inner development is diverted away from the direction which it should be taking.

Obviously a sixteen-year-old who has developed intellectually in the right way will suffer no great harm by playing an occasional computer game as a test of speed or skill.

18.6 Alcohol and drug addiction

One of the most painful experiences for parents is to discover that their child has become a drug-addict. How did it happen that we did not notice anything in good time? What have we done wrong? Why did it have to happen to *our* child?

Many young people today take drugs in the course of growing up. For most of them it is just an episode, but a few become dependent. There are many very different motives which impel young people to sample drugs. It may be for curiosity or so as not to lose a friend or be ostracized from a group. But often it is for clearly defined personal motives: escape from a world which has become unpleasant, escape from a disrupted home full of quarrels and marriage conflicts, escape from worries and dilemmas in school and from the fear of failure. The experiences which drugs can provide are equally varied. First there are the drugs which induce a state of euphoria and give a feeling of unbounded freedom and independence: to these belong cannabis (hashish), opium and its derivatives including the particularly dangerous heroin. Then there are the drugs called amphetamines which produce a bright wideawake awareness, such as cocaine. After the increased alertness and the accompanying feeling of lightness there follows a very deep sleep of exhaustion. A further group of drugs are the hypnotics which are used to provide tranquillization and sleep; the narcotics used in medicine, such as ether, as well as a whole series of sleep-inducing drugs, belong to this group. A final group is the hallucinogens which induce an abundance of experiences through heightened consciousness. The best known of these drugs is LSD which is also called the drug of initiation, because many of the experiences which its use occasions are described by people who through their own spiritual efforts have achieved a heightening of their normal consciousness. Among drug-addicts there are always those who started with a genuine thirst for knowledge, seeking to explore all the possible states of consciousness. Towards this knowledge two ways are available: one is through the drug whereby the individual's vitality is undermined and physical damage is suffered; the other is through spiritual effort which strengthens the soul and works harmoniously through the body.

What are the factors which predispose a child to addiction? It is often said that these factors cannot be clearly determined as drug addicts are to be found in all social levels. But if we look more closely, certain factors can be identified very clearly. Two elements always seem to operate together: one is a weakness of will in the child's personality and the other a lack of educational measures to strengthen the will. In individual cases one or other of these may dominate but usually they work together.

Children and adolescents who become dependent on alcohol and drugs are often more sensitive than others. They are receptive to what is beautiful and idealistic — and are therefore often inclined to be revolutionaries. But they cannot stand up sufficiently to the knocks of everyday life. Either they avoid problems or they try to solve them with violence, but they have difficulty in tackling them on a daily basis until they have really worked them out.

As a result, therapy has only a chance of being successful if the individual makes a great effort, most often in newly sought out surroundings. Here we can here mention only the most important preventive measures:

1. Provide loving interest in every stage of the child's development (see Chapter 16.6);
2. Try to establish the right balance between strictness and flexibility in upbringing. Draw up clear boundaries and limits within which the child can feel secure (see Chapter 16.4);
3. Help the child to cultivate good habits and keep to a regular daily routine, including regular meals. Limit the amount of sweets. Sugar can become the first addiction: quick energy, increased feeling of strength and self-assurance without much digestion (see Chapter 14);
4. Strengthen the child's imagination by telling fairy stories, reading good stories, legends and biographical accounts rather than letting him passively absorb ready-made pictures from comics and television. What can be enjoyed without effort also predisposes to addiction. The soul feels stimuli and receives pictures without doing any work itself; there is no active involvement and interaction with what has been absorbed (see Chapter 18.1);
5. Encourage the child to make music rather than be constantly and passively exposed to the desensitizing flood of radio and cassette;
6. Provide enough physical exercise corresponding to the child's age as a foundation for training of the will, for instance, playing out of doors, sport and walks;
7. Provide regular activities for training the will. The will is trained only by real activity, not by setting out to do something attractive and failing to achieve it;
8. Be aware of the use of alcohol in the home. Children will see that now and again a measured consumption of alcohol belongs to the world of grown-ups. If however the children see their parents and other adults in a state of abandon and irresponsibility they will not see why alcohol should

be allowed while other drugs are so strictly forbidden, especially as it is so well known that alcohol has hypnotically active and health-destroying properties. Here there is an inconsistency in our culture which reveals our general laxity and weakness of will and is in its own way related to the whole drug problem. While the child is growing and ideally up to the age of sixteen, alcohol should not be allowed at all. Strength and energy required for the training of the will derives from well developed healthily functioning metabolic organs. Even the slightest damage to the liver results in a weakening of the development of the will as the liver is the main metabolic organ. Consumption of alcohol while the body is growing not only impairs the functioning of the liver, but also the development of the liver as one of the organs which underpin the development of the will for later life.

These points show clearly how much certain aspects of our present day civilization predispose towards addiction. If we are to work against these tendencies, we must ourselves as adults tackle many of our favourite habits and assumptions even to the extent of distancing ourselves socially from our surroundings. The value of these protective measures for the physical and soul health of our growing children is immeasurable and, for the sake of the future of our growing adolescents, it is in many situations essential that these efforts should be made.

18.7 Psychological trauma

Psychological trauma involves deep impressions which the child is not able to absorb because of immaturity. Such impressions can imprint themselves deeply in the physical constitution and actually hinder the child's development. The younger the child is, the more deeply will the soul and spirit be influenced by physical events, and vice-versa. Every strong impression on the soul has its effect upon the bodily functions even to the extent of causing vomiting and incontinence. We shall now describe some typical disturbances in child development which can lead to a disposition to illness in later life.

Rage

A child exposed to outbursts of rage on the part of the father, mother, relative or even a teacher, will suffer repeated shocks. Fright leads to a quivering contraction which can even induce chattering of teeth and a fall in body temperature. It is obvious that frequent shocks can lead to the organism being ready to react by withdrawing into itself. This causes the metabolism to become sluggish because it requires a warm, pulsing, fully engaged consciousness free from fear, in order to develop fully. Rudolf Steiner, in *The Essentials of Education,* drew the attention of teachers to the fact that frequent shock not only causes children to become subservient and obsequious but also can cause the whole organism to be prone to metabolic and sclerotic disorders. When adult patients with rheumatism or diabetes are asked about their childhood experiences they often tell of an over-strict or intellectually taxing upbringing.

Depression

What are the physiological consequences for a child who is surrounded by adults who react to everything with disgruntled cheerlessness as if the world had nothing better to offer? Under this influence, a child will find it difficult to laugh, to talk happily or to have amusing thoughts, and will always be preoccupied with the serious side of things. There will be no healthy alternation between laughing and crying, no healthy balance and rhythm of feelings. The result is that the rhythmic functions of breathing and the circulation will be prone to suffer irregularities later in life. Various forms of heart and respiratory disorders can be the consequence.

Superficiality

Being constantly exposed to a superficial attitude of mind can also be harmful to the development of the child's physical-psychological makeup. If a child is always being offered something new but is then distracted at the very moment of really absorbed by it, the child will not develop any real powers of concentration. If there is nothing to counteract this influence, the personality will be marked by a lack of vitality and endurance with the result that in later life the individual will not be able to gather and direct energies purposefully towards any chosen ends.

Passivity

If a child is surrounded by an atmosphere of listlessness, inactivity or slow and sluggish reactions, there will be little stimulus for the child's own activity. As the growth forces which are released from the organism become available, the child will then be unable to direct them towards any definite intellectual outlet. The general tendency will be towards nervousness and aimlessness.

Divorce conflicts

Every child feels a natural love for both parents, regardless of their attitudes and behaviour. If the parents separate, the child will have a sense of being torn apart, even though on the surface there may be an apparent preference for one parent or the other. The consequences of this kind of conflict vary according to the age of the child. Under the age of seven, physical symptoms appear such as wetting and dirtying pants, nervousness, aggressiveness and irritability in various forms. In older children the problems are more of a psychological nature and can lead to a profound mistrust and questioning of human relationships.

Those who wish to spare their children such disruption and conflict will do all they can to reach an agreement over the future of the child. In no case should one parent sabotage the other's arrangements or allow the child things against the other's wishes. The parent who has the child least should keep informed about the situation at home and try to ensure regular contact is kept up through visits.

Lack of emotional contact

There are families which live together with very little mutual contact and communication. The home atmosphere tends to be very undemonstrative or even cold. When the child comes home from school, there is no friendly greeting or enquiry as to how the day went. In such homes, usually both parents go out to work and each has his and her own life and circle of friends outside the family. With such a surrounding framework of behaviour, the child is scarcely in a position to help to enliven the atmosphere. This so affects the child that problems of identity arise. All through life, the individual will be looking for an acceptable self and a viable role in society, and will have difficulty in forming a really open and deep relationships.

Fear

Fear always appears when we cannot understand the situation in which we find ourselves. Fear of the future and what it may bring in the way of pain, illness, poverty, misery, war and death, can permeate and destabilize the life of the soul. Fear, however, is reduced by our attempts to grasp and understand these things. An adult who has achieved a great trust in destiny will have a calming effect upon a child in times of danger; and the child by imitating this example will later be the more able to over-come fear through deeper insight. In childhood fear is usually aroused by the threat of unfamiliar things, dark-ness, noises or strange surroundings, and by experiences such as being abandoned and separated. A tenden-cy to fear is also induced by too early an intellectual education (see 18.4 above) or by parents' repeated en-joinders not to be afraid of the doctor, the dog, the noise, and so on. The parents themselves fear that the child might be afraid and so their words do not carry conviction. Leng-thy explanations of a situation stand in the way of a child's own, direct experience. The result is tension,, withdrawal, insecurity and timidity instead of the desired enlightenment and courage.

If a childhood is beset with fears, later life will be burdened with crises of self-confidence. Doubt and hypochondriac fears arise more easi-ly. These can destroy incipient human relationships and aggravate experi-ences of failure. By contrast, children who are privileged to grow up in an atmosphere of trust will derive a considerable strengthening of perso-nality for life.

18.8 Radioactive pollution

What is radioactivity?

Natural radioactivity is the characteristic of some extremely heavy substances to decay spontaneously and so to generate energy-filled rays. The naturally found radioactive substances lie deep below the surface of the earth hidden away in thick masses of rock. But since the development of uranium mining for industrial purposes, a totally new situation has been created for the world of living things: the introduction of radioactive elements into the air, water and earth.

Artificial radioactivity is brought about by bombarding with energy rays substances which are not naturally radioactive. These substances then become radioactive and unstable. If substances which have a particular function in the organism become radioactive in this way, they can produce a harmful effect upon life. The most notorious example is radioactive iodine accumulated in the thyroid gland.

Since the forties, with the continued programmes of atomic and nuclear bomb tests and the so-called "peaceful" use of nuclear energy, the amount of radioactive contamination of our living space is constantly on the increase. Plutonium, one of the deadliest radioactive by-products in existence, has not so far been found anywhere in nature. It exists only as a man-made by-product of uranium nuclear fission and serves as a substance in the production of nuclear weapons. Absorbed into the body from the air as aerosol in amounts as small as $\frac{1}{1000}$g it can lead to lung-cancer.

A third type of radiation is found in naturally occurring cosmic radiation: that is, energy rays coming from cosmic space. As these rays enter the earth's atmosphere they convert part of the nitrogen of the air into radioactive carbon. Small quantities of this carbon is found in the fossils of living creatures, information which is used to ascertain the age of fossils and archaeological finds. Cosmic radiation has accompanied life on earth over millions of years and has influenced the evolution of living creatures. This radiation is minimal but continuous and has helped living organisms to come to terms with radioactivity.

From these facts it becomes clear that humanity has always been exposed to very slight effects of natural radioactivity. However, no one can say what will be the long-term damage caused by the mounting radioactivity of our century. We do know that alterations in heredity, malformations and degeneration are typically harmful results of radiation. We also know that radiation can cause cancer and that severe exposure can cause inflammation especially of the mucous membrane. Since the discovery of radioactivity, research has constantly been carried out to find out how much exposure to radiation can be tolerated safely by humans and to establish safety limits. But it is still not known how increased exposure to radiation will affect future generations of humans or animals. So far as our present knowledge indicates, there would seem in reality to be no guaranteed safe level of radiation for it is the very nature of radiation to make matter unstable and to weaken the life-forces (regenerative processes) of the organism and with longer exposure to cause long-term damage. In addition stronger doses of radiation cause severe damage to the substance of the cell nucleus, that is the physical vehicle of genetic material with all its metabolic processes.

A great number of harmful effects of radiation are simply accepted and tolerated for economic and financial reasons by politicians and the industries responsible. But in time increasing numbers of individuals will start to consider more seriously the responsibility which each of us bears for the preservation of life upon earth. Those who have a sense of this responsibility feel themselves called upon to work at new concepts of values and aims. They will no longer consider the growth of industry and technology and a high standard of living as prime considerations. Many scientists, too, now take the view that science can continue to develop in a healthy fashion only if it is accompanied by an equally intensive moral development. This would entail a fundamental change in the manner in which knowledge is acquired as at present science is regarded as being purely objective and free of any moral criteria. Beginnings of a new scientific approach are to be found among those scientists who are doing research after the manner of Goethe. To acquire scientific knowledge without a love for the object in hand was for Goethe quite unthinkable. He said: "We can get to know only those things which we love." And what is morality other than true sympathy and interest in the human being and in the world?

Counteracting radioactivity

Most importantly, we must acquire an understanding of the growth forces in the living organism, forces which have already been described at various points in this book (see Index). In *The Fundamentals of Therapy*, Rudolf Steiner wrote: "It is of the greatest importance to know that the ordinary thinking powers of the human being are refined and formative forces of growth." In Steiner's understanding of the human body, the etheric body (see Chapter 6.14) as the vehicle of thought and growth processes can, because of its nature, be reinforced from two sides: from the natural side (regeneration and growth) and from the cultural side (thought activity).

External reinforcement

In other contexts we have already described some measures which can be taken to prevent illness. Some of these measures can be applied to acute or chronic injuries caused by radiation. These measures include the cultivation of rhythms and habits, the regulation of sense impressions, nutrition of quality, religious education and especially eurythmy. Eurythmy enables the "I" to act directly on the etheric body (see Chapter 16.8). Although eurythmy does not work on radioactivity in the body directly, it strengthens the regenerative forces and so acts indirectly. Everything in the organism right down to the life processes of single cells functions rhythmically and these rhythms can be encouraged and strengthened by the measures already described. As far as nutrition is concerned, try to obtain foods which have suffered least from radioactive contamination. Also you can stimulate the life forces of the organism by giving it germinating grains (cultivation is best carried out in clay bowls or flat plates which are obtainable from some health shops).

Medicinal support for the etheric body is also advisable, but this should be under a doctor's supervision. But in our opinion more important than all measures and all medicines is the overcoming of the attitude of mind that has led to the building and maintenance of atomic power stations. For the rest we should work to overcome the fear engendered by radioactivity. Fear consumes the life-forces and weakens the body. In general terms, we cannot stress too often the importance of cultivating the inner life of the soul.

Cultivating thought

At first sight it may seem strange to connect regeneration and growth with thought activity. If, however, we observe our thoughts we notice that in our thought activity we have a true mirror of all our life-functions. It is not for nothing that in ordinary speech we talk of thought-*life*. Whenever we assimilate a new idea or point of view our whole way of looking at things is changed and consequently also the whole interplay of our thoughts. We can only think in connections: we cannot think of "big" without having the idea of "little" as a contrast with it. Our life of thought is an extremely mobile organism of such connections. The more creatively a person thinks, the more readily he will make new thought connections and so come to new ideas. As the etheric body is a complete organism in itself, and as the bodily processes can influence thought activity and vice versa, we may well ask what kind of thought activity will stimulate regeneration and growth, and what kind of thought activity will encourage illness. In Chapter 7.1, we discussed how it has been known for centuries that idealistic and religious people have much better resistance to disease than timid people and those who are totally immersed in everyday activity. If we can give our thinking a spiritual content either by prayer, meditation, or by taking part in sacrament and church service, or by studying the Gospels, ancient wisdom or modern spiritual science (anthroposophy), then real strength can flow into our organism. Inner tranquillity, inner clarity, trust in existence, gratitude and worship warm and enrich the life of the soul and stimulate the life functions. The human being is neither a physically nor a spiritually enclosed system. In counterbalance to physical nutrition, to which at present our attention is predominantly directed, stands spiritual alimentation. Every idea for which we can feel enthusiasm, every ideal for which we strive gives our soul wings and strengthens us physically. Religious and meditative exercise enables us to find a connection to the beings of the spiritual world who lead and accompany human existence. They can help us when we seek them. Thus we find in the Gospel (Luke 11:9): "Ask and it will be given you, seek and you will find." Unlike in former times the spiritual world can now only open to the inner activity of the soul. To the same degree that the living environment of mankind is being harmed so it will be necessary to counteract the weakening of the body by constructive spiritual work. Then the dictum of Mark's Gospel (16:18) can be understood which says that poison cannot harm those who are united with Christ. The central reality of Christianity is the transformation of matter. Bread and wine become the body and blood of Christ: gifts filled with his spirit to strengthen mankind. In the man-made threat of radioactive fall-out we have a transformation of substance that does not heal, but destroys life.

The inner activity of thinking affects not only the human organism but also the earth as a whole. The more each single individual succeeds in discovering his affinity to the earth by inner activity, the more he will contribute not only to his own health, but also to the healing of the whole earth and its creatures.

To counter *knowledge* of the pollution threats around us, including radioactivity, we should consciously emphasize the *sense experience* of the purity of nature. This simple act of awareness will be of increasing importance in the future. We cannot see, hear, taste, smell or touch the harmful influences. Our eyes and ears bring to our consciousness a sense of the original beauty and divinity of nature. It is of the greatest importance for a child's development that it should learn to look at nature as presented by the senses without having the beauty of the impressions marred by negative thoughts. In promoting this awareness, it should be remembered always that, not only are we called upon to "know good and evil" as it stands in the Bible, but also to learn to direct the forces of good and evil in such a way as to serve the evolution of mankind.

18.9 Conclusion

The preceding description of all the environmental hazards confronting modern man with their harmful and weakening effects, could make depressing reading. We may ask ourselves how we can face up to these threats and difficulties and cope with them all?

It is important in the first place to understand that these influences will have their effect whether we are aware of them or not. Thus every effort that we make to help and protect our children's development will have some positive result. We should remember, too, that the child has actively chosen the time and environment for its own life and we should not fall into the trap of thinking that the only solution is to renounce the world as it is. Parents and children together must face the realities around them. As adults we can rise above complacency and passivity and begin to work on ourselves and on the world. These personal initiatives, freely undertaken, are the building-blocks of the future.

Appendix

In this appendix we have listed some suggestions for the use of compresses, baths and other external treatments, together with instructions for knitting the woollen clothes mentioned in the book. The reader will also find a table of average weights in the first nine years of childhood.

External treatments for home-nursing

There follow some general suggestions for treatment at home. We should emphasize that care must always be taken in following these suggestions. Further instructions can be found in *Caring for the Sick at Home.**

We recommend that fomentation cloths used for compresses are made of natural fibres, such as *wool* (hand-knitted, rib-patterned or garter-stitch, woven cloth, flannel or flannelette), *cotton* (gauze), *silk* or *linen*. In addition you will need untreated fleece-wool (or alternatively cotton-wool), two hot-water bottles and a lemon-squeezer.

Camomile compress for the ear

Take a handful of dried camomile flowers, tie them in a thin cloth, Place it between two plates and heat in a steam-bath. This kind of heating is best for preserving the etheric oils.

Test the warmed bag for heat first against your own cheek. Then lay the bag against the child's ear and secure with a woollen scarf or bonnet. Some fleece-wool (or cotton-wool) can also be put under the scarf or bonnet.

Onion bags for the ear

Cut up a medium-sized onion finely. Tie into a thin cloth, lay on the ear and secure with a woollen scarf or bonnet. Some fleece-wool (or cotton-wool) can also be laid under the scarf or bonnet.

If the cut-up onion is warmed in a frying-pan (without fat) it becomes even more effective.

* T. Bentheim, and others.

Throat compress with eucalyptus cream

Spread the cold eucalyptus cream (Weleda) in a rectangle on the middle of a thin cotton cloth. The cloth should be long enough to go round the neck three times, and wide enough to be folded and cover the neck.

Spread the eucalyptus cream wide enough to make it go right round the neck, keeping it a finger's width short of the spine at the back. Fold the cloth over the cream as in Figure 57.

The compress is now ready to be heated between two plates in a steam-bath.

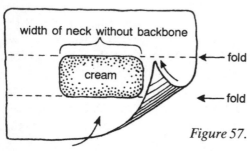

Figure 57.

Before applying the compress test it for warmth against the inside of your forearm. Then quickly lay the compress on the throat (without letting any creases form), draw tight, secure and wrap a woollen cloth around it.

The compress can now stay on during the night. By day it can be applied twice, each time remaining on until it cools.

Alternatively the tube of cream can be warmed up in hot water and then quickly applied to the cloth. The compress is then applied as above.

Throat compress with ointments

Archangelica or allium ointment (Weleda) can be used. Spread the ointment thickly on a cotton or linen cloth large enough to cover the whole neck except the spine. Lay this cloth with the ointment directly on to the skin, secure firmly with a larger cloth and wrap a woollen cloth round it.

To save ointment you can use the same cloth several times, each time adding only a little fresh ointment.

Throat compress with lemon juice

The lemon throat compress can be applied either cool (not cold) or warm according to the patient's preference.

Take a lemon (preferably one that has not been sprayed) and cut it in a bowl of water which completely covers the lemon. Squeeze it out by hand and make many cuts in the peel to release as much etheric oil as possible.

Fold a woollen or linen cloth so as to cover the throat and neck completely, except for the spine.

Dip the cloth into the lemon water and wring out well. Lay it on the neck without any creases, secure with a larger cloth and wrap tightly with a woollen cloth.

If an unsprayed lemon is not available use only the juice.

Throat compress with lemon slices

Cut an unsprayed lemon into slices. Wrap in a cloth and pound the slices (Figure 58).

Lay the compress containing the slices round the neck and secure firmly with a woollen scarf.

Throat compresses can also be made with pressed-out potato-peelings or quark (curd cheese).

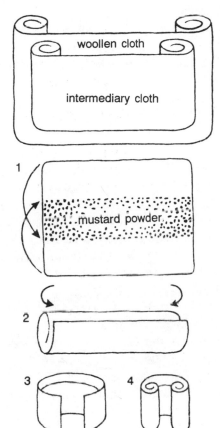

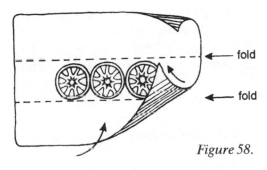

Figure 58.

Figure 59.

Mustard poultice on feet

Make a paste of ground mustard seeds and water, spread it thickly on two plasters the size of your palm, and lay one under the middle of each foot until they begin to burn. Remove the plasters and put on warm woollen socks.

Chest compress with mustard powder

Do all the preparations in a warm room. Spread a thick flannel or baize cloth on the bed over the place where the child's back will be. On top of it lay a towel. In colder weather put a woollen cap and pullover on the child in such a way that it can be rolled up from the bottom when necessary. The child sits in bed with the cloths behind him. Protect the nipples and armpits with vaseline and cover with a small cloth.

Spread the fomentation cloth out over a table. It should be about three times as wide as the length of the child's chest. The length should be a bit longer than the child's girth round the chest.

Place a bowl of lukewarm water ready.

Scatter a thin layer of mustard powder on the middle third of the fomentation cloth about a millimetre thick. Now fold the two other thirds over. The cloth should now be as wide as the length of the child's chest (Figure 59). Roll the two ends of the cloth inwards until they meet, forming two rolls. Dip the cloth in lukewarm water, press out briefly, lay the back of the cloth (with the rolls towards you) on the child's bare back, and unroll the cloth outwards in both directions, making sure that there are no creases, so that the ends overlap over the child's chest.

Now let the child (who has been sitting up all this while) lie on his back on the two prepared cloths.

Wrap the ends of the cloths over the compress, pull tight and secure. Now the child's pullover can be rolled down over all this. Wrap the child in a blanket and carry him to the open window so that while his breathing is stimulated he can breathe fresh air. Little children usually start to cry, but this only does the lungs good in this case. After a short while the chest will begin to feel burning warm, and after abut four minutes there will be a distinct reddening. Look under the compress and when you see the skin reddening remove the compress. If the reddening has not yet occurred you can extend the time once or twice by a couple of minutes up to a total of eight minutes. Then the compress must be removed.

The compress should be removed in the warm bed. Gently massage the reddened skin with a mild oil (for instance, massage balm). Also — and this is important — with the oil remove any excess mustard powder which may have got through the compress.

It is very important, particularly if you have little experience of this treatment, not to exceed the stated times, as there is a danger of causing burns. As every skin reacts differently you must stay with the child throughout the treatment. In some cases the child may feel a burning sensation much sooner and then the compress should be removed to check the skin.

If the skin did not turn red, check whether the mustard powder is too old. For best results use whole mustard seeds, coarsely ground just before making the compress; they can be ground in a hand coffee-grinder. Do not grind mustard seeds in an electric grinder, as there is a fire hazard when the flammable etheric oils are released. Freshly ground seeds will also give the strongest reaction of the skin, so take special care. Finally, be sure to use mustard-powder, not mustard-oil!

It is usual to make the compress once a day in the evening so that the child can go to sleep better afterwards. If the skin has become pimply the next day, use an oil compress (massage balm) only and repeat the mustard application one day later.

Chest compress with lavender oil

Instead of lavender oil (10%), eucalyptus (2%) or dwarf-pine oil can be used.

Soak a thin cotton cloth, wide enough to cover the chest, in the oil and warm in a plastic bag between two hot-water bottles. At the same time warm a pad of fleece-wool (or cotton-wool) which has been wrapped in gauze or muslin to prevent fluffing.

Apply the warm compress (without the plastic!) quickly to the chest and cover with the wool. Secure firmly and smoothly with a large cotton cloth or sheet round the trunk. Over this as a final covering use a woollen cloth or sleeveless woolly pullover. Check that the wool does not scratch or irritate.

This compress can be left on all night.

The cloth saturated with oil can be used again and again for about a week. Add only a little more oil each time.

A much cheaper method is to sprinkle a few drops of oil on a warmed cotton cloth, wrap it round the child, secure it and leave on all night.

Chest rub

Rub the chest with the selected oil with your hands warmed and cover the chest afterwards as described above in the chest compress. The effectiveness can be increased by applying a steam compress (see below).

Chest compress with quark (curd cheese)

Spread the quark about 1 cm (½″) thick on a thin cotton cloth enough to cover the part of the chest to be treated. Fold the cloth to make a pack so that there is only one layer of cloth between the quark and the skin.

Warm the compress between two hot-water bottles to room temperature, then apply it to the chest. Wrap a cotton or linen cloth over it right round the trunk. Make sure that there are no creases in either cloth. Secure with a woollen cloth.

If indicated by the doctor a cool compress can be applied.

Stomach compress with yarrow

To make the infusion, take a handful of yarrow to ½ litre (1 pint) of water, boil and allow to stand for ten minutes.

Meanwhile fold a cloth to the required width and lay inside a larger cloth to facilitate wringing out (Figure 60). Pour the tisane over it through a strainer. Pick up the larger cloth by the dry ends and wring out thoroughly. (If your taps are strong enough the cloth can be passed round the tap to facilitate wringing.)

Take the compress out of the wringing-cloth and apply as hot as

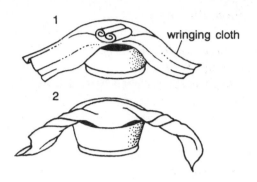

Figure 60.

possible. Secure with a cotton or linen cloth bound tightly round the body. Cover with a woollen cloth. The cloths should be much bigger than the compress to prevent cold areas arising along the edge.

Lay a loosely filled hot-water bottle over the cloths and keep in place with pyjamas. Leave the compress on for one hour or while warm.

Stomach compress with camomile

Proceed as above for the yarrow compress.

Stomach compress with oxalis essence

One tablespoonful of essence of wood sorrel (oxalis lotion, Weleda) to about ¼ litre (½ pint) hot water.

Stomach compress with caraway oil

Soak a thin cotton cloth in the caraway (or cumin balm) oil (Weleda), place in a plastic bag and warm between two hot-water bottles.

At the same time warm a pad of fleece-wool (or as a substitute cotton-wool or wadding) which has been wrapped in gauze to prevent fluffing.

Remove the cloth from the bag, apply and secure as for the yarrow compress (see above).

Stomach compress with copper ointment

Spread the copper ointment (0.4%) thinly on a cloth. Place the cloth on the affected part and secure as for the yarrow compress described above.

The cloth on which the ointment is spread can be used over and over again. Add fresh ointment two or three times a week.

Kidney compress with horsetail (equisetum)

The evening before you need the compress take a handful of horsetail (equisetum) and pour over it about ½ litre (1 pint) of cold water. Cover and leave to stand overnight. The following morning boil the brew for five to ten minutes.

While it is boiling fold a cloth to the right size and lay it inside a larger cloth to facilitate wringing out (Figure 60). Pour the infusion through a strainer on to the cloth. Take hold of the ends of the larger cloth and wring out thoroughly. If your taps are strong enough the cloth can be passed round the tap to facilitate wringing.

Remove the compress from the wringing-cloth and when it is not too hot lay it on to the middle of the back. Secure by wrapping a cotton or linen cloth tightly round the body.

For outer covering use a woollen cloth. Lay on a hot-water bottle (not too full) over this and hold in place with pyjamas.

Kidney compress with copper ointment 0.4%

Spread the copper ointment thinly on a cloth and lay it over the kidneys.

Secure with a cotton or linen cloth wrapped tightly round the body. Over this wrap a woollen cloth.

A well-secured ointment-compress can stay on for several hours. After removal wash the skin carefully with warm water.

The ointment compress can be used for about a week, adding some fresh ointment two to three times a week.

Bladder compress with eucalyptus oil 10%

Soak a thin cloth of the right size in eucalyptus oil. Lay the cloth over the bladder and cover with a second cloth or linen cloth. Secure with a woollen cloth wrapped smoothly and tightly round the body.

The compress can be used for about a week. Add fresh oil before each application.

Another method is to rub eucalyptus oil into the skin in the bladder region. Cover with a woollen cloth.

Leg compress

Only apply cool (not ice cold) leg compresses when the legs and feet are hot. *Never* apply a cold leg compress if the feet are cold or if the child is shivering even when there is high fever.

A rubber or plastic sheet should be used to protect the mattress. The legs must never be wrapped in a waterproof material. A woollen cloth will absorb the remains of any moisture very well and will protect the mattress without being airtight. A thick flannel or baize cloth between the woollen cloth and the damp compress is a good idea. While you are putting on the compress keep the patient lightly covered.

Dip two rolled up thin cotton or linen cloths in cool water and wring out thoroughly. A tablespoonful of lemon-juice or cider-vinegar can be added to the water.

Wind the cloths round each leg starting at the foot and finishing below the knee. Secure with a thick flannel or baize cloth. Wrap a woollen cloth tightly round each compress, or pull a big woollen sock over each leg.

With high fever the compress can be changed every ten minutes, as by that time the cloths will have warmed up. After the third change, leave off the compress for about half an hour.

If the feet go cold during this treatment remove the compress at once.

Mustard foot-bath

Take one to two handfuls of freshly ground mustard powder and put it into a pail filled with warm water (37–39°C, 98–102°F). The length of time for the foot-bath can be up to ten minutes. Prevent the water from cooling by wrapping a bath-towel round the pail or bath.

The bath-water must not come into contact with eyes, mouth or nose, so after the bath rinse the patient's legs and feet thoroughly and wash your own hands well.

The bath will cause the skin to turn very red, though this may only occur after several baths. As a rule give the patient only one bath per day.

Afterwards rub the legs with a good massage oil (for instance, Weleda massage balm).

Sweat-bath

Before the sweat-bath the child may be given a quick warm bath with a few drops of lemon in it.

Then give hot lime-blossom tea to drink. Cover the child up warmly in bed right up to the ears and even possibly wearing a dressing-gown. After half an hour to two hours, once the child has sweated properly (and perhaps slept), wash the patient down with a cool face-cloth and change the pyjamas.

Steam inhalation with camomile

This method requires great care, particularly with small children, because of the hot water.

Make some camomile tea in a wide saucepan or pudding basin. Place the hot open steaming saucepan on a narrow table. Seat yourself opposite the child with the table and the saucepan between you. *Take both the child's hands.* First blow the steam into each other's faces for fun, to get the child used to it. Then take a large towel to make a "circus tent" and lay it over both your heads, then play at breathing in through the nose and out through the mouth to see who can do it best! Bigger children, who can sit alone with the towel over them, will find the time pass more quickly with an egg-timer and a torch. Stop the inhalation once the steam decreases after about three to five minutes. Apply calendula or mercurialis ointment to the face and keep the child in a warm room for an hour.

Once again, be careful with the hot water to prevent scalding. And don't let the child catch a cold afterwards.

Herbal baths with leaves and blossoms

Camomile, nettles, and so on are suitable. For each full bath take two handfuls of the herb and pour on 1–2 litres (2–3 pints) of boiling water and cover. Allow to infuse for five minutes. Pour into the bath-water through a sieve. For a child's bath or a small bath take correspondingly less.

Herbal baths with equisetum or bark

Bark oak, elm, birch or similar can be used. Take two handfuls for each full bath and put in an old pot or saucepan. Add at least 2 litres (4 pints) of water and allow to soak overnight. Boil for ten minutes, and pour into the bath-water through a sieve. For a child's bath or small bath take correspondingly less.

Baths with essences or tinctures

Arnica or sloe are suitable. Take 1 teaspoonful to a child's bath, 1–3 tablespoons to a full bath. Length of time for bath two, five or ten minutes, as directed.

Enema

This treatment must be carried out with great care. Using an enema pack or syringe which can be bought at a chemist or surgical supply shop, about 300 to 800 ml (½ to 1½ pints) of water or warm camomile tea are introduced into the bowels.

Lay the child on its back or side. If the nozzle is a firm one (bone or metal) ease it into the rectum like a thermometer to a depth of 3 to 4 cm (1″ to 1½″). If you are using a tube, round at the end with vents at the side, it can be inserted up to 10 cm (4″). Tell the child to press against it. If the nozzle encounters an obstacles, withdraw it a little and push it in again at a slightly different angle until it goes in.

After opening the valve allow the fluid three minutes to run in. The child should try to keep the anal sphincter closed even when you are pulling out the tube. Only when there is a strong urge to evacuate (after about 3 to 5 minutes) set the child on the potty or lavatory.

A prepared enema in a tube is easier to use and so is in more general use; but it is not nearly as effective as an enema pack or syringe.

Knitting instructions

Baby's woollen pants

Size given is for about four months to fourteen months. (They tend to grow with the child!) For a smaller size use thinner knitting needles.

Materials
70 g (2.5 oz) pure untreated wool, double knitting thickness.
One pair each of No. 8 (4 mm) (5 US) and No. 10 (3.25 mm) (3 US) knitting needles.
One set of No. 10 (3.25 mm) (3 US) knitting needles.

Front
Cast on 60 sts. on No. 10 needles.
Work 16 rows K2, P2.
Change to No. 8 needles and work 48 rows in garter (plain) stitch.
Change back to No. 10 needles and knit 8 rows K2, P2.
Next 16 rows: K together the first two and the last two sts. of every row keeping K2, P2 rib intact. 28 sts.
Knit 5 more rows in K2, P2 and cast off.

Back
Work as front.

Finishing
Sew up side seams from waist down to where the ribbing starts.
Sew up seam between legs.
With set of No. 10 needles, pick up the end sts. around each leg (about 48 sts.).
Make a K2, P2 border of 6 rounds.
Cast off loosely.

Vest/Sleeveless pullover

Size given is for about 6 month to one year. (Larger size 4–6 years in parentheses.)

Materials
50 g (2 oz) (100 g, 4 oz) soft four-ply wool or silk.
One pair No. 9 (3.75 mm) (4 US) knitting needles.

Front
Cast on 50 (60) sts. and work 10 (14) rows in K2, P2.
Knit 40 (63) rows in st.st.
Work the next 18 (39) rows in K2, P2.
Next row, to shape neck opening:
Work 12 (14) sts. in K2, P2, cast off 26 (32) sts., work 12 (14) sts. in K2, P2.
Knit 6 (12) rows with the 12 (14) sts.

on each side, keeping the K2, P2 ribbing intact.
Cast off.

Back
Work as front.

Finishing
Press carefully. Join shoulder seams and side seams leaving an opening for the arms.

Baby's bonnet

Size given is for about birth to two months. (Larger size six to twelve months in parentheses.)

Materials
30 g (1 oz) of four-ply wool or cotton or silk.
One pair No. 11 (3 mm) (2 US) knitting needles. (Larger size: No. 8 (4 mm) (5 US) needles.

Method
Cast on 60 (80) sts. and work 7 (8) rows in K1, P1.
Carry on knitting in st.st. until work measures 10 cm (4″) (12.5 cm, 5″), ending on a right-side row.
Start to decrease as follows:
First row: * sl. 1, K1, psso, K8 *. Repeat from * to * to end of row, 54 sts. (72 sts)
Next and every alt. row: purl
Third row: * sl. 1, K1, psso, K7 *. Repeat from * to * to end of row.
Fifth row: * sl. 1, K1, psso, K6 *. Repeat from * to * to end of row. Continue in this way until you have 6 (8) sts. left.

Finishing
Break the yarn and thread through left over sts. Sew up back seam from back of hat to row at which decreasing started. Crochet two lengths of string for tying bonnet and sew one on to each front corner.

Knitting abbreviations
alt.   alternate
k.   knit
p.   purl
psso.   pass slip stitch over
rep.   repeat
sl.   slip
st(s).   stitch(es)
st.st.   stocking stitch

One-piece suit for eczema sufferers

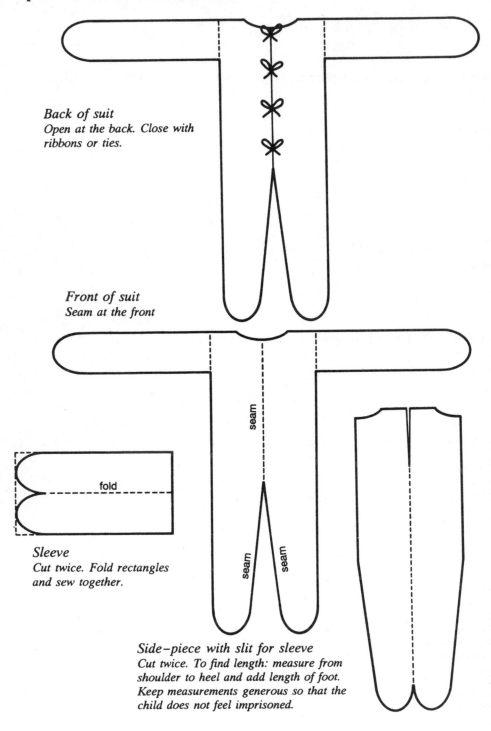

Back of suit
Open at the back. Close with
ribbons or ties.

Front of suit
Seam at the front

seam

Sleeve
Cut twice. Fold rectangles
and sew together.

fold

seam

seam

Side−piece with slit for sleeve
Cut twice. To find length: measure from
shoulder to heel and add length of foot.
Keep measurements generous so that the
child does not feel imprisoned.

Weight and height tables

Babies' and children's weights

Weight increase

From fourth week	Weekly between 150 and 250 g (5–10 oz)*
From fourth month	Weekly between 130 and 200 g (4–7 oz)
From eighth month	Monthly between 250 and 400 g (9–14 oz)

Birth weight should double during the fifth month, and treble after approximately 1 year.

* Prematurely born babies should show a higher increase in weight to begin with.

Weight and height proportions (approximate)

	Monthly increase	Height	Weight
At birth		50 cm (20″)	3.4 kg (7½ lb)
First 4 weeks	800 g (28 oz)		
2 months old	750 g (26 oz)		
5 months old	600 g (21 oz)	64 cm (25″)	7 kg (15 lb)
9 months old	400 g (14 oz)	70 cm (28″)	9 kg (20 lb)
1 year old	250 g (9 oz)	75 cm (30″)	10 kg (22 lb)
	Annual increase		
2 years old	2 kg (4 lb)	87 cm (2′ 10″)	12 kg (26 lb)
3 years old	2 kg (5 lb)	95 cm (3′ 1″)	14 kg (31 lb)
4 years old	2 kg (4 lb)	103 cm (3′ 5″)	16 kg (35 lb)
5 years old	2 kg (5 lb)	108 cm (3′ 7″)	18 kg (40 lb)
6 years old	3.5 kg (7 lb)	116 cm (3′ 10″)	21.5 kg (47 lb)
7 years old	2.5 kg (6 lb)	123 cm (4′)	24 kg (53 lb)
8 years old	3 kg (6 lb)	130 cm (4′ 3″)	27 kg (59 lb)
9 years old	2.5 kg (6 lb)	134 cm (4′ 5″)	29.5 kg (65 lb)

Up to puberty the increase is more or less constant, thereafter the growth and weight increase are individual.

Bibliography

Health and sickness

Arta (rehabilitation centre) *Rock Bottom: Beyond Drug Addiction*, Hawthorn Press, Stroud.

Bentheim, T, *Caring for the Sick at Home*, Floris Books, Edinburgh and Anthroposophic Press, New York.

Bos, Arie, *Aids: an Anthroposophical Art of Healing*, Hawthorn Press, Stroud.

Bott, Victor, *Anthroposophical Medicine*, Anthroposophic Press, New York.

Bühler, Walter, *Living with your Body: the Body as an Instrument of the Soul*, Rudolf Steiner Press, London.

Hauschka, M. *Fundamentals of Artistic Therapy*, Rudolf Steiner Press, London.

Holtzapfel, Walter, *Children's Destinies: the Three Directions of Human Development*, Mercury Press, New York.

---, *Our Children's Illnesses*, Mercury Press, New York.

Husemann, F. and Otto Wolff (Ed.) *The Anthroposophical Approach to Medicine*, (3 vols) Anthroposophic Press, New York.

Leroi, Rita, *Illness and Healing*, Temple Lodge Press, London.

Leviton, Richard *Anthroposophic Medicine Today*, Anthroposophic Press, New York.

Mees, L.F.S. *Blessed by Illness*, Anthroposophic Press, New York.

Steiner, Rudolf, *Health and Illness*, (2 vols) Anthroposophic Press, New York.

---, *Overcoming Nervousness*, Anthroposophic Press, New York.

Steiner, Rudolf, and Ita Wegman, *The Fundamentals of Therapy*, Rudolf Steiner Press, London.

Twentyman, Ralph, *The Science and Art of Healing*, Floris Books, Edinburgh.

Wolff, Otto, *Anthroposophically Orientated Medicine and its Remedies*, Mercury Press, New York.

Nutrition and bio-dynamics

Hauschka, Rudolf, *Nutrition*, Rudolf Steiner Press, London.

Koepf, Herbert, *Bio–Dynamic Agriculture: An Introduction*, Anthroposophic Press, New York.

---, *The Biodynamic Farm*, Anthroposophic Press, New York.

Kolisko, Eugen, *Nutrition*, (2 vols.) Kolisko Archive, Bournemouth.

Philbrick, John & Helen, *Gardening for Health and Nutrition*, Garber Communications, New York.

Podolinsky, Alex, *Bio Dynamic Agriculture: Introductory Lectures*, Gavemer Foundation, Sydney.

Schmidt, Gerhard, *The Dynamics of Nutrition*, Biodynamic Literature, Pennsylvania.

Steiner, Rudolf, *Nutrition and Health*, Anthroposophic Press, New York.

---, *Problems of Nutrition*, Anthroposophic Press, New York.

Storl, Wolf D. *Culture and Horticulture: a Philosophy of Gardening*, Biodynamic Literature, Pennsylvania.

General education

Britz–Crecelius, Heidi, *Children at Play --- Preparation for Life*, Floris Books, Edinburgh and Inner Traditions, Vermont.

Coplen, Dotty, *Parenting a Path through Childhood*, Floris Books, Edinburgh.

Elkind, David, *All Grown up and no Place to go*, Holt, New York.

---, *The Hurried Child: Growing up too Fast too Soon*, Holt, New York.

Gabert, Erich, *Educating the Adolescent*, Anthroposophic Press, New York.

---, *The Motherly and Fatherly Roles in Education*, Anthroposophic Press, New York.

Harwood, A.C. *The Recovery of Man in Childhood*, Rudolf Steiner Press, London.

---, *The Way of a Child*, Rudolf Steiner Press, London.

Heydebrandt, Caroline von, *Childhood*, Anthroposophic Press, New York.

Kane, Franklin G. *Parents as People: the Family as a Creative Process*, Aurora, Edmonton.

Koepke, Hermann, *Encountering the Self: Transformation and Destiny in the Ninth Year*, Anthroposophic Press, New York.

König, Karl, *Brothers and Sisters: the Order of Birth in the Family*, Floris Books, Edinburgh and Anthroposophic Press, New York.

Large, Martin, *Who's Bringing them up? Television and Child Development*, Hawthorn Press, Stroud.

Mander, Jerry, *Four Arguments for the Elimination of Television*.

Pearce, Joseph Chilton, *The Magical Child*, Bantam, New York.

Salter, Joan, *The Incarnating Child*, Hawthorn Press, Stroud.

Setzer, Valdemar, *Computers in Education*, Floris Books, Edinburgh.

Steiner, Rudolf, *Education as a Social Problem*, Anthroposophic Press, New York.

---, *The Education of the Child in the Light of Anthroposophy*, Rudolf Steiner Press, London.

---, *The Essentials of Education*, Rudolf Steiner Press, London.

---, *The Four Temperaments*, Rudolf Steiner Press, London.

---, *The Kingdom of Childhood*, Rudolf Steiner Press, London.

---, *A Modern Art of Education*, Rudolf Steiner Press, London.

Strauss, Michaela, *Understanding Children's Drawings*, Rudolf Steiner Press, London.

Babies and toddlers

Gibson, Margaret, *Becoming a Mother*, Hale & Iremonger, Sydney.

Glas, Norbert, *Conception, Birth and Early Childhood*, Anthroposophic Press, New York.

König, Karl, *The First Three Years of the Child*, Floris Books, Edinburgh and Anthroposophic Press, New York.

Linden, Wilhelm zur, *A Child is Born*, Rudolf Steiner Press, London.

Udo de Haes, Daniel, *The Young Child*, Floris Books, Edinburgh and Anthroposophic Press, New York.

Toys and activities

Berger, Thomas, *The Christmas Craft Book,* Floris Books, Edinburgh.

Jaffke, Freya, *Toymaking with Children,* Floris Books, Edinburgh.

Kraul, Walter, *Earth, Water, fire and air: Playful Explorations in the four Elements,* Floris Books, Edinburgh.

Leeuwen, M. van and J. Moeskops, *The Nature Corner: Celebrating the Year's Cycle with a Seasonal Tableau,* Floris Books, Edinburgh.

Müller, Brunhild, *Painting with Children,* Floris Books, Edinburgh.

Neuschütz, Karin, *The Doll Book,* Floris Books, Edinburgh and Larson Publications, New York.

Reinckens, Sunnhild, *Making Dolls,* Floris Books, Edinburgh.

Zimmermann, Erika, *Shadow Puppets for Children,* Floris Books, Edinburgh.

Fairy-tales and stories

Burnett, Francis Hodgson, *The Secret Garden,* Puffin, Harmondsworth.

Colum, Padraic, *The King of Ireland's Son,* Floris Books, Edinburgh.

Grimm, *The Complete Grimm's Fairy Tales,* Routledge & Kegan Paul.

Howden, Elizabeth, *The Blacksmith and the Fairies and other Scottish Folk-Tales,* Floris Books, Edinburgh.

Karadz[az]ic[aa], Vuk, *Nine Magic Pea-Hens and other Serbian Folk-Tales,* Floris Books, Edinburgh.

Lagerlöf, Selma, *Christ Legends,* Floris Books, Edinburgh.

Meyer, Rudolf, *The Wisdom of Fairy Tales,* Floris Books, Edinburgh and Anthroposophic Press, New York.

Sehlin, Gunhild, *Mary's Little Donkey,* Floris Books, Edinburgh.

Spink, Reginald, *Alexander and the Golden Bird and other Danish Folk-Tales,* Floris Books, Edinburgh.

Verschuren, I. *The Christmas Story Book,* Floris Books, Edinburgh.

---, *The Easter Story Book,* Floris Books, Edinburgh.

Waldorf (Rudolf Steiner) education

Aeppli, Willi, *Biography in Waldorf Education,* Anthroposophic Press, New York.

---, *Rudolf Steiner Education and the Developing Child,* Anthroposophic Press, New York.

---, *Teacher, Child and Waldorf Education,* Anthroposophic Press, New York.

Barnes, H. and others, *Introduction to Waldorf Education,* Mercury, New York.

Cusick, Lois, *Waldorf Parenting Handbook,* St George, New York.

Edmunds, Francis, *Rudolf Steiner Education,* Rudolf Steiner Press, London.

Murphy, Christine, *Emil Molt and the Beginnings of the Waldorf School Movement,* Floris Books, Edinburgh and Anthroposophic Press, New York.

Richards, Mary Caroline, *Towards Wholeness: Rudolf Steiner Education in America.*

Querido, René, *Creativity in Education: the Waldorf Approach,* St George, New York.

Rudel, Joan & Siegfried (Ed.) *Education toward Freedom,* Lanthorn, East Grinstead.

Spock, Marjorie, *Teaching as a Lively Art,* Anthroposophic Press, New York.

Steiner, Rudolf, *The Child's Changing Consciousness and Waldorf Education,* Rudolf Steiner Press, London.

———, *An Introduction to Waldorf Education,* Anthroposophic Press, New York.

Wilkinson, Roy, *Commonsense Schooling,* Henry Goulden, East Grinstead.

Eurythmy

Dubach, Annemarie, *Principles of Eurythmy,* Rudolf Steiner Press, London.

Spock, Marjorie, *Eurythmy,* Anthroposophic Press, New York.

Steiner, Rudolf, *Eurythmy as Visible Speech,* Rudolf Steiner Press, London.

———, *An Introduction to Eurythmy,* Anthroposophic Press, New York.

Festivals

Barz, Brigitte, *Festivals with Children,* Floris Books, Edinburgh.

Benesch, Friedrich, *Ascension,* Floris Books, Edinburgh.

———, *Easter,* Floris Books, Edinburgh.

———, *Whitsun,* Floris Books, Edinburgh.

Capel, Evelyn, *The Christian Year,* Floris Books, Edinburgh.

Carey, D. and J. Large, *Festivals, Family and Food,* Hawthorn Press, Stroud.

Cooper, S., C. Fynes-Clinton and M. Rowling, *The Children's Year,* Hawthorn Press, Stroud.

Jones, Michael (Ed.) *Prayers and Graces,* Floris Books, Edinburgh.

Lenz, Friedel, *Celebrating the Festivals with Children,* Anthroposophic Press, New York.

Steiner, Rudolf, *The Festivals and their Meaning,* Rudolf Steiner Press, London.

Religious education

Bittleston, Adam, *Meditative Prayers for Today,* Floris Books, Edinburgh.

Rittelmeyer, Friedrich, *Meditation: Guidance of the Inner Life,* Floris Books, Edinburgh.

Steiner, Rudolf, *Calendar of the Soul,* Anthroposophic Press, New York.

———, *Prayers for Mothers and Children,* Rudolf Steiner Press, London.

———, *Truth-Wrought Words,* Anthroposophic Press, New York.

———, *Verses and Meditations,* Rudolf Steiner Press, London.

Udo de Haes, Maarten, *Baptism in The Christian Community,* Floris Books, Edinburgh.

Social forms

Davy, Gudrun and Bons Voors, *Lifeways: Working with Family Questions,* Hawthorn Press, Stroud.

Lauer, H.E. *Aggression and Repression in the Individual and Society,* Rudolf Steiner Press, London.

Steiner, Rudolf, *The Renewal of the Social Organism,* Anthroposophic Press, New York.

———, *The Social Future,* Anthroposophic Press, New York.

———, *Towards Social Renewal,* Rudolf Steiner Press, London.

Voors, Tino and Chris Schaefer, *Vision in Action,* Hawthorn Press, Stroud.

Phases of life

Bittleston, Adam, *Counselling and Spiritual Development,* Floris Books, Edinburgh.

———, *Loneliness,* Floris Books, Edinburgh.

Capel, Evelyn, *In the Midst of Life,* Temple Lodge Press, London.

———, *Marriage,* Temple Lodge Press, London.

Glas, Norbert, *The Fulfilment of Old Age,* Anthroposophic Press, New York.

Howard, Alan, *Sex in the Light of Re-incarnation and Freedom,* St George, New York.

Keller, Helen, *The Story of my Life,* New York.

König, Karl, *The Human Soul,* Floris Books, Edinburgh.

Lauenstein, Diether, *Biblical Rhythms in Biography,* Floris Books, Edinburgh.

Lievegoed, Bernhard, *Man on the Threshold,* Hawthorn Press, Stroud.

———, *Phases: Crisis and Development in the Individual,* Rudolf Steiner Press, London.

———, *Phases of Childhood,* Floris Books, Edinburgh.

Lusseyran, Jacques, *And there was Light,* Floris Books, Edinburgh.

Mathews, M., S. Schaefer and B. Staley, *Ariadne's Awakening,* Hawthorn Press, Stroud.

Sleigh, Julian, *Crisis Points: Working through Personal Problems,* Floris Books, Edinburgh.

———, *Thirteen to Nineteen: Discovering the Light,* Floris Books, Edinburgh.

Staley, Betty,. *Between Form and Free-dom: A Practical Guide to the Teen-age Years,* Hawthorn Press, Stroud.

Treichler, Rudolf, *Soulways: The Develop-ing Soul ——— Life Phases, Thresholds and Biography,* Hawthorn Press, Stroud.

Pre-existence and reincarnation

Capel, Evelyn, *Reincarnation within Christianity,* Temple Lodge Press, London.

Drake, Stanley, *The Path to Birth,* Floris Books, Edinburgh.

Frieling, Rudolf, *Christianity and Reincar-nation,* Floris Books, Edinburgh.

Kolisko, Eugen, *Reincarnation and other Essays,* Kolisko Archive, Bournemouth.

Rittelmeyer, Friedrich, *Reincarnation,* Floris Books, Edinburgh.

Steiner, Rudolf, *Between Death and Re-birth,* Rudolf Steiner Press, London.

———, *Life between Death and Rebirth,* Anthroposophic Press, New York.

Death and caring for the dying

Drake, Stanley, *Though you Die,* Floris Books, Edinburgh.

Kübler-Ross, Elisabeth, *Death, the Final Stage of Growth,* Simon Schuster, New York.

———, *Living with Death and Dying,* Souvenir, London.

———, *On Children and Death,* Collier Macmillan, New York.

———, *On Death and Dying,* Tavistock Routledge, London.

———, *To Live until we say Good-bye,* Prentice Hall, London.

Moody, R.A. *Life after Life.*

Schilling, Karin von, *Where are You? Coming to Terms with the Death of my Child,* Anthroposophic Press, New York.

Handicapped children and curative education

Clarke, P., H. Kofsky and J. Lauruol, *To a Different Drumbeat: A Practical Guide to Parenting Children with Special Needs,* Hawthorn Press, Stroud.

Fischer, Berhard (Ed.) *Healing Education,* Freies Geistesleben, Stuttgart.

König, Karl, *Being Human: Diagnosis in Curative Education,* Camphill Press, Botton, and Anthroposophic Press, New York.

———, *In Need of Special Understanding,* Camphill Press, Botton.

Pietzner, Carlo, *Aspects of Curative Education,* Aberdeen University Press.

———, *Questions of Destiny: Mental Retardation and Curative Education,* Anthroposophic Press, New York.

Pietzner, Cornelius (Ed.) *A Candle on the Hill: Images of Camphill Life,* Floris Books, Edinburgh and Anthroposophic Press, New York.

Steiner, Rudolf, *Curative Education,* Rudolf Steiner Press, London.

Weihs, Anke, Joan Tallo and Wain Farrants, *Camphill Villages,* Camphill Press, Botton.

Weihs, Thomas, *Children in Need of Special Care,* Souvenir, London.

Rudolf Steiner and Anthroposophy

Davy, John (Ed.) *Work Arising from the Life of Rudolf Steiner,* Rudolf Steiner Press, London.

Easton, Stewart, *Man and World in the Light of Anthroposophy,* Anthroposophic Press, New York.

———, *The Way of Anthroposophy,* Rudolf Steiner Press, London.

———, *Rudolf Steiner: Herald of a New Epoch,* Anthroposophic Press, New York.

Edmunds, Francis, *From Thinking to Living: the Work of Rudolf Steiner,* Element, Dorset.

Hemleben, Johannes, *Rudolf Steiner: a Biography,* Henry Goulden, East Grinstead.

Hiebel, Friedrich, *Time of Decision with Rudolf Steiner,* Anthroposophic Press, New York.

Lissau, Rudi, *Rudolf Steiner, Life work, inner path and social initiatives,* Hawthorn Press, Stroud.

McDermott, Robert (Ed.) *The Essential Rudolf Steiner,* Harper & Row, San Francisco.

Nesfield–Cookson, Bernard, *Rudolf Steiner's Vision of Love,* Crucible, Wellingborough.

Rittelmeyer, Friedrich, *Rudolf Steiner enters my Life,* Floris Books, Edinburgh.

Seddon, Richard, *Rudolf Steiuner, Essential Readings,* Crucible, Wellingborough.

Shepherd, A.P. *Scientist of the Invisible,* Floris Books, Edinburgh.

Steiner, Rudolf, *Knowledge of the Higher Worlds: How is it Achieved?* Rudolf Steiner Press, London (*Knowledge of the Higher Worlds and its Attainment,* Anthroposophic Press, New York).

———, *Occult Science: an Outline,* Rudolf Steiner Press, London (*An Outline of Occult Science,* Anthroposophic Press, New York).

———, *The Philosophy of Freedom,* Rudolf Steiner Press, London (*The Philosophy of Spiritual Activity,* Anthroposophic Press, New York).

———, *Theosophy,* Rudolf Steiner Press, London.

Wachsmuth, Günther, *Life and Work of Rudolf Steiner,* Garber Communications, New York.

First Aid and Accident Prevention

Accidents to little children usually happen because they follow their natural urge to explore and have not yet learned to distinguish between what is dangerous and what is not. Then they are taken by surprise and accidents are often accompanied by shock. They will recover best in the hands of a capable adult who can deal calmly with the situation. Prompt action and calmness are the most important factors in first aid. Scolding or excessive worrying and comforting make it harder for the child, and do no good in serious accidents.

Emergency resuscitation

Artificial respiration
1. Check the child's breathing and remove any obvious obstacles to breathing.
2. Lay the child on its back and tip the head back by pressing on the forehead and lifting the chin.
3. Take a deep breath and blow gently into the child's mouth and nose until its chest rises. With an older child, pinch the nose and breath into the mouth only.
4. Remove your mouth to take another breath. The child's chest will fall.
5. Repeat three or four times rapidly. Check for pulse in the child's neck.
6. Continue at a rate which is like slightly fast breathing. Keep up the artificial respiration until the child breathes normally.
7. Make sure the child has medical attention.

Heart massage
1. Feel for the child's pulse in the carotid artery at the side of the neck. If the pulse has stopped, the child will be pale in colour, perhaps grey or blue, and the pupils will be dilated. Do not attempt heart massage if there is still a pulse.
2. Lay the child on its back and check the airways.
3. Push down lightly on the lower breastbone, keeping your arm straight. With a baby, press about twice per second. With an older child, press about once per second.
4. After fifteen compressions, give artificial respiration (see above).
5. If there is still no pulse, repeat steps 3 and 4.
6. Ensure the child gets medical attention as soon as possible.

Sudden choking, imminent suffocation

In babies or in children while not fully conscious, vomit or regurgitation can sometimes obstruct the windpipe. Breathing will be noisy and the child's lips may start to turn blue.

Sudden coughing or desire to vomit, wheezy and noisy breathing with a high-pitched or squeaky exhalation, indicate a foreign body in the windpipe. Small nuts, beads or bits of plastic toys are frequent causes. Round objects like marbles can totally block the air passages.

Action:

Observe the child's breathing closely and place your ear close to its mouth to feel whether breathing has stopped or not.

If the airway is partially or completely obstructed:

Call emergency services.

Do not turn the patient upside down. This may cause complete obstruction.

Do not stick your fingers blindly down the child's throat.

Do not carry out abdominal thrusts on an infant or child.

Attempt to clear the airway in the following way:

With **an infant**, support it on your arm with its head slightly down (*Figure 00). Support the head with your hand around the jaw and chest. Give four rapid blows between the shoulder blades. Turn the baby over onto its back, continuing to support the head and neck, and lay it on your thighs with the head again lower than the rest of the body. Give four chest thrusts with the heel of your hand.

With **an older child** with completely obstructed airway, kneel on the floor and lay the child across your thighs, keeping the head lower than the rest of the body (*Figure 00). Deliver four sharp back blows between the shoulder blades. Supporting the head and back, roll the child over and give four chest thrusts using the heel of the hand.

After any serious incident of this kind, the child should always be thoroughly checked by the doctor. If you suspect that a **foreign body is in the lung,** phone the doctor or take the child to the hospital.

Prevention:

Do not let very young children play with marbles, small toys or toys that have bits which can be broken or bitten off. Small children should only be given milled nuts, not whole ones.

Do not let children get too silly and giggly at meals.
Be aware that small children can strangle themselves with string or a necklace.
Keep an observant eye on a child's clothing and on objects within reach of children.
Remember that small children can suffocate while playing with plastic bags.

Drowning

Action:
Turn the child upside down to let the water run out.
If the breathing does not start again at once, give emergency resuscitation (see above).
Call emergency services as soon as possible.

Car accidents

If the injured child is still breathing, speaks or moves, lay him gently on his side, warmly wrapped, and stay with him till help comes. Paleness and vomiting may be caused by shock.

If the injured child is unconscious, but still breathing, leave him lying where he is until trained help comes, unless there is danger from fire or traffic. Meantime cover the child up warmly and stay with him if possible.

If the injured child is not breathing, give mouth-to-mouth resuscitation (see above). If neither heart-beat nor pulse can be detected, give heart massage(see above).

Wounds from which **blood is flowing** or spurting should be bound firmly with as clean a cloth as possible, but do not apply a tourniquet. Smaller cuts will stop bleeding by themselves.

Badly hurt parts of the body: do not move into another position. This applies specially to an injured back. Altering the injured child's position can cause damage.

In less serious cases get the child to move each limb carefully. In this way you can find out quickly if anything has been injured.

In all the above cases call an ambulance as quickly as possible.

Fainting

A wide variety of things can all cause fainting: standing for too long, a suffocating atmosphere, an acute virus infection, excessive pain, seeing blood.

Action:
Lay the unconscious child on the ground, loosen any tight clothing, and raise the legs. Hold smelling-salts or a cloth sprinkled with *eau de Cologne* in front of the child's nose or bathe his head with cold water. In restricted space, bend the child's head down between the knees.

Poisoning

Unusual sleepiness or excitement may lead one to suspect poisoning, and the child should be taken to the hospital as quickly as possible, or at least a doctor should be called.

Look around where the child has been for empty or opened bottles or packets which have contained medicines, drugs, solutions, alcohol, and so on, also any plants or berries which the child may have eaten. These and any vomit should be taken as evidence to the hospital with the child and shown to the doctor attending.

Action:
If **acid or alkaline substances** have been accidentally swallowed, do not attempt to make the child vomit. The same applies to metal polish, sprays petrol and several chemical cleaning products. In all these cases make the child drink *plenty of water* to dilute the solution.

With **pills, alcohol, and all non-corrosive poisons**, induce vomiting as soon as possible. We recommend the following procedure:

Give plenty of water to drink (1/2-1 litre, 1-2 pints). The water can be mixed with fruit juice to taste better.
Small children: lay over your knee. Older children: lay on their side.
With one hand open the mouth by pressing the cheeks between the teeth and push a finger of your other hand to touch the back of the throat or stick a spoon handle down the throat until vomiting occurs.

Acid or alkaline substance **in the eye**: Wash the eye out for ten minutes under running water, making sure that the eyelid is opened. Take the child straight to the hospital.

Concentrated acid **on the skin**: first carefully swab the acid away, then rinse the affected part thoroughly under running water and bathe with milk or soap. Finally treat as for burns.

Prevention:
To prevent such accidents, make sure that all dangerous liquids, poisons and medicines are well locked away and stored out of reach of children.

Scalds and burns

Action:
Pour cold water immediately over the affected parts and continue for some minutes until the pain eases off. Only then remove clothes where necessary to see where the child has been injured. With luck and prompt action the cold water, saturating the clothes or flowing into the shoes, will prevent blistering and damage to the tissue.

If the burns extend over more than five per cent of the body surface, the child must be taken to the hospital otherwise general complications can occur (to give some idea: a child's palm is about one per cent of the body surface). If blisters do form they should be covered with clean sterile gauze. Further treatment will be prescribed by the doctor. Minor burns can be treated at home with extract of nettle and arnica. This can be home-made, or *Combudoron* (Weleda) can be used (dilute 1 tablespoon in a cup of water), to keep the wound constantly moist.

Lesser injuries, accidents and minor shocks

Falling out of bed, or off a table
If a baby falls off a low bed on to the carpet, it is clearly unnecessary to take it to the doctor if:
it starts crying right away;
it is not sick;
no flat cushion-like swellings can be felt on its skull in the next thirty minutes or so;
and, once it has got over the fright, it is happy again.

But it is a different matter if a baby falls off a table, high-chair or out of a pram and lands head first on a stone or other hard floor. The doctor should see the child after a fall of this kind, in case of undisclosed injury.

If the baby **loses consciousness or starts vomiting**, or if a flat cushion-like swelling appears on the skull, it should be taken to the hospital immediately.

Bruising, jammed fingers
Action:
Press the ball of your thumb, a piece of ice, or a cold wet cloth on to the affected part immediately, and hold there for five minutes. Finger-nails that have been jammed or squashed should be held under the cold tap for three to five minutes.

Nosebleed
Action:
Sit the child upright on a chair with the head bent forward a little. Squeeze both nostrils tight shut. After five minutes (timed!) let go, let the child blow his nose gently and wait to see if fresh bleeding occurs.
Do not lay the child down with his head back, as is often suggested, because blood may flow back down the throat.

If the nosebleed does not stop after ten minutes, or if the nose has been hit so hard that the bridge of the nose is thickly swollen or misshapen, take the child to see a doctor.

Teeth knocked out
Take the child and the tooth/teeth straight to the dentist or dental clinic. With prompt action, a tooth can be successfully re-implanted.

Minor injuries
In a case of **limping**, before consulting the doctor examine the child's feet. There may be a weal, a sore from rubbing or pressure, or an injury, even a nail in the shoe. Is there anyone about with a limp that the child is imitating? A strained muscle can also be the cause of a limp.

Small cuts should be allowed to bleed for a bit, then apply a sterile plaster or gauze, if necessary. A smear of antiseptic cream may suffice.

Grazed knees should be cleaned gently with boiled water and cotton wool. Your own hands should be carefully washed beforehand and dried on a fresh towel. Allow the abrasion to dry in the air. To prevent the wound being chafed by clothing or exposed to further injury a bandage will nearly always be necessary. It is sufficient to change the bandage two or three times a week unless bleeding shows through, or it begins to smell, chafe, or signs of inflammation appear.

Slightly watery abrasions can be treated with a thin coating of *Calendula* ointment (Weleda). But for **very watery abrasions** apply a thick coating to prevent the wound sticking to the dressing.

Splinters, thorns and ticks should be removed from the skin immediately. For removing ticks we recommend that you put a drop of oil on the tick, wait for a moment, then using a tightly pressed wad of cotton-wool wind the tick out in an anti-clockwise direction. If you do not succeed in removing the tick completely, take the child to the doctor.

Gaping wounds or cuts, animal or human bites
After staunching the flow of blood, take the child straight to the doctor or to the hospital.

Insect bites and stings
After **a bee sting** remove the sting at once. If available press a freshly cut onion on to the sting, or failing that a wet compress which can be made with diluted nettle-arnica extract (Weleda *Combudoron*). If the insect has stung into a blood vessel or if the child has an allergy a general reaction can occur, in which case take the child to a doctor or hospital immediately. With **wasp stings** you should consider antitetanus injection (see Chapter 7.4).

Mosquito bites and gnat bites are not always recognized as such by parents, but a doctor will recognize them. On holiday where there are lots of mosquitoes a mosquito net should be hung over the bed. Midge-bites and many other insect bites are harmless but can be very itchy. Some relief can be obtained by bathing the bites with surgical spirit or Combudoron (Weleda).

Insect bites or stings at the back of the mouth or in the throat. Give the child a cold drink or ice to suck and take him straight to the doctor.

Jellyfish stings can be painful and if untreated can have effects lasting for up to twenty-four hours. Treatment with nettle-extract (Weleda *Combudoron*) is effective.

Prevention against tetanus (lockjaw)
This should be given where the child has a wound with dirt in it, and he has not been immunized against tetanus or where the child has been stung by a wasp or other insect which has contact with dirt. For further details see Chapter 7.4 on antitetanus immunization.

Index